MW01598961

Analysis of Correlated Data with SAS and R

THIRD EDITION

Analysis of Correlated Data with SAS and R

THIRD EDITION

Mohamed M. Shoukri
Mohammad A. Chaudhary

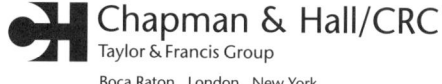

Chapman & Hall/CRC
Taylor & Francis Group
Boca Raton   London   New York

Chapman & Hall/CRC is an imprint of the
Taylor & Francis Group, an **informa** business

Chapman & Hall/CRC
Taylor & Francis Group
6000 Broken Sound Parkway NW, Suite 300
Boca Raton, FL 33487-2742

© 2007 by Taylor & Francis Group, LLC
Chapman & Hall/CRC is an imprint of Taylor & Francis Group, an Informa business

---

Library of Congress Cataloging-in-Publication Data

Shoukri, M. M. (Mohamed M.)
    Analysis of correlated data with SAS and R / by Mohamed M. Shoukri and Mohammad A. Chaudhary. -- 3rd ed.
       p. cm.
    Originally published: Statistical methods for health sciences. 2nd ed. Boca Raton, Fla. : CRC Press, c1999.
    Includes bibliographical references and index.
    ISBN 978-1-58488-619-8
    1. Epidemiology--Statistical methods. I. Chaudhary, Mohammad A. II. Shoukri, M. M. (Mohamed M.) Statistical methods for health sciences. III. Title.

RA652.2.M3S53 2007
614.4--dc22   2007000593

Visit the Taylor & Francis Web site at
http://www.taylorandfrancis.com

and the CRC Press Web site at
http://www.crcpress.com

*To the memory of my mother. To my wife, Sue, and my children,
Nader, Nadene, and Tamer*

— Mohamed M. Shoukri

To my mother, Nazir Begum, and my father, Siddiq Ahmed

— Mohammad A. Chaudhary

Contents

Preface to the First Edition

A substantial portion of epidemiologic studies, particularly in community medicine, veterinary herd health, field trials and repeated measures from clinical investigations, produce data that are clustered and quite heterogeneous. Such clustering will inevitably produce highly correlated observations; thus, standard statistical techniques in non-specialized biostatistics textbooks are no longer appropriate in the analysis of such data. For this reason it was our mandate to introduce to our audience the recent advances in statistical modeling of clustered or correlated data that exhibit extra variation or heterogeneity.

This book reflects our teaching experiences of a biostatistics course in the University of Guelph's Department of Population Medicine. The course is attended predominantly by epidemiology graduate students, as well as, students from Animal Science and researchers from disciplines which involve the collection of clustered and over-time data. The material in this text assumes that the reader is familiar with basic applied statistics, principles of linear regression and experimental design, but stops short of requiring a cognizance of the details of the likelihood theory and asymptotic inference. We emphasize the "how to" rather than the theoretical aspect; however, on several occasions the theory behind certain topics could not be omitted, but is presented in a simplified form.

The book is structured as follows: Chapter 1 serves as an introduction in which the reader is familiarized with the effect of violating the assumptions of homogeneity and independence on the ANOVA problem. Chapter 2 discusses the problem of assessing measurement reliability. The computation of the intraclass correlation as a measure of reliability allowed us to introduce this measure as an index of clustering in subsequent chapters. The analysis of binary data summarized in 2×2 tables is taken up in Chapter 3. This chapter deals with several topics including, for instance, measures of association between binary variables, measures of agreement and statistical analysis of medical screening tests. Methods of cluster adjustment proposed by Donald and Donner (1987), Rao and Scott (1992) are explained. Chapter 4 concerns the use of logistic regression models in studying the effects of covariates on the risk of disease. In addition to the methods of Donald and Donner, and Rao and Scott to adjust for clustering, we explain the Generalized Estimating Equations (GEE) approach proposed by Liang and Zeger (1986). A general background on time series models is introduced in Chapter 5. Finally, in Chapter 6 we show how repeated measures data are analyzed under the linear additive model for continuously distributed data and also for other types of data using the GEE.

We wish to thank Dr. A. Meek, the Dean of the Ontario Veterinary College, for his encouragement in writing this book; Dr. S. W. Martin, Chair of the Department of Population medicine, for facilitating the use of the departmental resources; the graduate students who took the course "Statistics for the Health Sciences"; special thanks to Dr. J. Sargeant for being so generous with her data and to Mr. P. Page for his invaluable computing expertise. Finally, we would like to thank J. Tremblay for her patience and enthusiasm in the production of this manuscript.

M.M. Shoukri
V.L. Edge
Guelph, Ontario
July 1995

Preface to the Second Edition

The main structure of the book has been kept similar to the first edition. To keep pace with the recent advances in the science of statistics, more topics have been covered. In Chapter 2 we introduce the coefficient of variation as a measure of reproducibility, and comparing two dependent reliability coefficients. Testing for trend using Cochran-Armitage chi-square, under cluster randomization has been introduced in Chapter 4. In this chapter we discussed the application of the PROC GENMOD in SAS, which implements the GEE approach, and "Multi-level analysis" of clustered binary data under the "Generalized Linear Mixed Effect Models," using Schall's algorithm, and GLIMMIX SAS macro. In Chapter 5 we added two new sections on modeling seasonal time series; one uses combination of polynomials to describe the trend component and trigonometric functions to describe seasonality, while the other is devoted to modeling seasonality using the more sophisticated ARIMA models. Chapter 6 has been expanded to include analysis of repeated measures experiment under the "Linear Mixed Effects Models," using PROC MIXED in SAS. We added Chapter 7 to cover the topic of survival analysis. We included a brief discussion on the analysis of correlated survival data in this chapter.

An important feature of the second edition is that all the examples are solved using the SAS package. We also provided all the SAS programs that are needed to understand the material in each chapter.

M.M. Shoukri, Guelph, Ontario
C.A. Pause, London, Ontario
July 1998

Preface to the Third Edition

It was brought to our attention by many of our colleagues that the title of the previous edition did not reflect the focus of the book, which was the analysis of correlated data. We therefore decided to change the title of the third edition to *Analysis of Correlated Data with SAS and R*. We believe that the change in the title is appropriate and reflects the main focus of the book.

The fundamental objectives of the new edition have been kept similar to those of the previous two editions. However, this edition contains major structural changes. The first chapter in the previous editions has been deleted and is replaced with a new chapter devoted to the issue of modeling and analyzing normally distributed variables under clustered sampling designs. A separate chapter is devoted to the analysis of correlated count data with extensive discussion on the issue of overdispersion. Multilevel analyses of clustered data using the "Generalized Linear Mixed Effects Models" fitted by the PROC GLIMMIX in SAS are emphasized. Chapter 6 has been expanded to include the analysis of repeated measures and longitudinal data when the response variables are normally distributed, binary and count. The "Linear Mixed Effects Models" are fitted using PROC MIXED and PROC GLIMMIX in SAS. An important feature of the third edition is the introduction of R codes for almost all the examples solved with SAS. The freeware R package can be downloaded from The Comprehensive R Archive Network (CRAN) at http://cran.r-project.org/ or at any of its mirrors. The reader of this book is expected to have prior working knowledge of SAS and R packages. Readers who have experience with S-PLUS will have no problem working with R. Readers completely new to R will benefit from the many tutorials available on the R web site.

The important features of the third edition are

1. We provide a large number of examples to cover the material, together with their SAS and the R codes.
2. In each chapter, we provide the reader with sample size requirements relevant to the topic discussed, with special emphasis on situations when the data are correlated either because the sampling units are physically clustered or because subjects are observed over time.
3. At the end of each chapter, a set of exercises is provided to enhance the understanding of the material covered.
4. We provide a CD that contains all the data along with the SAS and R codes.

Dr. Chaudhary's work was supported in part by the Bill and Melinda Gates Foundation as part of the Consortium to Respond Effectively to the AIDS-TB Epidemic (CREATE) project (19790.01).

M.M. Shoukri, London, Ontario, Canada
M.A. Chaudhary, Baltimore, Maryland

Authors

Mohamed M. Shoukri received his MSc and PhD degrees from the Department of Mathematics and Statistics, University of Calgary, Alberta, Canada. He held several faculty positions at various Canadian universities, and taught applied statistics at Simon Fraser University, the University of British Columbia, and the University of Windsor, and was a full professor with tenure at the University of Guelph, Ontario, Canada. His papers have been published in the *Journal of the Royal Statistical Society* (series C), *Biometrics, Journal of Statistical Planning and Inference, The Canadian Journal of Statistics, Statistics in Medicine, Statistical Methods in Medical Research*, and many other journals. He is a fellow of the Royal Statistical Society of London and an elected member of the International Statistical Institute. He is now principal scientist and the acting chairman of the Department of Biostatistics and Epidemiology at the Research Center of King Faisal Specialist Hospital.

Mohammad A. Chaudhary is an associate scientist (biostatistics) at the Department of International Health, Johns Hopkins Bloomberg School of Public Health. He received his PhD degree in biostatistics from the University of North Carolina at Chapel Hill and his master degrees from Islamia University and the University of Southampton. He has taught at Islamia University, Punjab University, and at the University of Memphis while he was a postdoctoral fellow at St. Jude Children Research Hospital. Before joining his current position, he served as a scientist (biostatistics) at King Faisal Specialist Hospital and Research Center, Riyadh. His papers have published in *Statistics in Medicine, Journal of Statistical Planning and Inference, Computer Methods and Programs in Medicine, Biometrical Journal, Journal of Statistical Research, Cancer Research, Lancet*, and other biomedical research journals. His current research interests include statistical computing and the design and analysis of randomized clinical trials evaluating novel interventions for the prevention of TB and HIV-AIDS.

1

Analyzing Clustered Data

CONTENTS

1.1 Introduction

Clusters are aggregates of individuals or items that are the subject of investigation. A cluster may be a family, school, herd of animals, flock of birds, hospital, medical practice, or an entire community. Data obtained from clusters may be the result of an intervention in a randomized clinical or a field trial. Sometimes interventions in randomized clinical trials are allocated to groups of patients rather than to individual patients. This is called cluster randomization or cluster allocation, and is particularly common in human and animal health research. There are several reasons why investigators wish to randomize clusters rather than the individual study subjects. The first being the intervention may naturally be applicable to clusters. For example, Murray et al. (1992) evaluated the effect of school-based interventions in reducing adolescent tobacco use. A total of 24 schools (of various sizes) were randomized to an intervention condition (SFG = smoke-free generation) or to a control condition (EC = existing curriculum). The number (and proportion) of children in each school who continued to use smokeless tobacco after 2 years of follow-up is given in Table 1.1.

It would be impossible to assign students to intervention and control groups because the intervention is through the educational program that is received by all students in a school.

TABLE 1.1

Smokeless Tobacco Use among Schoolchildren

Control (EC)	Intervention (SFG)
5/103	0/42
3/174	1/84
6/83	9/149
6/75	11/136
2/152	4/58
7/102	1/55
7/104	10/219
3/74	4/160
1/55	2/63
23/225	5/85
16/125	1/96
12/207	10/194

Second, even if individual allocation is possible, there is the possibility of contamination. For example, in a randomized controlled intervention trial the purpose was to reduce the rate of cesarean section. The intervention was that each physician should consult with his/her fellow physician before making the decision to operate, and the control was to allow the physician to make the decision without consulting his/her colleague. Ten hospitals were randomized to receive the intervention, while ten other hospitals were kept as controls. In this example, cluster randomization is desired even if the randomization by the physician is possible, because of the possibility of significant crossover contamination. Because the physicians work together, it is likely that a physician in the control group, who did not receive the intervention, might still be affected by it via interactions with colleagues in the intervention group.

Third, cluster allocation is sometimes cheaper or more practical than individual allocation. Many public health interventions are relatively less costly when implemented at an organizational level (e.g., community) than at an individual level.

Similar to cluster randomization, cluster allocation is common in observational studies. In this case, it is sometimes more efficient to gather data from organizational units such as farms, census tracts, or villages rather than from individuals (see Murray et al., 1992).

1.1.1 The Basic Feature of Cluster Data

When subjects are sampled, randomized, or allocated by clusters, several statistical problems arise. Observations within a cluster tend to be more alike than observations selected at random. If observations within a cluster are correlated, one of the assumptions of estimation and hypothesis testing is violated. Because of this correlation, the analyses must be modified to take into account the cluster design effect. When cluster designs are used, there are two sources of variations in the observations. The first is the one between subjects within a cluster, and the second is the variability among clusters. These two sources of variation cause the variance to inflate and must be taken into account in the analysis.

The effect of the increased variability due to clustering is to increase the standard error of the effect measure, and thus widen the confidence interval and inflate the type I error rate, compared to a study of the same size using individual randomization. In other words, the effective sample size and consequently the power are reduced. Conversely, failing to account for clustering in the analysis will result in confidence intervals that are falsely narrow and the *p*-values falsely small. Randomization by cluster accompanied by an analysis appropriate to randomization by individual is an exercise in self-deception (Cornfield, 1978).

Failing to account for clustering in the analysis is similar to another error that relates to the definition of the unit of analysis. The unit of analysis error occurs when several observations are taken on the same subject. For example, a patient may have multiple observations (e.g., systolic blood pressure) repeated over time. In this case, the repeated data points cannot be regarded as independent, since measurements are taken on the same subject. For example, if five readings of systolic blood pressure are taken from each of the 15 patients, assuming 75 observations to be independent is wrong. Here, the patient is the appropriate unit of analysis and is considered as a cluster.

To recognize the problem associated with the unit of analysis, let us assume that we have *k* clusters each of size *n* units (the assumption of equal cluster size will be relaxed later on). The data layout (Table 1.2) may take the form:

TABLE 1.2

Data Layout

			Clusters			
Units	1	2	......	i	......	k
1	Y_{11}	y_{21}	....	y_{i1}	....	y_{k1}
2	y_{12}	Y_{22}	....	y_{i2}	....	y_{k2}
$\vdots$	$\vdots$	$\vdots$	....	$\vdots$	....	$\vdots$
j	Y_{1j}	y_{2j}	....	y_{ij}	....	y_{kj}
$\vdots$	$\vdots$	$\vdots$	....	$\vdots$	....	$\vdots$
n	y_{1n}	y_{2n}	....	y_{in}	....	y_{kn}
Total	$y_{1.}$	$y_{2.}$	....	$y_{i.}$	....	y_{k}
Mean	$\bar{y}_1$	$\bar{y}_2$	....	$\bar{y}_i$		$\bar{y}_k$

The grand sample mean is denoted by $\bar{y} = \frac{1}{nk} \sum_{i=1}^{k} \sum_{j=1}^{n} \bar{y}_{ij}$.

If the observations within a cluster are independent, then the variance of the *i*th cluster mean is

$$V(\bar{y}_i) = \frac{\sigma_y^2}{n} \qquad (1.1)$$

where $\sigma_y^2 = E(y_{ij} - \mu)^2$ and μ is the population mean. Assuming that the variance is constant across clusters, the variance of the grand mean is

$$V(\bar{y}) = \frac{\sigma_y^2}{nk} \tag{1.2}$$

Now, if k clusters are sampled from a population of clusters, and because members of the same cluster are similar, the variance within the cluster would be smaller than would be expected if members were assigned at random. To articulate this concept, we first assume that the jth measurement within the ith cluster y_{ij} is such that $y_{ij} = \mu + b_i + e_{ij}$, where

$$b_i \equiv \text{random cluster effect and}$$
$$e_{ij} \equiv \text{within cluster deviation from cluster mean}$$

so that $E(b_i) = 0$, $V(b_i) = \sigma_b^2$, $E(e_{ij}) = 0$, $V(e_{ij}) = \sigma_e^2$, and b_i and e_{ij} are independent of each other. Under this setup, we can show that

$$V(y_{ij}) = \sigma_b^2 + \sigma_e^2 \equiv \sigma_y^2 \tag{1.3}$$

$$\text{Cov}(y_{ij}, y_{il}) = \sigma_b^2 \quad j \neq l \tag{1.4}$$

Therefore, the correlation between any pair of observations within a cluster is

$$\text{Corr}(y_{ij}, y_{il}) = \rho = \frac{\sigma_b^2}{\sigma_b^2 + \sigma_e^2} \tag{1.5}$$

This correlation is known as the intracluster correlation (ICC). Therefore,

$$\sigma_e^2 = \sigma_y^2(1 - \rho) \tag{1.6}$$

Equation 1.4 shows that if the observations within a cluster are not correlated ($\rho = 0$), then the within-cluster variance is identical to the variance of randomly selected individuals. Since $0 \leq \rho < 1$, the within-cluster variance σ_e^2 is always less than σ_y^2.

Simple algebra shows that

$$V(\bar{Y}_i) = \frac{\sigma_y^2}{n}[1 + (n - 1)\rho] \tag{1.7}$$

and

$$V(\bar{\bar{Y}}) = \frac{\sigma_y^2}{nk}[1 + (n - 1)\rho] \tag{1.8}$$

Note that for binary response, σ^2 is replaced with $\pi(1 - \pi)$. The quantity $[1 + (n - 1)\rho]$ is called the variance inflation factor (VIF) or the "design effect" (DEFF) by Kerry and Bland (1998). It is also interpreted as the relative efficiency of the cluster design relative to the random sampling of subjects and is the ratio of Equation 1.8 to Equation 1.2:

$$\text{DEFF} = [1 + (n - 1)\rho] \qquad (1.9)$$

The DEFF represents the factor by which the total sample size must be increased if a cluster design is to have the same statistical power as a design in which individuals are sampled or randomized. If the cluster sizes are not equal, which is commonly the case, the cluster size n should be replaced with $n' = \sum_{i=1}^{k} n_i^2 / N$, where $N = \sum_{i=1}^{k} n_i$.

Since ρ is unknown, we estimate its value from the one-way ANOVA layout (Table 1.3):

TABLE 1.3

ANOVA Table

SOV	DF	Sum of square	Mean square
Between clusters	$k - 1$	BSS	$\text{BMS} = \dfrac{\text{BSS}}{k - 1}$
Within clusters	$N - k$	WSS	$\text{WMS} = \dfrac{\text{WSS}}{N - k}$
Total	$N - 1$		

where $\text{BSS} = n\sum_i^k (\bar{y}_i - \hat{\mu})^2$, $\text{WSS} = \sum_i^k \sum_j^n (y_{ij} - \bar{y}_i)^2$, and the ICC is estimated by

$$\hat{\rho} = \frac{\text{BMS} - \text{WMS}}{\text{BMS} + (n_0 - 1)\text{WMS}} = \frac{\hat{\sigma}_b^2}{\hat{\sigma}_b^2 + \hat{\sigma}_e^2}$$

where $\hat{\sigma}_b^2 = (\text{BMS} - \text{WMS})/n_0$ and $\hat{\sigma}_e^2 = \text{WMS}$ are the sample estimates of σ_b^2 and σ_e^2, respectively.

$$n_0 = \bar{n} - \frac{\sum_{i=1}^{k}(n_i - \bar{n})^2}{k(k - 1)\bar{n}} \qquad \bar{n} = \frac{N}{k} \qquad (1.10)$$

Note that when $n_1 = n_2 = \cdots = n_k$, then $n_0 = \bar{n} = n$.

If $\hat{\rho} > 0$, then the variance in a cluster design will always be greater than a design in which subjects are randomly assigned so that, conditional on the cluster size, the confidence interval will be wider and the p-values larger. We note further that, if the cluster size (n) is large, the DEFF would be large even for small values of $\hat{\rho}$. For example, an average cluster size of 40 and ICC $= 0.02$ would give DEFF of 1.8, implying that the sample size of a cluster-randomized design should be 180% as large as the estimated sample size of an individually randomized design to achieve the same statistical power.

We have demonstrated that applying conventional statistical methods to cluster data assuming independence between the study subjects is wrong, and one has to employ appropriate approach that duly accounts for the correlated nature of cluster data. The complexity of the approach depends on the complexity of design. For example, the simplest form of cluster data is the one-way layout, where subjects are nested within clusters. Conventionally, this design has two levels of hierarchy: subjects at the first level and clusters at the second level. For example, the sib-ship data (will be shown below) have two levels: the first is observations from sibs and the second is formed by the family identifiers. Data with multiple levels of hierarchy, such as animals within the farms, farms nested within regions, may also be available, and one must account for the variability at each level of hierarchy.

We shall now review some of the studies reported in the medical literature that must be included under "cluster randomization trials" where we clearly identify what is meant by "cluster."

Russell et al. (1983) investigated the effect of nicotine chewing gum as a supplement to the general practitioners' advice against smoking. Subjects were assigned by week of attendance (in a balanced design) to one of three groups: (a) nonintervention controls, (b) advice and booklet, and (c) advice and booklet plus the offer of nicotine gum. There were six practices, with recruitment over 3 weeks, 1 week to each regime. There were 18 clusters (practices) and 1938 subjects. The unit of analysis will be subject nested within practice.

1. In a trial of clinical guidelines to improve general-practice management and referral of infertile couples, Emslie et al. (1993) randomized 82 general practices in Grompian region and studied 100 couples in each group. The outcome measure was whether the general practitioner had taken a full sexual history and examined and investigated both partners appropriately, so that the general practitioner would be the unit of analysis.

2. A third example is the Swedish two-county trial of mammographic screening for breast cancer. In this study, clusters (geographical areas) were randomized within strata, comprising 12 pairs of geographical clusters in Ostergotland county and 7 triplets in Kopperberg county. The strata were designed so that clusters within a stratum were similar in socioeconomic terms. It should be noted that for randomization or allocation by cluster, there is a price to be paid at the analysis stage. We can no longer think of our trial subjects as independent individuals, but must do the analysis at the level of the sampling unit. This is because we have two sources of variation, one between subjects within a cluster and the other between clusters; and the variability between clusters must be taken into account. Clustering leads to a loss of power and a need to increase the sample size to cope up with the loss. The excess variation resulting from randomization being at the cluster level rather than the individual level was neglected by Tabar

et al. (1985). They claimed (without supporting evidence) that such excess variation was negligible. This study was later analyzed by Duffy et al. (2003) who used hierarchical modeling to take clustering into account and found an evidence for an effect. Taking account of the cluster randomization, there was a significant 30% reduction in breast cancer mortality. They concluded that mammographic screening does indeed reduce mortality from breast cancer and that the criticisms of the Swedish two-county trial were unfounded. The fact is that the criticism was founded, because it was wrong to ignore clustering in such a study. Getting the same answer when we do it correctly is irrelevant.

There are several approaches that can be used to allow for clustering ranging from simple to quite sophisticated:

1. Whether the outcome is normally distributed or not, group comparisons may be achieved by adjusting the standard error of the "effect measure" using the DEFF. These are generally approximate methods, but more realistic than ignoring the within-cluster correlation.
2. Multilevel or hierarchical or random effects modeling.
3. When covariates adjustment are required within the regression analyses, the "generalized estimating equation" (GEE) approach is used.
4. Bayesian hierarchical models.

The focus in this book will be on the statistical analysis of correlated data using the first three approaches.

1.1.2 Sample and Design Issues

As we have seen, the main reasons for adopting trials with clusters as the sampling unit are:

- Evaluation of interventions, which by their nature have to be implemented at community level, e.g., water and sanitation schemes, and some educational interventions, e.g., smoking cessation project.
- Logistical convenience, or to avoid the resentment or contamination that might occur if unblended interventions were provided for some individuals, but not others in each cluster.

It might be desirable to capture the mass effect on disease of applying an intervention to a large proportion of community or cluster members, for example, due to "an overall reduction in the transmission of an infectious agent" (Hayes and Bennett, 1999).

The within-cluster correlation can come about by any of several mechanisms, including shared exposure to the same physical or social environment, self-selection in belonging to the cluster or the group, or sharing ideas or diseases among members of the group.

As we see from Equation 1.9, the DEFF is a function of the cluster size and the ICC. The values of ρ tend to be larger in small groups such as a family, and smaller in large groups such as a county or a village because the degree of clustering often depends on the interaction of group members; family members are usually more alike than individuals in different areas of a large geographic region. Unfortunately, the influence of ρ on study power is directly related to cluster size. Studies with a few large clusters are often very inefficient.

Example 1.1 Comparison of Means

We assume in this example that k clusters of n individuals are assigned to each of an experimental group E and a control group C. The aim is to test the hypothesis $H_0: \mu_E = \mu_C$, where μ_E and μ_C are the means of the two groups, respectively, of a normally distributed response variable Y having common but unknown variance σ^2.

Unbiased estimates of μ_E and μ_C are given by the usual sample means $\bar{y}_E$ and $\bar{y}_C$, where

$$\bar{y}_E = \frac{1}{nk} \sum_{i=1}^{k} \sum_{j=1}^{n} y_{ij}$$

and

$$V(\bar{y}_E) = \frac{\sigma^2}{nk}[1 + (n-1)\rho] \tag{1.11}$$

with similar expression for $V(\bar{y}_C)$.

For sample size determination, expression 1.11 implies that the usual estimate of the required number of individuals in each group should be multiplied by the inflation factor or DEFF $= [1 + (n-1)\rho]$ to provide the same statistical power as would be obtained by randomizing nk subjects to each group when there is no clustering effect. More formally, let $z_{\alpha/2}$ denote the value of a standardized score cutting of $100\alpha/2\%$ of each tail of a standard normal distribution and z_β denote the value of a standardized score cutting of the upper $100\beta\%$. Then the test $H_0: \mu_E = \mu_C$ versus $H_1: \mu_E \neq \mu_C$ has a power of $100(1-\beta)\%$ when performed at the $100\alpha\%$ level of significance; the number of individuals n required in each group is given by

$$n' = 2(z_{\alpha/2} + z_\beta)^2 \sigma^2 [1 + (n-1)\rho]/\delta^2 \tag{1.12}$$

where δ is a "meaningful difference" specified in advance by the investigator. Alternatively, Equation 1.12 may be written as

$$n' = (z_{\alpha/2} + z_\beta)^2 [1 + (n-1)\rho]/\Delta^2 \tag{1.13}$$

where $\Delta = \dfrac{\mu_E - \mu_C}{\sigma\sqrt{2}} = \dfrac{\delta}{\sigma\sqrt{2}}$.

At $\rho = 0$, formula 1.12 reduces to the usual sample size specification given by Snedecor and Cochran (1981). When $\rho = 1$, there is variability within the cluster, and the usual formula applies with n as the number of clusters that must be sampled from each group. In most epidemiologic applications, however, values of ρ tend to be no greater than 0.6, and advance estimates may also be available from previous data. Obtaining an estimate of ρ is no different in principle from the usual requirement imposed on the investigator to supply an advance estimate of the population variance σ^2. In the case of unequal cluster sizes, we may replace n in the right-hand side of Equation 1.12 or 1.13 by the average cluster size, $\bar{n}$ (or by n_0). A conservative approach would be to replace n by n_{max}, the largest expected cluster size in the sample.

We now consider a test of significance on $\bar{y}_E - \bar{y}_C$. Note that in most applications, the clusters are likely to be of unequal size n_i, $i = 1, 2, \ldots, k$. In this case, formula 1.11 generalizes to

$$V(\bar{y}_E) = \frac{\sigma_e^2}{N}\left[1 + \left(\frac{\sum n_i^2}{N}\right)\frac{\sigma_b^2}{\sigma_e^2}\right] \tag{1.14}$$

An estimate $\hat{V}(\bar{y}_E)$ of $V(\bar{y}_E)$ may be calculated by substituting $\hat{\sigma}_b^2$ and $\hat{\sigma}_e^2$ (defined earlier), the sample estimates of σ_b^2 and σ_e^2, respectively, in Equation 1.14.

A large sample test on $H_0: \mu_E = \mu_C$ may be obtained by calculating

$$Z = \frac{\bar{y}_E - \bar{y}_C}{[\hat{V}(\bar{y}_E) + \hat{V}(\bar{y}_C)]^{1/2}} \tag{1.15}$$

(See Donner et al., 1981.)

Example 1.2

The milk yield data from 10 Ontario farms, 5 large and 5 small farms, are analyzed. Each farm provided 12 observations representing the average milk yield per cow per day for each month. For the purpose of this example, we shall ignore the sampling time as a factor and consider each farm as a cluster size of 12. The following SAS code shows how to read in the data and run the general linear model.

```
data milk;
input farm milk size $;
cards;
1   32.33   L
1   29.47   L
1   30.19   L
. . .
10   24.12   S
;

proc sort data=milk; by size;
```

```
proc glm data = milk;
class farm;
model milk = farm;
run;
```

The ANOVA results from the SAS output are given below:

Source	DF	Sum of Squares	Mean Square
Model	9	905.122484	100.569165
Error	110	734.014075	6.672855

$$\hat{\sigma}_e^2 = 6.67$$

$$\hat{\sigma}_b^2 = \frac{100.57 - 6.67}{12} = 7.83$$

Therefore, the estimated ICC is $\hat{\rho} = \frac{7.83}{7.83 + 6.67} = 0.54$.

An important objective of this study was to test whether average milk yield in large farms differs significantly from the average milk yield of small farms. That is to test $H_0: \mu_s = \mu_1$ versus $H_1: \mu_s \neq \mu_1$.

The ANOVA results separately for each farm size (small and large) are now produced. The SAS code is

```
proc glm data = milk;
class farm;
model milk = farm;
by size;
run; quit;
```

Large farm size

Source	DF	Sum of Squares	Mean Square
Model	4	283.4424600	70.8606150
Error	55	407.2490000	7.4045273

Small farm size

Source	DF	Sum of Squares	Mean Square
Model	4	379.2289833	94.8072458
Error	55	326.7650750	5.9411832

For large farms, since $\bar{y}_l = 28.00$, $k = 5$, $n = 12$, $N = 60$

$$\hat{\sigma}_{el}^2 = 7.40, \quad \hat{\sigma}_{bl}^2 = \frac{70.86 - 7.4}{12} = 5.29$$

$$\hat{\sigma}_{bl}^2 / \hat{\sigma}_{el}^2 = 0.71$$

then $\hat{V}(\bar{y}_l) = \frac{7.40}{60}[1 + (12)(0.71)] = 1.17$.

For small farms

$$\bar{y}_s = 25.32, k = 5, n = 12, N = 60$$

$$\hat{\sigma}_{es}^2 = 5.94, \hat{\sigma}_{bs}^2 = \frac{94.81 - 5.94}{12} = 7.4$$

$$\frac{\hat{\sigma}_{bs}^2}{\hat{\sigma}_{es}^2} = 1.24$$

$$\hat{V}(\bar{y}_s) = \frac{5.94}{60}[1 + (12)(1.24)] = 1.57$$

$$Z = \frac{28 - 25.32}{(1.17 + 1.57)^{1/2}} = 1.61$$

p-value $= 0.10$, and there is no sufficient evidence in the data to support H_0. The R code to read in the milk data and produce the ANOVA results:

```
milk <- read.table("x:/xxx/milk.txt",header=T)

# ANOVA results overall
anova(lm(milk ~ factor(farm), data=milk))

# ANOVA results for large farms
anova(lm(milk ~ factor(farm), data=milk[milk$size=='L',]))

# ANOVA results for small farms
anova(lm(milk ~ factor(farm), data=milk[milk$size=='S',]))
```

1.2   Regression Analysis for Clustered Data

A fundamental question in many scientific investigations is concerned with how and to what extent a response variable is related to a set of independent variables. For example, a health economist may be interested in the relationship between the effect of intervention and the cost of its administration, a clinical nutritionist in the relationship between obesity and hypertension, or a radiologist in the relationship between the ultrasound diagnosis of cancer and the tumor size. The list of situations of this kind in biomedical research is endless, let alone other areas of applications.

Suppose for a given situation, the actual mathematical relationship between the response variable "Y" and a set of independent variables is known. The investigator is then in a position to understand the factors that control the direction of the response. Unfortunately, there are few situations in practice in which the true mathematical model connecting the response to the independent variables is known. Consequently, one is forced to combine practical experience and mathematical theory to develop an approximate model that characterizes the main features of the behavior of the response variable.

Regression analysis is among the most commonly used methods of statistical analysis to model the relationship between variables. Its objective is to describe the relationship of response with independent or explanatory variables. In its very general form, a regression model is written as

$$Y = X\beta + e \qquad (1.16)$$

where Y is the $(n \times 1)$ vector of dependent variable values, X an $(n \times (p+1))$ matrix containing the values of the independent variables, β the $((p+1) \times 1)$ vector of parameters, and e the $(n \times 1)$ vector of error components. It is well known that the method of least squares is the most preferred method of estimation of the parameter of the regression model. There are fundamental assumptions that should be satisfied to use this method to estimate the parameter vector β:

(a) The components of Y are uncorrelated with each other.
(b) The error components e are assumed to be uncorrelated with mean 0 and common variance σ^2.
(c) The vector of error components e is uncorrelated with the matrix X.

Under the above conditions and provided that $(X^T X)^{-1}$ exists, the least squares estimate of β is

$$\hat{\beta} = (X^T X)^{-1} X^T Y \qquad (1.17)$$

Equation 1.17 is important in regression analysis since it provides the estimates of β once we are sure that conditions (a, b, c) are satisfied and the matrix X is specified.

In addition to the linear models (Equation 1.16), regression models include logistic models for binary responses, log-linear model for counts, and survival analysis for time to events. In this chapter, we discuss the linear-normal model for continuous responses when the basic assumption that all the observations are independent, or at least uncorrelated, is violated. Recall that the assumption of zero correlation would mean that knowing one subject's response provides no information regarding the status of another subject in the same study. However, the assumption of independence may not hold if the subjects belong to the same cluster as has been already demonstrated. As an example of a regression problem when clusters of subjects are sampled together is Miall and Oldham's arterial blood pressure levels family study. Owing to their common household environment and their shared genetic makeup, we would expect a family member to have a greater chance of having elevated blood pressure levels if his/her sibling had the same. Data from this study can be usefully thought of as being "clustered" into families. Blood pressure levels from different families are likely to be independent; those from the same family are not. This dependence among observations from the same cluster must be accounted for in assessing the relationships between risk factors and health outcomes.

Another example cited by Liang and Zeger (1993) is the growth study of Hmong refugee children. In this example, 1000 Hmong refugee children receiving health care at two Minnesota clinics between 1976 and 1985 were examined for their growth patterns. The objective was to study the patterns of growth and its association with age at entry into the United States. It is believed that stature is influenced by both genetic and environmental factors. When the offending environmental factors are removed, the growth process progresses at a faster rate. To study the growth, repeated measurements of height of each child were recorded. The number of visits per child ranged from 1 to 15 and averaged 5. The correlation between repeated observations on height for each child may be a nuisance but cannot be ignored in regression analysis.

The above two examples have common features, although they address questions with different scientific objectives. Data in the above two studies are organized in clusters. For family study, the clusters are formed by families, and in the second example a cluster comprises the repeated observations for a child. Another aspect of similarity between the two studies is that one can safely assume that the response variables (blood pressure in the family study and height in the growth study) are normally distributed. The two studies also differ in the structure of the within-cluster correlation. For example, in the family study one may assume that the correlation between the pairs of sibs within the family is equal, that is, we may assume a constant within-cluster correlation. For repeated measures longitudinal study, the situation is different. Although the repeated observations are correlated, this correlation may not be constant across time (cluster units). It is common sense to assume that observations taken at adjacent time points are more correlated than observations that are taken at separated time points.

In the remainder of this chapter, we shall focus on regression analysis of clustered data assuming common or fixed within-cluster correlation and the response variable is normally distributed. Other types of response variables and different correlation structures will be discussed in detail in subsequent chapters.

Within the framework of linear regression, we illustrate an answer to the question: what happens when the conventional linear regression is used to analyze clustered data?

Let Y_{ij} denote the score on the jth offspring in the ith family; X_i the score of the ith parent, where $j = 1, 2, \ldots, n_i$, $i = 1, 2, \ldots, k$; n_i the number of offspring in the ith family; and k the total number of families. We assume that the regression of Y on X is given by

$$Y_{ij} = \mu_y + \beta(X_i - \mu_x) + E_{ij} \tag{1.18}$$

where $\mu_y = E(Y_{ij})$, $\mu_x = E(X_i)$, β is the regression coefficient of Y on X, and E_{ij} is the deviation of the jth offspring of the ith parent. We further assume that

$$\text{Cov}(Y_{ij}, Y_{il}) = \begin{cases} \rho\sigma^2 & j \neq l \\ \sigma^2 & j = l \end{cases}$$

Under this model, Kempthorne and Tandon (1953) showed that the minimum variance unbiased estimator of β is given by

$$b_1 = \frac{\sum_{i=1}^{k} w_i(x_i - \hat{x})\bar{y}_i}{\sum w_i(x_i - \hat{x})^2} \tag{1.19}$$

and

$$V(b_1) = \frac{\sigma^2(1 - \rho)}{\sum w_i(x_i - \hat{x})^2}$$

where $w_i = n_i/(1 + n_i\rho_e)$, $\rho_e = (\rho - \beta^2)/(1 - \beta^2)$, $\bar{y}_i = \sum_j y_{ij}/n_i$, and $\hat{x} = \sum w_i x_i / \sum w_i$.

The most widely used estimator for β ignores the ICC ρ and is given by the usual estimator:

$$b = \frac{\sum_{i=1}^{k} n_i(\bar{y}_i - \bar{y})(x_i - \bar{x})}{\sum_{i=1}^{k} n_i(x_i - \bar{x})^2} \tag{1.20}$$

where $\bar{y} = \sum n_i\bar{y}_i/N$, $\bar{x} = \sum n_i x_i/N$, and $N = n_1 + n_2 + \cdots + n_k$.

$$V(b) = \frac{\sigma^2(1 - \rho) \sum n_i(1 + n_i\rho_e)(x_i - \bar{x})^2}{\left[\sum n_i(x_i - \bar{x})^2\right]^2} \tag{1.21}$$

If $\rho_e = 0$, then $w_i = n_i$ and $\text{var}(b) = \text{var}(b_1) = \sigma^2(1 - \rho)/\sum n_i(x_i - \bar{x})^2$, which means that b_1 is fully efficient.

Therefore,

$$\frac{V(b)}{V(b_1)} = \left[\frac{\sum n_i(1 + n_i\rho_e)(x_i - \bar{x})^2}{\sum n_i(x_i - \bar{x})^2}\right]$$

or equivalently

$$\frac{V(b)}{V(b_1)} = 1 + \frac{\rho_e \sum n_i^2(x_i - \bar{x})^2}{\sum n_i(x_i - \bar{x})^2} \tag{1.22}$$

Assuming $\rho_e > 0$, b is always less efficient.

The most important message of Equation 1.22 is that ignoring within-cluster correlation can lead to a loss of power when both within-cluster and cluster-level covariate information are being used to estimate the regression coefficient.

To analyze clustered data, one must therefore model both the regression of Y on X and the within-cluster dependence. If the responses are independent of each other, then ordinary least squares can be used, which produces regression estimators that are identical to the maximum likelihood in the case of normally distributed responses. In this chapter we consider two different modeling approaches: marginal and random effects. In marginal models, the regression of Y on X and the within-cluster dependence are modeled separately. The random effects models attempt to address both issues simultaneously through a single model. We shall explore both modeling strategies for a much wider class of distributions named "generalized linear models" (GLM) that includes the normal distribution as a special case.

1.3 Generalized Linear Models

GLM are a unified class of regression methods for continuous and discrete response variables. There are two components in a GLM, the systematic component and the random component. For the systematic component, one relates Y to X assuming that the mean response $\mu = E(Y)$ satisfies $g(\mu) = X_1\beta_1 + X_2\beta_2 + \cdots + X_p\beta_p$, which may conveniently be written as

$$g(\mu) = X^T\beta \tag{1.23}$$

Here, $g(.)$ is a specified function known as the "link function." The normal regression model for continuous data is a special case of Equation 1.23, where $g(.)$ is the identity link. For binary response variable Y, the logistic regression is a special case of Equation 1.23 with the logit transformation as the link. That is,

$$g(\mu) = \log \frac{\mu}{1 - \mu} = \log \frac{P(Y = 1)}{P(Y = 0)} = X^T\beta$$

When the response variable is count, we assume that

$$\log E(Y) = X^T\beta$$

To account for the variability in the response variable that is not accounted for by the systematic component, GLM assume that Y has the probability density function given by

$$f(y) = \exp[(y\theta - b(\theta))/\phi + C(y, \phi)] \tag{1.24}$$

which is a general form of the exponential family of distributions. This includes among others, the normal, binomial, and Poisson as special cases. It can be easily shown that

$$E(Y) = b'(\theta)$$

and

$$V(Y) = \phi b''(\theta)$$

For the normal distribution:

$$\theta = \mu \text{ (identity link)}$$
$$b(\theta) = \mu^2/2, \quad \phi = \sigma^2$$

Hence, $b'(\theta) = \mu$ and $b''(\theta) = 1$, indicating that ϕ is the variance.
For the Poisson distribution:

$$\theta = \ln \mu \text{ (log-link)}$$
$$b(\theta) = \mu = e^{\theta}, \quad \phi = 1$$
$$b'(\theta) = e^{\theta} = \mu$$
$$b''(\theta) = e^{\theta} = \mu$$

Hence, $E(Y) = V(Y) = \phi\mu$.

The scale parameter ϕ in Equation 1.24 is called the over-dispersion parameter. If $\phi > 1$, then the variance of the counts is larger than the mean.

When the link function in Equation 1.23 and the random component are specified by the GLM, we can estimate the regression parameters β by solving the estimating equation:

$$U = \sum_{i=1}^{p} \left(\frac{\partial \mu_i(\beta)}{\partial \beta} \right)^T V^{-1}(Y_i)[Y_i - \mu_i(\beta)] = 0 \qquad (1.25)$$

The above equation provides valid estimates when the responses are independently distributed. For clustered data, the GLM and hence Equation 1.25 are not sufficient, since the issue of within-cluster correlation is not addressed. We now discuss the two modeling approaches commonly used to analyze clustered data.

1.3.1 Marginal Models (Population Average Models)

As already mentioned, in a marginal model, the regression of Y on X and the within-cluster dependence are modeled separately. We assume:

1. The marginal mean or "population average" of the response, $\mu_{ij} = E(Y_{ij})$, depends on the explanatory variables X_{ij} through a link function $g(\mu_{ij}) = X_{ij}^T \beta$, where g is a specified link function.
2. The marginal variance depends on the marginal mean through $V(Y_{ij}) = \phi V(\mu_{ij})$, where $V(.)$ is a known variance function, such as $V(\mu_{ij}) = \phi$ for normally distributed response and $V(\mu_{ij}) = \mu_{ij}$ for count data similar to the GLM setup.

3. $\text{Cov}(Y_{ij}, Y_{il})$, the covariance between pairs within clusters, is a function of the marginal means and another additional parameter α, i.e.,

$$\text{Cov}(Y_{ij}, Y_{il}) = \gamma(\mu_{ij}, \mu_{il}, \alpha)$$

where $\gamma(.)$ is a known function.

1.3.2 Random Effects Models

There are several names given to these types of models: multilevel, hierarchical, random coefficients, or mixed effects models. The fundamental feature of these models is the assumption that parameters vary from cluster to cluster, reflecting natural heterogeneity due to unmeasured cluster-level covariates.

The general setup for the random effects GLM was described by Zeger and Karim (1991) as follows:

1. Conditional on random effects b_i, specific to the ith cluster, the response variable Y_{ij} follows a GLM with

$$g[E(Y_{ij}|b_i)] = X_{ij}^T\beta + Z_{ij}^T b_i \qquad (1.26)$$

where Z_{ij}, a $q \times 1$ vector of covariates, is a subset of X_{ij}.

2. Conditional on b_i, $Y_i = (Y_{i1}, Y_{i2}, \ldots, Y_{in})^T$ are statistically independent.

3. The b_i's are independent observations from a distribution $F(., \alpha)$, indexed by some unknown parameter α. The term "random effect" was assigned to the variable b_i, because we treat b_i as a random sample from F. The random effects b_i are not related to X_{ij}.

1.3.3 Generalized Estimating Equation (GEE)

The GEE provides a tool for practical statistical inference on the β coefficient under the marginal model when the data are clustered. The regression estimates are obtained by solving the equation:

$$U_1(\beta, \alpha) = \sum_{i=1}^{k} \left(\frac{\partial \mu_i}{\partial \beta}\right)^T \text{Cov}^{-1}(Y_i, \beta, \alpha)[y_i - \mu_i(\beta)] = 0 \qquad (1.27)$$

where $\mu_i(\beta) = E(Y_i)$, the marginal mean of Y_i. One should note that $U_1(.)$ has the same form of $U(.)$ in Equation 1.25, except that Y_i is now $n_i \times 1$ vector, which consists of the n_i observations of the ith cluster, and the covariance matrix $\text{Cov}(Y_i)$, which depends on β and α, a parameter that characterizes the within-cluster dependence.

For a given α, the solution $\hat{\beta}$ to Equation 1.27 can be obtained by an iteratively reweighted least squares calculations. The solution to these equations is a consistent estimate of β, provided that $\mu_i(\beta)$ is correctly specified. The consistency property follows because $\left(\frac{\partial \mu_i}{\partial \beta}\right)^T \text{Cov}^{-1}(Y_i)$ does not depend on the Y_i's, so Equation 1.27 converges to 0 and has consistent roots as long as $E(Y_i - \mu_i(\beta)) = 0$ (see Liang and Zeger (1986) and Zeger and Liang (1986)).

If a $\sqrt{k}$ consistent estimate of α is available, $\hat{\beta}$ are asymptotically normal, even if the correlation structure is misspecified. Liang and Zeger (1986) proposed a "robust" estimate of the covariance matrix of $\hat{\beta}$ as

$$V(\hat{\beta}) = A^{-1}MA^{-1}$$

where

$$A = \sum_{i=1}^{k} \widetilde{D}_i^T \widetilde{V}_i^{-1} \widetilde{D}_i$$

$$M = \sum_{i=1}^{k} \widetilde{D}_i^T \widetilde{V}_i^{-1} \text{Cov}(Y_i) \widetilde{V}_i^{-1} \widetilde{D}_i$$

$$\text{Cov}(Y_i) = (Y_i - \mu_i(\widetilde{\beta}))(Y_i - \mu_i(\widetilde{\beta}))^T$$

where $\sim$ denotes evaluation at $\widetilde{\beta}$ and $\widetilde{\alpha}(\widetilde{\beta})$.

Liang and Zeger (1986) proposed a simple estimator for α based on Pearson's residuals

$$\hat{r}_{ij} = \frac{y_{ij} - \mu_{ij}(\beta)}{\sqrt{\text{var}(y_{ij})}}$$

For example, under common correlation structure that $\text{Cor}(y_{ij}, y_{il}) = \alpha$ for all i, j, and l, an estimate of α is

$$\hat{\alpha} = \frac{\sum_{i=1}^{k} \sum_{j=1}^{n_i} \sum_{l=j+1}^{n_i-1} \hat{r}_{ij}\hat{r}_{il}}{\left[\sum_{i=1}^{k} \binom{n_i}{2} - p\right]} \tag{1.28}$$

where p in the denominator of Equation 1.28 is the number of regression parameters.

One of the limitations of the above approach is that estimation of β and α from Equations 1.27 and 1.28 are done as if (β, α) are independent of each other. Consequently, very little information from β is used when estimating α. This can lead to a significant loss of information on α. To improve on the efficiency of estimating β, Prentice (1988) and Liang et al. (1992) discussed estimating $\theta = (\beta, \alpha)$ jointly by solving

$$U_2(\beta, \alpha) = \sum_{i=1}^{k} \left(\frac{\partial \mu_i^*}{\partial \beta}\right) [\text{Cov}(Z_i, \delta)]^{-1} (Z_i - \mu_i^* \theta) = 0$$

where

$$Z_i = (Y_{i1}, \ldots, Y_{in_i}, Y_{i1}^2, \ldots, Y_{in_i}^2, Y_{i1}Y_{i2}, Y_{i1}Y_{i3}, \ldots, Y_{i'n_{i'}-1}Y_{in_i})^T$$

where $\mu_i^* = E(Z_i, \theta)$, which is completely specified by the modeling assumptions of the GLM. They called this expanded procedure that uses both the Y_{ij}'s and $Y_{ij}Y_{il}$ the GEE2.

GEE2 seems to improve the efficiency of both β and α. On the other hand, the robustness property for β of GEE is no longer true. Hence, correct inferences about β require correct specification of the within-cluster dependence structure. The same authors suggest using a sensitivity analysis when making inference on β. That is, one may repeat the procedure with different models for the within-cluster dependence structure to examine the sensitivity of $\tilde{\beta}$ to choose the dependence structure.

1.4 Fitting Alternative Models for Clustered Data

Example 1.3

We will use a subset of the data from a survey conducted by Miall and Oldham (1955) to assess the correlations in systolic and diastolic blood pressures among family members living within 25 miles of Rhonda Fach Valley in South Wales. The purpose of the following analysis is to illustrate the effect of the within-cluster correlation in the case of the normal linear regression model. The part of the data that we use for this illustration consists of the observations made on siblings and their parents. Each observation consists of systolic and diastolic blood pressures to the nearest 5 or 10 mmHg. In this analysis, we will not distinguish among male and female siblings. The following variables will be used to run a few models in this section.

familyid:	Family ID
subjid:	Sibling ID
sbp:	Sibling systolic blood pressure
msbp:	Mother systolic blood pressure
age:	Sibling age
armgirth:	Sibling arm girth
cenmsbp:	Mother systolic blood pressure centered
cenage:	Sibling age centered within the family
cengirth:	Sibling arm girth centered within the family

The records with missing values of sibling age, mother systolic blood pressure, sibling arm girth, and sibling systolic blood pressure are deleted. The dataset consists of 488 observations on 154 families. The family size ranges from 1 to 10. We begin by first analyzing the data using the GEE approach. This is followed by a series of models using the multilevels modeling approach. All models are fitted using the SAS procedures GENMOD for the GEE and the MIXED for the multilevels approach. The equivalent R code (R 2.3.1—A Language and Environment Copyright 2006, R Development Core Team) is also provided.

The SAS code to read in the data and fit this model is

```
data fam;
input familyid subjid sbp age armgirth msbp;
datalines;
1   1     85    5   5.75    120
1   2    105   15   8.50    120
. . . . . .

200  5   135   40   12.50   255
213  1   120   64   11.00   110
;


* Computing the overall mean for msbp;
proc means data=fam noprint; var msbp; output out=msbp mean=
mmsbp; run;


* Computing cluster-specific means for age and armgirth;
proc means data=fam noprint; class familyid; var age armgirth;
output out=fmeans mean=mage marmgirth; run;
data fmeans; set fmeans; if familyid=. then delete; drop _TYPE_ _FREQ_;
run;


* Centering msbp at overall mean and age and armgirth at cluster-specific
means;
data family; merge fam fmeans; by familyid; if _n_=1 then set
msbp(drop=_TYPE_ _FREQ_);
cenage=age-mage; cengirth=armgirth-marmgirth; cenmsbp=
msbp-mmsbp;
keep familyid subjid sbp age armgirth msbp cenage cengirth cenmsbp;


proc genmod data=family;
class familyid;
model sbp = msbp cenage cengirth/dist = n lnk=id;
repeated subject = familyid /type = cs corrw;
run;
```

The following is the partial output showing the analysis of the GEE parameter estimates:

Analysis of GEE Parameter Estimates

			Empirical Standard Error Estimates			
Parameter	Estimate	Standard Error	95% Confidence Limits		Z	Pr > |Z|
Intercept	119.0985	0.9198	117.2957	120.9013	129.48	<0.0001
cenmsbp	0.2024	0.0349	0.1340	0.2707	5.80	<0.0001
cenage	0.1802	0.1984	−0.2086	0.5690	0.91	0.3636
cengirth	3.5445	0.8263	1.9249	5.1641	4.29	<0.0001

This model treats the within-cluster correlation as nuisance. It is assumed that the within-subject correlation structure is exchangeable or compound symmetry. The estimated working correlation under the common (compound symmetry) structure is 0.328. The analysis indicates that the arm girth and the mother systolic blood pressure are significant predictors of the sibling systolic blood pressure levels.

We now illustrate the application of the random effects model to analyze clustered data. We followed an informative strategy given by Singer (1998) for fitting multilevel data. Therefore, we shall present three nested random effects models and discuss the relative advantages of each model.

PROC MIXED for Clustered Data

Here we illustrate how two levels of clustered data are analyzed using PROC MIXED in SAS (SAS Institute 1995, and 1996). By two levels we mean a situation where subjects are nested within organizational units. The subjects in the dataset are the siblings and the clusters are the families. We are interested in examining the behavior of a level 1 outcome (siblings outcome) as function of level 1 and level 2 (family) covariates. The siblings-level outcomes are the systolic blood pressures (sbp), and the covariates measured at the siblings level are age (cenage) and arm girth (cengirth). There are several family-level outcomes, but we shall restrict to the systolic blood pressure of the mother (cenmsbp).

The first baseline model is called an "unconditional means" model, which examines the variability in sbp across families.

Model 1: Unconditional Mean Model

Under this model, we express sbp (y_{ij}) as a one-way random effects model

$$y_{ij} = \mu + b_i + e_{ij}$$

$b_i \approx N(0, \sigma_b^2)$ and $e_{ij} \approx N(0, \sigma_e^2)$

The model has one fixed effect (μ) and two variance components—one representing the variation between family means (σ_b^2) and the other variation among siblings within families (σ_e^2).

The SAS code to fit this model is

```
proc mixed data=family noclprint noitprint;
class familyid;
model sbp=/bw;
random familyid;
run;
```

The selected output is shown below.

Covariance Parameter Estimates

Cov Parm	Estimate
familyid	106.98
Residual	166.22

Solution for Fixed Effects

Effect	Estimate	Standard Error	DF	T-Value	Pr > |t|
Intercept	118.67	1.0554	487	112.44	<0.0001

The mixed procedure produces a set of information: the "familyid" estimate is an estimate of the parameter (σ_e^2), while the "residual" estimate is an estimate of the parameter (σ_b^2). The maximum likelihood estimate of the ICC is

$$\hat{\rho} = \frac{\hat{\sigma}_b^2}{(\sigma_b^2 + \sigma_e^2)} = \frac{106.98}{(106.98 + 166.22)} = 0.39$$

This tells us that there is a great deal of clustering of systolic blood pressure levels of siblings within families.

There is another approach that generalizes more easily to data with multiple levels. This approach expresses the subject-level outcome y_{ij} using a pair of linked models: one at the subject level (level 1) and another at the family level (level 2). At level 1, we express y_{ij} as the sum of an intercept for the subject's family (β_{i0}) and random error (e_{ij}):

$$y_{ij} = \beta_{i0} + e_{ij} \quad \text{where } e_{ij} \approx N(0, \sigma_e^2).$$

At the higher level (family level), we express the family-level intercept as the sum of an overall mean (β) and random deviation (u_{i0}) so that

$$\beta_{i0} = \beta + u_{i0} \quad \text{where } u_{i0} \approx N(0, \tau_0)$$

Therefore,

$$y_{ij} = \beta + u_{i0} + e_{ij}$$

The SAS code for this model is

```
proc mixed data=family noclprint noitprint covtest;
class familyid;
model sbp =/s ddfm=bw;
random intercept/sub = familyid;
run;
```

The parameter estimates under this model are the same as in the previous model. The purpose of the *covtest* option in the "proc mixed" statement is to test the hypothesis for the variance components.

Model 2: Including a Family-Level Covariate

In this model, we include the mother's systolic blood pressure score (msbp) as a predictor of the siblings score. Following Singer (1998), the msbp is centered at the overall mean so that it has mean 0 and allows a meaningful interpretation of the intercept. For this model we write

$$y_{ij} = \beta_{i0} + e_{ij}$$
$$\beta_{i0} = \gamma_{00} + \gamma_{01}x_i + u_{i0}$$

where

$$e_{ij} \approx N(0, \sigma_e^2), \quad u_{i0} \approx N(0, \sigma_0^2).$$

Therefore, $y_{ij} = (\gamma_{00} + \gamma_{01}x_i) + (u_{i0} + e_{ij})$, where $x_i = \text{msbp} - \text{mean(msbp)} = \text{cenmsbp}$.

The above model has two components, a fixed part enclosed in the first bracket and a random part enclosed in the second bracket. The SAS code to fit this model is

```
proc mixed data=family noclprint noitprint;
class familyid;
model sbp = cenmsbp/s ddfm=bw notest;
random intercept/subject = familyid;
run;
```

Note that there is another option in the "model" statement, which is ddfm = bw. This allows SAS to use the "between/within" method for computing the denominator degrees of freedom for tests of fixed effects. See SAS documentation or Littell et al. (1996) for details.

The SAS output is

Covariance Parameter Estimates

Cov Parm	Subject	Estimate
Intercept	familyid	67.4679
Residual		163.89

Solution for Fixed Effects

Effect	Estimate	Standard Error	DF	t-Value	Pr > |t|
Intercept	119.11	0.9161	152	130.01	<0.0001
cenmsbp	0.2005	0.02748	152	7.29	<0.0001

Note that there are two fixed effects to be estimated: the intercept and the covariate (MSBP). The null hypothesis, which states that there is no relationship between mother's systolic blood pressure levels and the siblings, is not supported by the data. Also note that the variance components estimates are 67.47 and 163.89 for τ_0 and σ_e^2, respectively. These estimates under the present model have different interpretations. In model 1, there were no covariates, so these were unconditional components. After adding the mother's blood pressure as a covariate, these are now conditional components. Note that the conditional within-family component is slightly reduced (from 166.22 to 163.89). The variance component representing variation between families τ_0 or σ_b^2 has diminished markedly (from 106.98 to 67.47). This tells us that the cluster- or family-level covariate (mother's systolic blood pressure) explains a large percentage of the family-to-family variation. One way of measuring how much variation exists in family mean blood pressures as explained by the mother's blood pressure levels is to compute how much the variance component for this term τ_0 has diminished between the two models. Following Bryk and Raudenbush (1992), we compute this as $(106.98 - 67.47)/106.98 = 36.9\%$. This is interpreted by saying that about 36% of the explainable variation in the sibling's mean systolic blood pressure levels is explained by the mother's systolic blood pressure levels.

Model 3: Including Sib-Level Covariate
The simplest model may be written as

$$y_{ij} = \beta_{i0} + \beta_{11}Z_{ij} + e_{ij}$$

Here, Z_{ij} is the age of the jth subject within the ith family centered at its mean value. The other terms are defined as before. Let

$$\beta_{i0} = \beta_{00} + u_{i0}$$
$$\beta_{i1} = \beta_{11} + u_{i1}$$

Hence,

$$y_{ij} = \beta_{00} + u_{i0} + (\beta_{11} + u_{i1})Z_{ij} + e_{ij}$$
$$= (\beta_{00} + \beta_{11}Z_{ij}) + (u_{i0} + u_{i1}Z_{ij} + e_{ij})$$

where $e_{ij} \approx N(0, \sigma_e^2)$, $u_i = (u_{i0}, u_{i1}) \approx \text{BIVN}(0, \sum)$, and e_{ij} is independent of the bivariate normal random vector u_i. The Σ is a 2×2 symmetric matrix whose elements are $\delta_{00} = V(u_{i0})$, $\delta_{11} = V(u_{i1})$, and $\delta_{01} = \text{Cov}(u_{i0}, u_{i1})$. The SAS code to fit this model is

```
proc mixed data=family noclprint noitprint;
class familyid;
model sbp= cenmsbp/s ddfm=bw notest;
random intercept cenage/ subject=familyid type=un;
run;
```

Notice that the random statement has two random effects—one for intercept and one for the Z-slope. There is also an additional option in the random statement, "type=un," indicating that an unstructured specification for the covariance of u_i is assumed. Partial SAS output is shown below.

Covariance Parameter Estimates

Cov Parm	Subject	Estimate
UN(1,1)	familyid	78.9632
UN(2,1)	familyid	4.3682
UN(2,2)	familyid	1.0199
Residual		133.16

Solution for Fixed Effects

Effect	Estimate	Standard Error	DF	t-Value	Pr > |t|
Intercept	118.43	0.8977	152	131.92	<0.0001
cenmsbp	0.1973	0.02687	152	7.34	<0.0001

We shall start by first interpreting the fixed effects. The estimate of the intercept 118.43 indicates the estimated average sibling systolic blood pressure levels after controlling for the mother's systolic blood pressure. The estimate of the cenmsbp indicates that the average slope representing the relationship between siblings' blood pressure and the mother's systolic blood pressure is 0.20. The standard errors of these estimates are very small, resulting in small, *p*-values. We conclude that, on average, there is a statistically significant relationship between siblings' systolic blood pressures and the mother's systolic blood pressure.

The covariance parameter estimates tell us how much these intercepts and slopes vary across families. The $\hat{\delta}_{00} = 78.96$ represents the variability in the intercepts, $\hat{\delta}_{11} = 4.37$ the variability in the slopes, and $\hat{\delta}_{01} = 1.02$ the covariance between intercepts and slopes. We can say that the intercepts vary considerably; in other words, families do differ in average systolic blood pressure levels after controlling for the effects of the mother's blood pressure levels. We also note that the slopes do not considerably vary between the families, and there is no evidence that the effects of mother's blood pressure on sibling systolic blood pressure differ between the families.

Finally, we compare the residual error variance of the unconditional model to that of the present model. Recall that the estimated variance of the unconditional model was 166.22. Here we have the conditional estimate of 133.16. Inclusion of the sibling's age is therefore explained as $(166.22 - 133.16)/166.22 = 20.0\%$ of the explainable variation within families.

**Model 4: Including One Family-Level Covariate and Two
Subject-Level Covariates**

Following Singer (1998), it is always helpful to write the outcome variable as a function of the covariates measured at the lowest (subject) level. Thereafter, we write the slopes and the intercepts as functions of the higher level (in our example, a family).

$$y_{ij} = B_{i0} + B_{i1}Z_{ij} + B_{i2}a_{ij} + e_{ij}$$

$$B_{i0} = \gamma_{00} + \gamma_{01}x_i + u_{i0}$$

$$B_{i1} = \gamma_{10} + \gamma_{11}x_i + u_{i1}$$

$$B_{i2} = \gamma_{20} + \gamma_{21}x_i + u_{i2}$$

where Z_{ij} is the centered arm girth of the jth subject within the ith family, a_{ij} the centered age of the jth subject within the ith family, and x_i the centered mother's systolic blood pressure in the ith family.

Hence,

$$y_{ij} = \gamma_{00} + \gamma_{01}x_i + u_{i0} + Z_{ij}(\gamma_{10} + \gamma_{11}x_i + u_{i1}) + a_{ij}(\gamma_{20} + \gamma_{21}x_i + u_{i2}) + e_{ij}$$

Simplifying, we get

$$y_{ij} = \lfloor \gamma_{00} + \gamma_{01}x_i + \gamma_{10}Z_{ij} + \gamma_{20}a_{ij} + \gamma_{11}x_iZ_{ij} + \gamma_{21}x_ia_{ij} \rfloor + \lfloor u_{10} + Z_{ij}u_{i1} + a_{ij}u_{iz} + e_{ij} \rfloor$$

Terms in the first bracket should appear in the model statement, while those in the second bracket should appear in the random statement.

The SAS code to fit the model is

```
proc mixed data=family covtest noclprint noitprint;
class familyid;
```

```
model sbp=cenmsbp cenage cengirth cenmsbp*cenage cenmsbp*cengirth/s
ddfm=bw notest;
random cenage cengirth/subject=familyid type=un;
run;
```

The variable cengirth has a zero variance component; we fit the model after removing cengirth from the random statement. The results are given below.

Covariance Parameter Estimates

Cov Parm	Subject	Estimate	Standard Error	Z-Value	Pr > |Z|
UN(1,1)	familyid	81.8458	15.4989	5.28	<0.0001
UN(2,1)	familyid	4.7531	1.7062	2.79	0.0053
UN(2,2)	familyid	0.6185	0.3115	1.99	0.0235
Residual		124.29	11.2232	11.07	<0.0001

Solution for Fixed Effects

Effect	Estimate	Standard Error	DF	t-Value	Pr > |t|
Intercept	119.07	0.9208	152	129.32	<0.0001
cenmsbp	0.2043	0.02777	152	7.36	<0.0001
cenage	0.02669	0.1624	330	0.16	0.8695
cengirth	4.2129	0.7010	330	6.01	<0.0001
cenmsbp*cenage	0.008845	0.004130	330	2.14	0.0330
cenmsbp*cengirth	−0.02641	0.01736	330	−1.52	0.1292

Interpretation of the above output has been left as an exercise to the reader.

The R code reads the data; computes the centered variables cenage, cengirth, and cenmsbp; and fits the alternative models discussed in this example. Note that the packages "nlme" and "gee" should be installed and loaded for functions "lme" and "gee", respectively, to run.

```
fam <-read.table("x:/xxx/familydata.txt",header=T)
cenage = unlist(tapply(fam[,4], fam[,1], scale, scale=FALSE))
cengirth = unlist(tapply(fam[,5], fam[,1], scale, scale=FALSE))
cenmsbp = scale(fam[,6], center=TRUE, scale=FALSE)
family = data.frame(fam, cenage, cengirth, cenmsbp)

# Generalized estimating equations (GEE)
fam.gee <- gee(sbp ~ cenmsbp+cenage+cengirth, familyid, data=family,
family=gaussian, corstr="exchangeable")
summary(fam.gee)

# Unconditional mean model—Mixed Model 1
fam.lme1 <- lme(fixed=sbp ~ 1, random=~1 | familyid, data=family)
summary(fam.lme1)
```

# Mixed model including one cluster-level covariate, cenmsbp—Mixed Model 2
fam.lme2 <- lme(fixed = sbp ~ cenmsbp, random=~1 | familyid, data = family)
summary(fam.lme2)

# Mixed model including sib-level covariate, cengirth—Mixed Model 3
fam.lme3 <- lme(fixed = sbp ~ cenmsbp, random=~ cenage | familyid, data = family)
summary(fam.lme3)

# Mixed model including one sibling-level covariate, cengurth—*Mixed Model 4
fam.lme4 <- lme(fixed = sbp ~ cenmsbp + cenage + cengirth + cenmsbp* cenage + cenmsbp*cengirth, random=~ cenage −1 | familyid, data = family)
summary(fam.lme4)

Appendix

1. Linear combinations of random variables

Let $x = (x_i, x_2, \ldots, x_k)$ be a set of random variables such that $E(x_i) = \mu_i$, $V(x_i) = \sigma_i^2$, and $Cov(x_i, x_j) = c_{ij}$. We define a linear combination of the random variable x as

$$y = \sum_{i=1}^{k} w_i x_i$$

where $w_1, w_2, \ldots, w_k$ are constants.

$$E(y) = \sum_{i=1}^{k} w_i \mu_i \tag{A.1}$$

and

$$V(y) = \sum_{i=1}^{k} w_i^2 \sigma_i^2 + \sum_{\substack{i=1 \\ i \neq j}}^{k} \sum_{j=1}^{k} w_i w_j c_{ij} \tag{A.2}$$

2. Consider two linear combinations $y_s = \sum_{i=1}^{k} a_{si} x_i$ and $y_t = \sum_{i=1}^{k} a_{ti} x_i$. Then the covariance between y_s and y_t is

$$Cov(y_s, y_t) = \sum_{i=1}^{k} \sum_{j=1}^{k} a_{si} a_{tj} Cov(x_i, x_j) \tag{A.3}$$

3. The delta method

Let $g(.)$ be a differentiable function of x. Then to the first order of approximation

$$E[g(x)] = g(E(x))$$

and

$$V[g(x)] = \left(\frac{\partial g}{\partial x}\right)_{x=\mu}^2 V(x) \tag{A.4}$$

In general, if g is a differentiable function of $x_1, x_2, \ldots, x_k$, then to the first approximation

$$V[g(x_1, x_2, \ldots, x_k)] \approx \sum_{i=1}^{k} \left(\frac{\partial \dot{g}}{\partial x_i}\right)^2 V(x_i) + \sum_{i=1 \neq j=1}^{k} \left(\frac{\partial \dot{g}}{\partial x_i}\right)\left(\frac{\partial \dot{g}}{\partial x_j}\right) \mathrm{cov}(x_i, x_j) \tag{A.5}$$

where the (.) on top of $\partial g/\partial x_i$ means that they are evaluated at μ.

If we have two differentiable functions $g_1(x_1, \ldots, x_k)$ and $g_2(x_1, \ldots, x_k)$, then to the first order of approximation

$$\mathrm{Cov}(g_1, g_2) = \sum_{i=1}^{k} \sum_{j=1}^{k} \left(\frac{\partial \dot{g}_1}{\partial x_i}\right)\left(\frac{\partial \dot{g}_2}{\partial x_j}\right) \mathrm{Cov}(x_i, x_j) \tag{A.6}$$

Exercises

1.1 Suppose that we have k clusters, each of size n, and that the model generating the data is the one-way random effects:

$$y_{ij} = \mu + b_i + e_{ij}, \quad b_i \approx N(0, \sigma_b^2), \quad e_{ij} \approx N(0, \sigma_e^2)$$

Under the same model assumptions, and given that

$$\mathrm{var}(\hat{\sigma}_e^2) = \frac{2\sigma_e^4}{k(n-1)}$$

$$\mathrm{var}(\hat{\sigma}_b^2) = \frac{2}{n^2}\left[\frac{(n\sigma_b^2 + \sigma_e^2)^2}{k-1} + \frac{\sigma_e^4}{k(n-1)}\right]$$

and $\mathrm{cov}(\hat{\sigma}_e^2, \hat{\sigma}_b^2) = -2\sigma_e^4/kn(n-1)$,
use the delta method to show that

$$\mathrm{var}(\hat{\rho}) = \frac{2(1-\rho)^2(1+(n-1)\rho)^2}{kn(n-1)}$$

1.2   Under the same assumptions of exercise 1.1, it is known that

$$MSB \approx (n\sigma_b^2 + \sigma_e^2)\chi_{k-1}^2$$
$$MSW \approx \sigma_e^2 \chi_{k(n-1)}^2$$

On defining upper and lower points of the *F*-distribution as F_u and F_l by

$$\Pr[F_l \leq F_{k(n-1)}^{k-1} \leq F_u] = 1 - \alpha$$

construct an exact $(1 - \alpha)100\%$ confidence interval on $\rho = \sigma_b^2/(\sigma_b^2 + \sigma_e^2)$.

1.3   Suppose that we have a two-arm cluster randomized clinical trial as described in this chapter. Let $\theta = \mu_E/\mu_C$. Use the delta method to find a first-order approximation to the maximum likelihood of θ. Hence, find an approximate $(1 - \alpha)100\%$ confidence interval on θ assuming that the number of clusters is the same in each arm.

1.4   Suppose that we have H treatment groups and k_h clusters are randomized in the hth group $(h = 1, 2, \ldots, H)$ with n_{hj} denoting the jth cluster size within the hth group $(j = 1, 2, \ldots, k_h)$. It is required to test the hypothesis $H_0: \mu_1 = \mu_2 = \cdots = \mu_H$. Cochran (1937) suggested that for individual randomization, the statistic

$$G_H^2 = \sum_{h=1}^{H} w_i \bar{y}_i (\bar{y}_{h'} - \bar{\bar{y}})^2$$

has approximately χ^2 distribution with $(H - 1)$ degrees of freedom. Here $\bar{y}_{h'}$ is the hth group mean,

$$\bar{\bar{y}} = \frac{\sum_{i=1}^{H} w_i \bar{y}_i}{\sum_{i=1}^{H} w_i}$$

and $w_i = [\text{var}(\bar{y}_i)]^{-1}$
   For the case of cluster randomization,
   (i) What is w_i and $\text{var}(\bar{\bar{y}})$.
   (ii) Show that G_H is equivalent to Z given in Equation 1.15. State your assumptions.

1.5   Under the one-way random effects, define the within-cluster coefficient of variation as $\theta = \sigma_e/\mu$, and its maximum likelihood estimator as $\hat{\theta} = (MSW)^{\frac{1}{2}}/\bar{y}$. Use the delta method to derive a first-order approximation to the variance of $\hat{\theta}$. Assume the data are normally distributed.

1.6 Run a sequence of models using SAS programs and R programs on 13 families, a subset of Miall and Oldham's data provided below:

FID	SID	FBP	MBP	SBP	AGE	SEX	ARMGIRTH
1	1	104.47	103.70	94.30	3.66	1	5.90
1	2	104.47	103.70	96.51	15.47	0	11.00
1	3	104.47	103.70	96.51	15.43	1	9.80
1	4	104.47	103.70	102.00	17.16	0	10.00
1	5	104.47	103.70	92.00	2.00	1	3.20
1	6	104.47	103.70	103.00	12.28	1	8.00
1	7	104.47	103.70	91.90	2.11	1	3.30
2	1	109.48	102.55	96.70	4.35	0	5.90
2	2	109.48	102.55	95.00	8.57	0	8.60
2	3	109.48	102.55	104.80	9.51	0	6.70
2	4	109.48	102.55	96.00	7.14	1	6.00
2	5	109.48	102.55	90.00	1.28	1	2.30
3	1	107.44	103.02	94.00	5.46	1	5.90
3	2	107.44	103.02	96.52	15.70	1	10.50
3	3	107.44	103.02	102.00	9.16	0	8.00
3	4	107.44	103.02	100.00	20.92	0	11.39
3	5	107.44	103.02	94.00	6.34	1	8.00
3	6	107.44	103.02	93.00	2.42	1	4.20
4	1	111.68	106.51	97.00	4.44	0	4.99
4	2	111.68	106.51	96.49	14.26	0	7.90
4	3	111.68	106.51	101.00	17.44	0	9.00
4	4	111.68	106.51	105.00	9.17	1	7.00
4	5	111.68	106.51	96.60	4.71	0	6.00
4	6	111.68	106.51	108.00	12.47	0	7.80
4	7	111.68	106.51	99.00	6.36	1	6.00
5	1	110.18	107.44	89.00	1.48	1	3.00
5	2	110.18	107.44	97.99	11.01	1	4.50
5	3	110.18	107.44	93.00	3.09	1	5.00
5	4	110.18	107.44	10.00	12.09	1	7.50
5	5	110.18	107.44	110.00	9.70	1	9.10
5	6	110.18	107.44	96.48	15.46	1	9.90
5	7	110.18	107.44	92.00	8.30	1	7.00
5	8	110.18	107.44	96.48	14.42	0	9.50
6	1	109.98	108.09	98.17	11.42	0	7.50
6	2	109.98	108.09	95.00	5.07	1	5.40
6	3	109.98	108.09	104.30	12.75	1	9.60
6	4	109.98	108.09	96.47	13.43	1	8.00
6	5	109.98	108.09	95.50	8.54	0	6.60
6	6	109.98	108.09	104.00	9.03	0	5.90
7	1	110.18	108.15	90.00	6.89	1	7.40
7	2	110.18	108.15	104.20	16.84	0	10.20
7	3	110.18	108.15	96.90	6.83	0	6.70
7	4	110.18	108.15	97.99	11.51	0	7.80
7	5	110.18	108.15	98.00	6.04	1	7.50
7	6	110.18	108.15	96.60	7.25	1	6.80
7	7	110.18	108.15	98.00	5.67	1	5.00
7	8	110.18	108.15	96.91	18.03	0	10.60

(Continued)

(*Continued*)

FID	SID	FBP	MBP	SBP	AGE	SEX	ARMGIRTH
8	1	108.69	103.60	95.90	7.00	1	6.60
8	2	108.69	103.60	101.50	17.55	1	11.40
8	3	108.69	103.60	96.00	8.67	1	5.50
8	4	108.69	103.60	96.90	5.39	0	5.60
8	5	108.69	103.60	98.60	8.49	1	7.50
8	6	108.69	103.60	96.98	20.70	1	11.00
8	7	108.69	103.60	96.94	11.80	0	7.50
9	1	113.43	104.33	96.51	14.03	0	9.90
9	2	113.43	104.33	96.51	15.30	0	8.00
9	3	113.43	104.33	96.51	13.92	1	7.00
9	4	113.43	104.33	98.27	11.48	0	8.00
9	5	113.43	104.33	97.12	9.85	1	7.00
10	1	111.52	108.42	96.47	15.05	0	10.50
10	2	111.52	108.42	97.00	5.75	1	7.00
10	3	111.52	108.42	106.50	9.57	1	8.00
10	4	111.52	108.42	97.73	12.06	0	9.50
11	1	112.62	103.85	98.19	18.61	0	10.00
11	2	112.62	103.85	96.51	14.45	1	9.50
11	3	112.62	103.85	96.98	10.99	1	8.50
12	1	107.28	112.91	96.00	4.54	0	5.00
12	2	107.28	112.91	104.00	12.94	0	7.90
13	1	111.84	108.56	96.00	4.00	0	5.50
13	2	111.84	108.56	98.31	10.65	0	7.00
13	3	111.84	108.56	97.00	8.53	0	7.00
13	4	111.84	108.56	98.31	10.17	0	8.00
13	5	111.84	108.56	99.00	5.49	0	4.99

2

Analysis of Cross-Classified Data

CONTENTS

2.1   Introduction

There are two broad categories of investigative studies that produce statistical data: the first is *designed controlled experiments* and the second is *observational studies*. The controlled experiments are conducted to achieve the following two major objectives: (a) to clearly detect with reasonable power the effects of the treatment (or combination of treatments) structure and (b) to ensure maximum control on the experimental error. There are several advantages of studies run under controlled experiments, the most important being that it permits one to disentangle a complex causal problem by proceeding in a step-wise fashion. As suggested by Schlesselman (1982), within an experimental procedure the researcher can decompose the main problem and explore each component by a series of separate experiments with comparatively simple causal assumptions.

Observational studies are those that are concerned with investigating relationships among characteristics of certain populations where the groups to be compared have not been formed by random allocation. A frequently used example to illustrate this point is that of establishing a link between smoking cigarettes and contracting lung cancer. This cannot be explored using random allocation of patients to smoking and nonsmoking conditions for obvious ethical and practical reasons. Therefore, the researcher must rely on observational studies to provide evidence of epidemiological and statistical associations between a possible risk factor and a disease.

One of the most common and important questions in observational investigation involves assessing the occurrence of the disease under study in the presence of a potential risk factor. The most frequently employed means of presenting statistical evidence is the 2×2 table. The following section is devoted to assessing the significance of association between disease and a risk factor in a 2×2 table.

2.2   Measures of Association in 2 × 2 Tables

In this section, an individual classified as *diseased* will be denoted by D and by $\overline{D}$ if *not diseased*. Exposure to the risk factor is denoted by E and $\overline{E}$ for *exposed* and *unexposed*, respectively. Table 2.1 illustrates how a sample of size n is cross-classified according to the above notation.

There are, in practice, several methods of sampling by which the above table of frequencies can be obtained. The three most common methods are the cross-sectional study (historical cohort), the cohort study (prospective design), and the case–control study (retrospective design). These are described here with regard to the 2×2 table analysis.

TABLE 2.1

Cross-Classified Data in a 2×2 Table

	Disease		
Exposure	D	$\overline{D}$	Total
E	n_{11}	n_{12}	$n_{1.}$
$\overline{E}$	n_{21}	n_{22}	$n_{2.}$
Total	$n_{.1}$	$n_{.2}$	n

2.2.1 Cross-Sectional Sampling

This method calls for the selection of a total of n subjects from a large population after which the presence or absence of disease and the presence or absence of exposure is determined for each subject. Only the sample size can be specified prior to the collection of data. With this method of sampling, the issue of association between disease and exposure is the main concern. In the population from which the sample is drawn, the unknown proportions are denoted as in Table 2.2.

TABLE 2.2

Model 2×2 for Cross-Sectional Sampling

	Disease		
Exposure	D	$\overline{D}$	Total
E	p_{11}	p_{12}	$p_{1.}$
$\overline{E}$	p_{21}	p_{22}	$p_{2.}$
Total	$p_{.1}$	$p_{.2}$	1

The exposure and disease would be independent of each other if and only if $p_{ij} = p_{i.} p_{.j}$ $(i, j = 1, 2)$. Assessing independence based on the sample outcome is determined by how close the value of n_{ij} is to $e_{ij} = n\hat{p}_{i.}\hat{p}_{.j}$ (the expected frequency under independence), where $\hat{p}_{i.} = n_{i.}/n$ and $\hat{p}_{.j} = n_{.j}/n$ are the maximum likelihood estimators of $p_{i.}$ and $p_{.j}$, respectively.

There are two commonly used measures of distance between n_{ij} and e_{ij} and the χ^2 and the Wilks likelihood ratio test statistics. Historically, emphasis has been placed on large sample χ^2 methods for the analysis of contingency tables with arbitrary number of rows and columns. In more recent years, with the advance of computational power, there has been an increased interest in the exact methods.

In choosing an appropriate statistical method for categorical data analysis, one should consider the measurement scale of the response variable as well as the independent variable. As we have already indicated, statistical analyses of contingency tables involve the analysis of two-way tables for the assessment of significance of the association between two variables. We note that statistics exist for situations in which both the exposure variable and the response variable are nominal, when only the response is ordinal or when both variables are ordinal. We first introduce the Pearson χ^2 statistic:

$$\chi^2 = \sum_i \sum_j \frac{(n_{ij} - e_{ij})^2}{e_{ij}}$$

which with Yates's continuity correction becomes

$$\chi^2 = \sum_i \sum_j \frac{(|n_{ij} - e_{ij}| - 0.5)^2}{e_{ij}}$$

The hypothesis of independence is rejected for values of χ^2 that exceed $\chi^2_{\alpha,1}$ (the cut-off value of χ^2 at α-level of significance and one degree of freedom). The second is Wilks statistic,

$$G^2 = 2 \sum_i \sum_j n_{ij}(\ln n_{ij} - \ln e_{ij})$$

This statistic is called the likelihood-ratio chi-squared statistic. As for the Pearson χ^2 statistic, larger values of G^2 lead to the rejection of the null hypothesis of independence.

When independence holds, the Pearson χ^2 statistic and the likelihood ratio statistic G^2 have asymptotic (i.e., in large samples) chi-squared distribution with one degree of freedom.

It is not simple to determine the sample size needed for the χ^2 distribution to approximate the exact distributions of χ^2 and G^2 well. For a fixed number of cells (the case being discussed here), χ^2 converges to the χ^2 distribution more quickly than the G^2 and the approximation is usually poor for G^2 when $n < 20$. Further guidelines regarding sample-size considerations and the validity of χ^2 and G^2 are given in Agresti (1990, p. 246).

The most commonly used measures of association between disease and exposure are the relative risk and the odds ratio. To explain how these measures are evaluated, some changes in notations in Table 2.1 would be appropriate and are shown in Table 2.3.

TABLE 2.3

Additional Notations for the 2 × 2 Cross-Classified Data

Exposure	Disease		Total
	D	$\bar{D}$	
E	$n_{11} = y_1$	$n_{12} = n_1 - y_1$	n_1
$\bar{E}$	$n_{21} = y_2$	$n_{22} = n_2 - y_2$	n_2
Total	$y.$	$n - y.$	N

The following estimates obtained using the entries in Table 2.3 are important:

1. Estimated risk of disease among those exposed to the risk factor:

$$\Pr\left[\frac{D}{E}\right] = \frac{y_1}{n_1} \equiv \hat{p}_1$$

where Pr denotes the probability of the event.

2. Estimated risk of disease among those not exposed to the risk factor:

$$\Pr\left[\frac{D}{\overline{E}}\right] = \frac{y_2}{n_2} \equiv \hat{p}_2$$

3. The *relative risk* (RR) measured as the risk of disease for those exposed to the risk factor relative to those not exposed:

$$\text{RR} = \frac{y_1/n_1}{y_2/n_2}$$

The relative risk represents how much it is more (or less) likely that disease occurs in the exposed group compared to the unexposed group. For RR > 1, the association between exposure and disease is positive and negative for RR < 1.

4. The fourth and probably the most extensively used measure is the *odds ratio*. Let T_1 and T_2 denote the occurrence of disease in the exposed and the unexposed groups, respectively. The odds of disease in the exposed group may be expressed as

$$\text{odds}(T_1) = \frac{\Pr[T_1]}{1 - \Pr[T_1]} = \frac{\Pr[\text{disease}|\text{exposed}]}{1 - \Pr[\text{disease}|\text{exposed}]}$$

$$= \frac{y_1/n_1}{1 - y_1/n_1} = \frac{y_1}{n_1 - y_1}$$

Similarly, the odds of disease in the unexposed group would be

$$\text{odds}(T_2) = \frac{\Pr[T_2]}{1 - \Pr[T_2]} = \frac{\Pr[\text{disease}|\text{unexposed}]}{1 - \Pr[\text{disease}|\text{unexposed}]}$$

$$= \frac{y_2/n_2}{1 - y_2/n_2} = \frac{y_2}{n_2 - y_2}$$

The estimated odds ratio usually denoted by OR or $\hat{\psi}$ would then be the ratio of these two odds, thus

$$\hat{\psi} = \frac{\text{odds}(T_1)}{\text{odds}(T_2)} = \frac{y_1(n_2 - y_2)}{y_2(n_1 - y_1)} \tag{2.1}$$

The odds ratio is an important estimator in at least two contexts. One is that in the situation of rare diseases, the odds ratio approximates relative risk, and secondly, it can be determined from either cross-sectional, cohort, or case–control studies as will be illustrated later in this chapter.

2.2.2 Cohort and Case–Control Studies

In a cohort study, individuals are selected for observation and followed over time. Selection of subjects may depend on the presence or absence of exposure to risk factors that are believed to influence the development of the disease.

This method entails choosing and studying a predetermined number of individuals, n_1 and n_2, who are exposed and who are not exposed, respectively. This method of sampling forms the basis of prospective or cohort study and the retrospective studies. In prospective studies n_1 individuals with, and n_2 individuals without, a suspected risk factor are followed over time to determine the number of individuals who develop the disease. In retrospective case–control studies, n_1 individuals having the disease (cases) and n_2 individuals not having the disease (controls) would be investigated in terms of past exposure to the suspected antecedent risk factor.

The major difference between the cohort and case–control sampling methods is in the selection of study subjects. A prospective cohort study selects individuals who are initially disease-free and follows them over time to determine how many become ill. This would determine the rates of disease in the absence or presence of exposure. By contrast, the case–control method selects individuals on the basis of the presence or absence of disease.

Recall that the odds ratio has been defined in terms of the odds of disease in exposed individuals relative to the odds of disease in the unexposed. An equivalent definition can be obtained in terms of the odds of exposure conditional on the disease, so that the odds of exposure among diseased and not diseased are

$$\text{odds}_D(E) = \frac{\Pr[E|D]}{1 - \Pr[E|D]} = \frac{y_1}{y_2}$$

$$\text{odds}_{\overline{D}}(E) = \frac{\Pr[E|\overline{D}]}{1 - \Pr[E|\overline{D}]} = \frac{n_1 - y_1}{n_2 - y_2}$$

The odds ratio of exposure in diseased individuals relative to the nondiseased is

$$\hat{\psi} = \frac{\text{odds}_D(E)}{\text{odds}_{\overline{D}}(E)} = \frac{y_1(n_2 - y_2)}{y_2(n_1 - y_1)} \tag{2.2}$$

Thus, the exposure odds ratio defined by Equation 2.2 is equivalent to the disease odds ratio defined by Equation 2.1. This relationship is quite important in the design of case–control studies.

2.2.3 Statistical Inference on Odds Ratio

Cox (1970) indicated that the statistical advantage of the odds ratio is that it can be estimated from any of the study designs that were outlined in the previous section (cross-sectional survey, prospective cohort study, and the retrospective case–control study).

A problem that is frequently encountered when an estimate of odds ratio is constructed is the situation where $n_{12} n_{21} = 0$, in which case ψ is undefined. To allow for estimation under these conditions, Haldane (1956) suggested adding a correction term, $\delta = 0.5$, to all four cells in the 2×2 tables, to modify the estimator proposed earlier by Woolf (1955). The odds ratio estimate is then given by

$$\hat{\psi}_{H} = \frac{(n_{11} + 0.5)(n_{22} + 0.5)}{(n_{12} + 0.5)(n_{21} + 0.5)}$$

Adding $\delta = 0.5$ to all cells gives a less-biased estimate than if it is added only as necessary, such as when a zero cell occurs (Walter, 1985). Another estimator of ψ was given by Jewell (1984, 1986), which is

$$\hat{\psi}_{J} = \frac{n_{11} n_{22}}{(n_{12} + 1)(n_{21} + 1)}$$

The correction of $\delta = 1$ to the n_{12} and n_{21} cells is intended to reduce the positive bias of the uncorrected estimator ψ and also to make it defined for all possible tables. Walter and Cook (1991) conducted a large-scale Monte-Carlo simulation study to compare among several point estimators of the odds ratio. Their conclusion was that for sample size $n = 25$, ψ_{J} has lower bias, mean-square error, and average absolute error than the other estimators included in the study. Approximate variances of $\hat{\psi}$, $\hat{\psi}_{H}$, and $\hat{\psi}_{J}$ are given by

$$\text{var}(\hat{\psi}) = (\hat{\psi})^2 \left[\frac{1}{n_{11}} + \frac{1}{n_{12}} + \frac{1}{n_{21}} + \frac{1}{n_{22}} \right]$$

$$\text{var}(\hat{\psi}_{H}) = \hat{\psi}_{H}^2 \left[\frac{1}{n_{11} + 0.5} + \frac{1}{n_{12} + 0.5} + \frac{1}{n_{21} + 0.5} + \frac{1}{n_{22} + 0.5} \right]$$

$$\text{var}(\hat{\psi}_{J}) = \hat{\psi}_{J}^2 \left[\frac{1}{n_{11}} + \frac{1}{n_{12}} + \frac{1}{n_{21} + 1} + \frac{1}{n_{22} + 1} \right]$$

Before we deal with the problem of significance testing of the odds ratio, there are several philosophical points of view concerning the issue of "statistical" significance as opposed to "scientific" significance. It is known that the general approach to test the association between disease and exposure is to contradict the null hypothesis H_0: $\psi = 1$. The p-value of this test is a summary measure of the consistency of the data with the null hypothesis. A small p-value provides the evidence that the data are not consistent with the null hypothesis (in this case implying a significant association). As indicated by

Oakes (1986), the p-value should be considered only as a guide to interpretation. The argument regarding the role played by the p-value in significance
tests dates back to Fisher (1932). He indicated that the null hypothesis cannot
be affirmed as such but is possibly disproved. On the other hand, scientific
inference is concerned with measuring the magnitude of an effect, regardless
of whether the data are consistent with the null hypothesis. Therefore, the
construction of a confidence interval on ψ is very desirable as an indication of
whether or not the data contain adequate information to be consistent with
the H_0, or to signal departures from the H_0 that are of scientific importance.

2.2.3.1 Significance Tests

The standard chi-square test for association in a 2×2 table provides an
approximate test on the hypothesis H_0: $\psi = 1$. Referring to the notation in
Table 2.3, the χ^2 statistic is given by

$$\chi^2 = \frac{n \left(|y_1(n_2 - y_2) - y_2(n_1 - y_1)| - n/2\right)^2}{n_1 n_2 y_. (n - y)} \tag{2.3}$$

Under H_0, the above statistic has an approximate χ^2 distribution with one
degree of freedom and is used in testing the two-sided alternative. However,
if there is interest in testing the null hypothesis of no association against a
one-sided alternative, the standard normal approximation $Z_\alpha = \pm\sqrt{\chi^2}$ can
be used. In this case, the positive value is used for testing the alternative,
H_1: $\psi > 1$, and the negative values to test H_1: $\psi < 1$. Quite frequently, the
sample size may not be sufficient for the asymptotic theory of the χ^2 statistic
to hold. In this case an exact test is recommended.

When large sample methods cannot be justified, owing either to small samples or highly skewed observed table margins, exact methods are employed.
These are based on the enumeration of a reference set of tables with the margins fixed to the totals observed in the data. The p-values are evaluated by
summing probabilities associated with tables from the reference set identified
as more extreme than the table observed.

We shall now illustrate the computation of the p-value based on Fisher's
exact test. First, let $p_{11} \equiv p_1$ and $p_{21} \equiv p_2$ be the proportion of diseased individuals in the population of exposed and unexposed, respectively. Suppose
two independent samples of sizes n_1 and n_2 are taken from the exposed and
the unexposed population. Referring to Table 2.3, it is clear that y_1 and y_2
are independent binomially distributed random variables with parameters
(n_1, p_1) and (n_2, p_2). Hence their joint probability distribution is

$$p(y_1, y_2) = \binom{n_1}{y_1}\binom{n_2}{y_2} p_1^{y_1} q_1^{n_1 - y_1} p_2^{y_2} q_2^{n_2 - y_2} \tag{2.4}$$

Under the transformation $y_. = y_1 + y_2$, Equation 2.4 can be written as

$$p(y_., y_1 | \psi) = \binom{n_1}{y_1} \binom{n_2}{y_. - y_1} \psi^{y_1} q_1^{n_1} p_2^{y_.} q_2^{n_2 - y_.}.$$

where $\psi = \frac{p_1 q_2}{q_1 p_2}$ is the population odds ratio. Clearly $\psi = 1$, if and only if $p_1 = p_2$. Conditional on the sum $y_.$, the probability distribution of y_1 is

$$p(y_1 | y_., \psi) = c(y_., n_1, n_2; \psi) \binom{n_1}{y_1} \binom{n_2}{y_. - y_1} \psi^{y_1} \tag{2.5}$$

where

$$c^{-1}(y_., n_1, n_2; \psi) = \sum_x \binom{n_1}{x} \binom{n_2}{y_. - x} \psi^x$$

Under the hypothesis: $\psi = 1$, Equation 2.5 becomes the hypergeometric distribution:

$$p(y_1 | y_., 1) = \frac{\binom{n_1}{y_1} \binom{n_2}{y_. - y_1}}{\binom{n_1 + n_2}{y_.}}, \quad y_1 = 0, 1, \ldots, y_. \tag{2.6}$$

The exact p-value of the test on the hypothesis $\psi = 1$ is calculated from Equation 2.6 by summing the probabilities of obtaining all tables with the same marginal totals, with y_1 observed as extreme as that obtained from the sample.

Example 2.1
Researchers in veterinary microbiology conducted a clinical trial on two drugs used for the treatment of diarrhea in calves. Colostrum-deprived calves are given a standard dose of an infectious organism (strain B44 *Escherichia coli*) at two days of age, and then the therapy is instituted as soon as the calves begin to show diarrhea (Table 2.4). The following data were obtained from the trial:

TABLE 2.4

Data in Diarrhea in Calves

	Died	Lived	Total
Drug (1)	7	2	9
Drug (2)	3	5	8
Total	10	7	17

Since

$$P(y_1 | y_., 1) = \frac{\binom{9}{y_1} \binom{8}{10 - y_1}}{\binom{17}{10}}$$

we have

y_1	0	1	2	3	4	5	6	7	8	9
$p(y_1\|y_.,1)$	0	0	0.0018	0.0345	0.1814	0.363	0.302	0.104	0.013	0.0004

The more extreme configurations correspond to $y_1 = 8$ and 9. Therefore, the one-tailed p-value of Fisher's exact test is $p = 0.0004 + 0.013 + 0.104 = 0.1174$. The two-tailed p-value is obtained by adding the probabilities of all the table configuration as probable as the observed one or less, which is

$$p = 0 + 0.0004 + 0.013 + 0.104 + 0.0345 + 0.0018 = 0.1537$$

The probabilities of tables corresponding to $y_1 = 4$, 5, and 6 are not included because they are less extreme or more probable than the observed configuration. We conclude that no significant association between treatment and mortality can be justified by the data.

From the properties of the hypergeometric distribution, if $E(y_.|y_1,1)$ and $V(y_.|y_1,1)$ denote the mean and variance of Equation 2.6, they are, respectively, given by

$$E(y_1|y_.,1) = \frac{n_1 y_.}{n_1 + n_2} \tag{2.7}$$

$$V(y_1|y_.,1) = \frac{n_1 n_2 y_. (n_1 + n_2 - y_.)}{(n_1 + n_2)^2 (n_1 + n_2 - 1)} \tag{2.8}$$

As an approximation to the tail area required to test $H_0: \psi = 1$, we refer to the table of standard normal distribution:

$$Z = \frac{|y_1 - E(y_1|y_.,1)| - \frac{1}{2}}{\sqrt{V(y_1|y_.,1)}} \tag{2.9}$$

From the above example, $y_1 = 7$ and the estimates of $E(y_.|y_1,1)$ and $V(y_.|y_1,1)$ are 5.29 and 1.03, respectively. Hence, $z = 1.19$ and $p = 0.12$ indicating no significant association.

The following SAS code reads the count data and computes the χ^2 and the Fisher exact tests along with other statistics.

```
data calves;
input drug dead count @@;
cards;
1 1 7 1 2 2 2 2 1 3 2 2 5
;

proc format;
value drugf 1='Drug 1'
    2='Drug 2';
```

value deadf 1='Died'
    2='Lived';

proc freq;
weight count;
tables drug*dead/nocol nopercent chisq exact measures;
format drug drugf. dead deadf.; run;

Partial SAS output is shown below.

Statistic	DF	Value	Prob
χ^2	1	2.8367	0.0921
Likelihood ratio χ^2	1	2.9151	0.0878
Continuity adj. χ^2	1	1.4175	0.2338
Mantel-Haenszel χ^2	1	2.6698	0.1023
Phi coefficient		0.4085	
Contingency coefficient		0.3782	

Fisher's Exact Test

Cell (1,1) frequency (F)	7
Left-sided Pr $\leq F$	0.9866
Right-sided Pr $\geq F$	0.1170
Table probability (P)	0.1037
Two-sided Pr $\leq P$	0.1534

The corresponding R code is

```
x <- matrix(c(7, 3, 2, 5), nc = 2)
chisq.test(x,correct=FALSE)
fisher.test(x)
```

2.2.3.2 *Interval Estimation*

To construct an approximate confidence interval on ψ, it is assumed that when n is large, $(\hat{\psi} - \psi)$ follows a normal distribution with mean 0 and variance $V(\hat{\psi})$. An approximate $(1 - \alpha)100\%$ confidence interval is

$$\hat{\psi} \pm Z_{\alpha/2}\sqrt{V(\hat{\psi})}$$

To avoid asymmetry, Woolf (1955) proposed constructing confidence limits on $\beta = \ln \psi$. He showed that

$$V(\hat{\beta}) = V(\hat{\psi})/\hat{\psi}^2 = \frac{1}{y_1} + \frac{1}{n_1 - y_1} + \frac{1}{y_2} + \frac{1}{n_2 - y_2} \tag{2.10}$$

and the lower and upper confidence limits on ψ are given, respectively, by

$$\hat{\psi}_L = \hat{\psi} \exp\left[-Z_{\alpha/2}\sqrt{V(\hat{\beta})}\right]$$

$$\hat{\psi}_U = \hat{\psi} \exp\left[+Z_{\alpha/2}\sqrt{V(\hat{\beta})}\right]$$

2.3 Analysis of Several 2 × 2 Contingency Tables

Consider k pairs of mutually independent binomial variables y_{i1} and y_{i2} with corresponding parameters p_{i1} and p_{i2} and sample sizes n_{i1} and n_{i2}, where $i = 1, 2, \ldots, k$. This information has a k 2×2 table representation (Table 2.5) as follows.

TABLE 2.5

2 × 2 Contingency Table for the ith Pair

	Disease		
Exposure	D	$\overline{D}$	Total
E	y_{i1}	$n_{i1} - y_{i1}$	n_{i1}
$\overline{E}$	y_{i2}	$n_{i2} - y_{i2}$	n_{i2}
Total	$y_{i.}$	$n_i - y_{i.}$	n_i

There is a considerable literature on the estimation and significance testing of odds ratios in several 2×2 tables (Thomas and Gart, 1977; Fleiss, 1979; Gart and Thomas, 1982). The main focus of such studies was to address the following questions:

1. Does the odds ratio vary considerably from one table to another?
2. If no significant variation among the k odds ratios is established, is the common odds ratio statistically significant?
3. If no significant variation among the k odds ratios is established, how can we construct confidence intervals on the common odds ratio after pooling information from all tables?

Before addressing these questions, the circumstances under which several 2×2 tables are produced will now be explored in more detail.

One very important consideration is the effect of confounding variables. In a situation where a variable is correlated with both the disease and the exposure factor, "confounding" is said to occur. Failure to adjust for this effect would bias the estimated odds ratio as a measure of association between the disease and exposure variables.

If we assume for simplicity that the confounding variable has several distinct levels, then one way to control for its confounding effect is to construct a 2×2 table for the disease and exposure variable, at each level of the confounder. Epidemiologists name this procedure "stratification." Example 2.2 illustrates this idea.

Example 2.2

The following data are from a case–control study on enzootic pneumonia in pigs by Willeberg (1980). Under investigation is the effect of ventilation systems where exposure (E) denotes those farms with fans. The data are given in Table 2.6.

TABLE 2.6

Classification of Diseased and Exposed Pigs in Enzootic
Pneumonia Study

		Disease		
	Fan	D	$\bar{D}$	Total
Exposure	Yes (E)	91	73	164
	No ($\bar{E}$)	25	60	85
	Total	116	133	249

$$\hat{\psi} = 2.99$$

$$\ln \hat{\psi} = 1.095$$

$$\sqrt{\text{var}(\hat{\beta})} = \left[\frac{1}{91} + \frac{1}{73} + \frac{1}{25} + \frac{1}{60} \right]^{1/2} = 0.285$$

and 95% confidence limits are

$$\hat{\psi}_L = 2.99e^{-(1.96)(0.285)} = 1.71$$

$$\hat{\psi}_U = 2.99e^{(1.96)(0.285)} = 5.23$$

A factor that is not taken into account in analyzing data is the size of the farms involved in the study. In attempting to filter out the effect of farm size (if it is present) on the disease, two groups are formed, large and small farms. By stratifying this possible confounder into large and small farms, the data are arranged in Table 2.7 and the odds ratios are given in Table 2.8.

Now it is evident that the relationship between the disease and the exposure factor is not clear, and this could be due to the possible confounding effect of farm size. For farms of large size, the estimated odds ratio of disease-risk association is $\hat{\psi} = 2.99$, which is identical to the estimate obtained from Table 2.6. However, it is not statistically significant ($p = 0.10$, two-sided). It follows that pooling the data from large and small farms to form a single 2×2

TABLE 2.7

Stratification by Farm Size

Farm Size	Fan	Disease	
		D	*D̄*
Large	Yes (*E*)	61	17
	No (*Ē*)	6	5
Small	Yes (*E*)	30	56
	No (*Ē*)	19	55

TABLE 2.8

Odds Ratios and Confidence Intervals after Stratification by Farm Size

Farm Size	$\hat{\psi}_i$	$\hat{\beta}_i$	SE $(\hat{\beta}_i)$	95% CI
Large	2.99	1.095	0.665	(0.67, 13.2)
Small	1.55	0.438	0.349	(0.74, 3.26)

table can produce misleading results. Therefore, the subgroup-specific odds ratio may be regarded as descriptive of the effects. Now, in the context of multiple tables, the three questions posed previously will be addressed.

Note: The SAS and R codes given in Example 2.1 produce the odds ratio and the confidence intervals.

2.3.1 Test of Homogeneity

This is a reformulation of the question "Does the odds ratio vary considerably across tables?" This is equivalent to testing the hypothesis H_0: $\psi_1 = \psi_2 = \cdots = \psi_k = \psi$. Woolf (1955) proposed a test that is based on the estimated log odds ratios ($\hat{\beta}_i$) and their estimated variances. Since the estimated variance of $\hat{\beta}_i$ is

$$V(\hat{\beta}_i) = w_i^{-1} = \frac{1}{y_{i1}} + \frac{1}{n_{i1} - y_{i1}} + \frac{1}{y_{i2}} + \frac{1}{n_{i2} - y_{i2}}$$

an estimate of $\ln \psi$ is constructed as

$$\hat{\beta} = \ln \hat{\psi} = \frac{\sum_{i=1}^{k} w_i \hat{\beta}_i}{\sum_{i=1}^{k} w_i}$$

Furthermore, it can be shown that

$$V(\hat{\beta}) = \frac{1}{\sum_{i=1}^{k} w_i}$$

To assess the homogeneity (i.e., constancy of odds ratios) the statistic

$$\chi_w^2 = \sum_{i=1}^{k} w_i(\hat{\beta}_i - \hat{\beta})^2$$

has approximately a χ^2 distribution with $k-1$ degrees of freedom. Large values of χ_w^2 provide an evidence against the homogeneity hypothesis.

Example 2.2 (Continued)

This example applies Woolf's method to the summary estimates from Table 2.6 to test for a difference between the odds ratios of the two groups.

The χ^2 value is calculated as follows:

$$\hat{\beta}_1 = 1.095 \qquad \hat{\beta}_2 = 0.438$$

$$w_1 = 2.26 \quad w_2 = 8.20 \quad \sum w_i = 10.46$$

$$\hat{\beta} = \frac{\sum w_i \beta_i}{\sum w_i} = 0.58$$

$$\chi_w^2 = \sum_{i=1}^{k} w_i(\hat{\beta}_i - \hat{\beta})^2 = 0.764$$

From the value of χ^2 with one degree of freedom, we can see that there is no significant difference between the odds ratios of the two groups.

If we intend to find a summary odds ratio from several 2×2 tables, it is useful to test for interaction. Consider the summary calculations in Table 2.8. The odds ratios for the two strata are 2.99 and 1.55. If the underlying odds ratios for individual strata are really different, it is questionable if a summary estimate is appropriate. In support of this, the implication of a significant value of χ_w^2 should be stressed. A large value of χ_w^2 indicates that the homogeneity of ψ_i's is not supported by the data and that there is an interaction between the exposure and the stratification variable. Thus, in the case of a significant value of χ_w^2, one should not construct a single estimate of the common odds ratio.

2.3.2 Significance Test of Common Odds Ratio

Recall that inference on the odds ratio can be based on the total y. conditional on the marginal totals of the 2×2 table. From Cox and Snell (1989), the inference on the common odds ratio ψ is based on the conditional distribution of $T = \sum_{i=1}^{k} y_{.i}$, given the marginal total of all tables.

Now, we know that under H_0: $\psi = 1$ the distribution of $y_{.i}$ (the total of diseased in the ith table) for a particular i is given by the hypergeometric distribution (Equation 2.6), and the required distribution of T is the convolution of k of these distributions. It is clear that this is impracticable for exact calculation of confidence limits. However, we can test the null hypothesis that $H_0: \psi = 1$ by noting from Equations 2.7 and 2.8 that the mean and variance of T are given, respectively, as

$$E(T|\psi = 1) = \sum_{i=1}^{k} \frac{n_{i1} y_{.i}}{n_{i1} + n_{i2}} \tag{2.11}$$

$$V(T|\psi = 1) = \sum_{i=1}^{k} \frac{n_{i1} n_{i2} y_{.i}(n_{i1} + n_{i2} - y_{.i})}{(n_{i1} + n_{i2})^2 (n_{i1} + n_{i2} - 1)} \tag{2.12}$$

where $y_{.i}$ is the observed number of diseased in the ith table. A normal approximation, with continuity correction, for the distribution of T will nearly always be adequate. Cox and Snell (1989) indicate that the approximation is good even for a single table and will be improved by convolution. The combined test of significance from several 2×2 contingency tables is done by referring

$$\chi_1^2 = \frac{\left(|T - E(T|\psi = 1)| - \frac{1}{2}\right)^2}{V(T|\psi = 1)} \tag{2.13}$$

to the χ^2 table with one degree of freedom.

Another form of the one degree of freedom χ^2 test on $H_0: \psi = 1$ was given by Mantel and Haenszel (1959) as

$$\chi_{mh}^2 = \frac{\left[\sum_{i=1}^{k} \dfrac{y_{i1}(n_{i2} - y_{i2}) - y_{i2}(n_{i1} - y_{i1})}{n_i}\right]^2}{\sum_{i=1}^{k} \dfrac{n_{i1} n_{i2} y_{.i}(n_i - y_{.i})}{n_i^2(n_i - 1)}} \tag{2.14}$$

where $n_i = n_{i1} + n_{i2}$ and $y_{.i} = y_{i1} + y_{i2}$.

In Example 2.4, we consider the data in Table 2.5 and calculate both Cox and Snell, and Mantel and Haenszel formulations.

Example 2.2 (Continued)

As a test of significance of the common odds ratio using the data in Table 2.7, we have $T = 91$, $E(T|\psi = 1) = 85.057$, and $V(T|\psi = 1) = 10.3181$. Hence, $\chi_1^2 = 2.872$ and the combined odds ratio is nonsignificant. Using Mantel and Haenszel χ_{mh}^2 formula, we get $\chi_{mh}^2 = 2.882$, which is quite similar to the value obtained using the Cox and Snell method with similar conclusions.

The following SAS code analyzes these data.

```
data willeberg;
input farms fan disease count @@;
```

```
cards;
1 1 1 61 1 1 2 17 1 2 1 6  1 2 2 5
2 1 1 30 2 1 2 56 2 2 1 19 2 2 2 55;

proc format;
value farmsf 1='Large'
      2='Small';
value fanf 1='Yes'
      2='No';
value diseasef 1='Disease'
      2='No Disease';

proc freq;
weight count;
tables farms*fan*disease/nocol nopercent cmh measures;
format farms farmsf. fan fanf. disease diseasef.; run;
```

Partial SAS output below shows the odds ratios stratified by farm size with confidence intervals, the common odds ratios and confidence intervals, and the Breslow–Day test for the homogeneity of odds ratios. Unfortunately, SAS does not support the Woolf (1955) and Cox and Snell (1989) tests for the homogeneity of odds ratios.

Farm Size: Large

Estimates of the Relative Risk (Row1/Row2)

Type of Study	Value	95% Confidence Limits	
Case–control (odds ratio)	2.9902	0.8126	11.0035
Cohort (col1 risk)	1.4338	0.8255	2.4901
Cohort (col2 risk)	0.4795	0.2216	1.0375

Farm Size: Small

Estimates of the Relative Risk (Row1/Row2)

Type of Study	Value	95% Confidence Limits	
Case–control (odds ratio)	1.5508	0.7820	3.0751
Cohort (col1 risk)	1.3586	0.8379	2.2031
Cohort (col2 risk)	0.8761	0.7140	1.0750

Estimates of the Common Relative Risk (Row1/Row2)

Type of Study	Method	Value	95% Confidence Limits	
Case–control (odds ratio)	Mantel–Haenszel	1.7624	0.9587	3.2396
	Logit	1.7875	0.9751	3.2767

Breslow–Day Test for
Homogeneity of the Odds Ratios

χ^2	0.7759
DF	1
Pr > ChiSq	0.3784

The following R code reads the grouped data in an array "willeberg" as
required for the Mantel–Haenszel test function in R. χ^2 and the Fisher exact
tests are then computed separately for large and small farms' data followed
by Mantel–Haenszel test and the exact conditional tests for the homogeneity
of odds ratios across the strata. The exact conditional test suggests that the
odds ratios are homogeneous (p-value = 0.09). However, if odds ratios turn
out to be different, then the traditional approach would be using the Woolf
(1955) test for interaction. The "woolf" function that computes this test is run
on the current dataset again, indicating that there is no interaction by the
stratifying factor, and therefore the Mantel–Haenszel test is admissible.

```
willeberg=array(c(61, 6, 17, 5, 30, 19, 56, 55),
dim = c(2, 2, 2),
dimnames = list(
Fan = c("Yes", "No"),
Disease = c("Disease", "No Disease"),
Farm.Size = c("Large", "Small")))

apply(willeberg, 3, function(x) chisq.test(x))
apply(willeberg, 3, function(x) fisher.test(x))

mantelhaen.test(willeberg)
mantelhaen.test(willeberg,exact=TRUE)
*********
woolf <- function(x) {
x <- x + 1 / 2
k <- dim(x)[3]
or <- apply(x, 3, function(x) (x[1,1]*x[2,2])/(x[1,2]*x[2,1]))
w <- apply(x, 3, function(x) 1 / sum(1 / x))
1 - pchisq(sum(w * (log(or) - weighted.mean(log(or), w)) ^ 2), k - 1)
}
woolf(willeberg)
```

2.3.3 Confidence Interval on the Common Odds Ratio

Mantel and Haenszel (1959) suggested a highly efficient estimate of the
common odds ratio from several 2×2 tables as

$$\hat{\psi}_{mh} = \frac{\sum_{i=1}^{k} \dfrac{y_{i1}(n_{i2} - y_{i2})}{(n_{i1} + n_{i2})}}{\sum_{i=1}^{k} \dfrac{y_{i2}(n_{i1} - y_{i1})}{(n_{i2} + n_{i2})}} \tag{2.15}$$

Note that $\hat{\beta}_{mh} = \ln \hat{\psi}_{mh}$ can be regarded as a special form of weighted means, based on the linearizing approximation near $\beta_{mh} = 0$. This equivalence has been used to motivate various estimates of the variance of $\hat{\beta}_{mh}$. Robins et al. (1986) constructed an estimate of the variance as

$$V(\hat{\beta}_{mh}) = \frac{1}{2} \left\{ \sum \frac{A_i C_i}{C_.^2} + \sum \frac{(A_i D_i + B_i C_i)}{(C.D.)} + \sum \frac{B_i D_i}{D_.^2} \right\} \qquad (2.16)$$

where

$$A_i = (y_{i1} + n_{i2} - y_{i2})/(n_{i1} + n_{i2})$$
$$B_i = (y_{i2} + n_{i1} - y_{i1})/(n_{i1} + n_{i2})$$
$$C_i = y_{i1}(n_{i2} - y_{i2})/(n_{i1} + n_{i2})$$
$$D_i = y_{i2}(n_{i1} - y_{i1})/(n_{i1} + n_{i2})$$

and

$$C_. = \sum C_i \quad D_. = \sum D_i$$

Using the results from the previous example (Example 2.2), we find that $\hat{\psi}_{mh} = 1.76$, and the 95% confidence limits for ψ_{mh} are $(0.96, 3.24)$.

Hauck (1979) derived another estimator of the large sample variance of $\hat{\psi}_{mh}$ as

$$\hat{V}_{mh} = \frac{\hat{\psi}_{mh}^2 \left(\sum_{i=1}^{k} \hat{w}_i^2 \hat{b}_i \right)}{\left(\sum \hat{w}_i \right)^2} \qquad (2.17)$$

where

$$\hat{w}_i = (n_{i1}^{-1} + n_{i2}^{-1})^{-1} \hat{p}_{i2}(1 - \hat{p}_{i1})$$

$$\hat{b}_i = \frac{1}{n_{i1}\hat{p}_{i1}\hat{q}_{i1}} + \frac{1}{n_{i2}\hat{p}_{i2}\hat{q}_{i2}}$$

and

$$\hat{p}_{ij} = \frac{y_{ij}}{n_{ij}} \quad j = 1, 2 \qquad \hat{q}_{ij} = 1 - \hat{p}_{ij}$$

2.4 Analysis of 1:1 Matched Pairs

The *matching* of one or more control to each case means that the two are paired based on their similarities with respect to some characteristic(s). Pairing individuals can involve attributes such as age, weight, farm, parity, type of hospital of admission, and breed. These are just a few examples.

It is important to note that since cases and controls are believed to be similar on the matching variables, their differences with respect to disease may be attributed to different extraneous variables. It was pointed out by Schlesselman (1982, p. 105) that "if the cases and controls differ with respect to some exposure variable, suggesting an association with the study disease, then this association cannot be explained in terms of case–control differences on the matching variables." The main objective of matching is in removing the bias that may affect the comparison between the cases and controls. In other words, matching attempts to achieve comparability on the important potential confounding variables (a confounder is an extraneous variable that is associated with the risk factor and the disease of interest). This strategy of matching is different from what is called "adjusting." Adjusting attempts to correct for differences in the cases and controls during the data analysis step, as opposed to matching, which occurs at the design stage.

In this section, we investigate the situation where one case is matched with a single control, where the risk factor is dichotomous. As before, we denote the presence or absence of exposure to the risk factor by E and $\bar{E}$, respectively. In this situation, responses are summarized by a 2×2 table, which exhibits two important features. First, all probabilities or associations may show a symmetric pattern about the main diagonal of the table. Second, the marginal distributions may differ in some systematic way.

Subsections 2.4.1 and 2.4.2 will address the estimation of the odds ratio and testing the equality of the marginal distributions under the 1:1 matched case–control design.

2.4.1 Estimating the Odds Ratio

Suppose that one has matched a single control to each case and that the exposure under study is dichotomous. Denoting the presence or absence of exposure by E and $\bar{E}$, respectively, there are four possible outcomes for each case–control pair.

To calculate ψ_{mh} for matched pair data, in which each pair is treated as a stratum, we must first change the matched pair table to its unpaired equivalent resulting in four possible outcomes (Tables 2.9 through 2.12).

TABLE 2.9

Outcome (1)

		Paired		Unpaired Equivalent	
		Control			
		E	$\bar{E}$	Case	Control
Case	E	1	0	E $1\,(y_1)$	$1\,(n_1 - y_1)$
	$\bar{E}$	0	0	$\bar{E}$ $0\,(y_2)$	$0\,(n_2 - y_2)$

$y_1(n_2 - y_2) = y_2(n_1 - y_1) = 0.$

TABLE 2.10

Outcome (2)

		Paired			Unpaired Equivalent	
		Control			Case	Control
		E	$\bar{E}$			
Case	E	0	0	E	0 (y_1)	1 $(n_1 - y_1)$
	$\bar{E}$	1	0	$\bar{E}$	1 (y_2)	0 $(n_2 - y_2)$

$y_1(n_2 - y_2) = 0$ and $y_2(n_1 - y_1) = 1$.

TABLE 2.11

Outcome (3)

		Paired			Unpaired Equivalent	
		Control			Case	Control
		E	$\bar{E}$			
Case	E	0	0	E	1 (y_1)	0 $(n_1 - y_1)$
	$\bar{E}$	1	0	$\bar{E}$	0 (y_2)	1 $(n_2 - y_2)$

$y_1(n_2 - y_2) = 1$ and $y_2(n_1 - y_1) = 0$.

TABLE 2.12

Outcome (4)

		Paired			Unpaired Equivalent	
		Control			Case	Control
		E	$\bar{E}$			
Case	E	0	0	E	0 (y_1)	0 $(n_1 - y_1)$
	$\bar{E}$	0	1	$\bar{E}$	1 (y_2)	1 $(n_2 - y_2)$

$y_1(n_2 - y_2) = y_2(n_1 - y_1) = 0$.

Since $\psi_{mhp} = \left[\sum y_{i1}(n_{i2} - y_{i2})/n_i \right] / \left[\sum y_{i2}(n_{i1} - y_{i1})/n_i \right]$ and $n_i = 2$, then

$$\hat{\psi}_{mhp} = \frac{\text{number of pairs with } y_{i1}(n_{i2} - y_{i2}) = 1}{\text{number of pairs with } y_{i2}(n_{i1} - y_{i1}) = 1}$$

For the following matched pairs table (Table 2.13), the odds ratio estimate would be $\hat{\psi}_{mhp} = g/h$.

It was shown (see Fleiss, 1981) that for the matched pairs, the variance of the odds ratio estimate is

$$\text{var}(\hat{\psi}_{mhp}) = \left(\frac{g}{h}\right)^2 \left(\frac{1}{g} + \frac{1}{h}\right)$$

TABLE 2.13

Matched Pairs Table

		Control		
		E	$\bar{E}$	Total
Case	E	$f\ (p_{11})$	$g\ (p_{12})$	$f+g\ (p_{1.})$
	$\bar{E}$	$h\ (p_{21})$	$i\ (p_{22})$	$h+i\ (p_{2.})$
Total		$f+h(p_{.1})$	$g+i\ (p_{.2})$	$f+g+h+i$

For the test of the hypothesis $H_0: \psi_{mhp} = 1$, the statistic

$$\chi^2_{(1)} = \frac{(g-h)^2}{g+h}$$

follows χ^2 distribution asymptotically with one degree of freedom. A better approximation includes a correction factor so that the statistic becomes

$$\chi^2_{(1)} = \frac{(|g-h|-1)^2}{g+h}$$

The implication of a large value of this $\chi^2_{(1)}$ is that the cases and the controls differ with regard to the distribution of the risk factor.

2.4.2 Testing the Equality of Marginal Distributions

When $p_{1.} = p_{.1}$, then $p_{2.} = p_{.2}$ and there is marginal homogeneity. When $(p_{1.} - p_{.1}) = (p_{2.} - p_{.2})$, then the marginal homogeneity is equivalent to symmetry of probabilities of the main diagonal, that is $p_{12} = p_{21}$. Naturally, a test of marginal homogeneity should then be based on

$$D = \hat{p}_{1.} - \hat{p}_{.1} = \frac{(g-h)}{n}$$

From Agresti (1990, p. 348), it can be shown that

$$V(D) = \frac{1}{n}\left[p_{1.}(1-p_{1.}) + p_{.1}(1-p_{.1}) - 2(p_{11}\,p_{22} - p_{12}\,p_{21})\right] \tag{2.18}$$

Note that the dependence on the sample marginal probabilities resulting from the matching of cases and controls is reflected in the term $2(p_{11}\,p_{22} - p_{12}\,p_{21})$. Moreover, dependent samples usually show positive association between responses, that is, $\psi = p_{11}\,p_{22}/p_{12}\,p_{21} > 1$, or equivalently, $p_{11}\,p_{22} - p_{12}\,p_{21} > 0$.

From Equation 2.18 this positive association implies that the variance of D is smaller than when the samples are independent. This indicates that matched studies that produce dependent proportions can help improve the precision of the test statistic D.

For large samples, $D = \hat{p}_{1.} - \hat{p}_{.1} = (g - h)/n$ has a sampling distribution that is approximately normal. A $(1 - \alpha)$ 100% confidence interval on $p_{1.} - p_{.1}$ is

$$D \pm Z_{\alpha/2} \sqrt{\hat{V}(D)}$$

where

$$\hat{V}(D) = \frac{1}{n}[\hat{p}_{1.}(1 - \hat{p}_{1.}) + \hat{p}_{.1}(1 - \hat{p}_{.1}) - 2(\hat{p}_{11}\hat{p}_{22} - \hat{p}_{12}\hat{p}_{21})]$$

The test statistic

$$Z = \frac{D}{\sqrt{\hat{V}(D)}}$$

is used to test the hypothesis $H_0: p_{1.} = p_{.1}$. Under H_0, it can be shown that the estimated variance of D is

$$\hat{V}(D/H_0) = \frac{g + h}{n^2}$$

The test statistic simplifies to $Z_0 = (g - h)/\sqrt{(g + h)}$. The square of Z_0 gives the one degree of freedom χ^2 test on $H_0: \psi = 1$, referred to as McNemar's test.

Example 2.3
To illustrate McNemar's test, the following hypothetical data from a controlled trial with matched pairs are used. The null hypothesis being tested is $H_0: \psi = 1$.

		Control	
		E	$\bar{E}$
Case	E	15	20
	$\bar{E}$	5	85

$$\hat{\psi} = \frac{20}{5} = 4$$

$$SE(\hat{\psi}) = \frac{20}{5}\left[\frac{(20 + 5)}{(20)(5)}\right]^{1/2} = 2$$

$$\chi^2_{(1)} = \frac{(|20 - 5| - 1)^2}{25} = 7.84$$

Based on the calculated value of the χ^2, the data do not support the null hypothesis, meaning that there is a significant difference ($p < 0.05$) in the rate of exposure among the cases and the controls.

For 2×2 matched pair data, SAS PROC FREQ computes the uncorrected McNemar test by using "agree" option in the "table" statement and prints the kappa coefficient, its asymptotic standard error, and the confidence interval.

The following R code prints the 2×2 table and computes the continuity-corrected McNemar test.

```
paired <- matrix(c(15, 5, 20, 85),nr = 2,
dimnames = list("Case" = c("Present", "Absent"),
"Control" = c("Present", "Absent")))
paired
mcnemar.test(paired,correct=TRUE)
```

2.5   Statistical Analysis of Clustered Binary Data

In this section, we review methods that have been proposed for comparing the overall proportion of successes among individuals in several groups (treatments) when the clusters are the sampling units. The methods are illustrated by several examples.

Example 2.4

The data in this example were given by Williams (1975) taken from Weil (1970) and give the results from an experiment comparing two treatments. One group of 16 pregnant female rats was fed a control diet during pregnancy and lactation, while the diet of a second group of 16 pregnant females was treated with a chemical. For each cluster (litter or cluster comprises the pups born to a female rat), the number n of pups alive at 4 days and the number y of pups that survived at 31-day lactation period were recorded. The data are given as fraction y/n in Table 2.14.

TABLE 2.14

Weil's Data

Control	13/13	12/12	9/9	9/9	8/8	8/8	12/13	11/12
	9/10	9/10	8/9	11/13	4/5	5/7	7/10	7/10
Treatment	12/12	11/11	10/10	9/9	10/11	9/11	9/11	8/9
	8/9	4/5	7/9	4/7	5/10	3/6	3/10	0/7

The purpose of the experiment was to determine if the chemical treatment significantly affects the survival rate among the pups. That is, we need to test $H_0: P_1 = P_2$, where P_i is the true proportion of successes in group $i(=1,2)$.

The clustering of responses within litters that invalidates the standard χ^2 test may be adjusted for, allowing a modified version of this test procedure to be applied (Donner, 1982; Donner and Donald, 1987). For completeness of the presentation we use the following notations:

We assume that k_1 clusters have been randomly assigned to the treatment group and k_2 clusters to the control group. The sizes of the clusters in the treatment group are denoted by n_{1j}, where $j = 1, 2, \ldots, k_1$, and the control group by n_{2j}, where $j = 1, 2, \ldots, k_2$. The total number of individuals in each group is denoted by $N_1 = \sum_{j=1}^{k_1} n_{1j}$ for the treatment and $N_2 = \sum_{j=1}^{k_2} n_{2j}$ for the control group. In a completely randomized design with binary response, $\hat{P}_{ij} = Y_{ij}/n_{ij}$ denotes the cluster-specific success rate. We further define

$$Y_i = \sum_{j=1}^{k_i} Y_{ij} \quad \hat{P}_i = \frac{Y_i}{N_i}$$

$$\hat{P} = \frac{\sum_{i=1}^{2} Y_i}{N}$$

where

$$N = N_1 + N_2 \quad k = \sum_{i=1}^{2} k_i$$

The rates $\hat{P}_i$ and $\hat{P}$ denote the event rates as computed overall for clusters in group i and the overall event rate observed in the study, respectively.

Letting $\bar{n}_{ai} = \sum_{j=1}^{k_i} n_{ij}^2/N_i$, the analysis of variance estimator of the intraclass correlation coefficient (ICC) ρ is defined as

$$\hat{\rho} = \frac{\text{MSB} - \text{MSW}}{\text{MSB} + (n_0 - 1)\text{MSW}}$$

where

$$\text{MSB} = \sum_{i=1}^{2} \sum_{j=1}^{k_i} n_{ij} \frac{(\hat{P}_{ij} - \hat{P}_i)^2}{(k-2)} \quad \text{MSW} = \sum_{i=1}^{2} \sum_{j=1}^{k_i} n_{ij} \hat{P}_{ij\cdot} \frac{(1 - \hat{P}_{ij})}{(N-k)}$$

and

$$n_0 = \frac{(N - \sum_{i=1}^{k} \bar{n}_{ai})}{(k-2)}$$

The mean squares MSB and MSW measure the variation in responses between and within clusters, respectively.

The unadjusted Pearson χ^2 statistic for testing $H_0: P_1 = P_2$ is

$$\chi_P^2 = \sum_{i=1}^{k} N_i \frac{(\hat{P}_i - \hat{P})^2}{\hat{P}(1 - \hat{P})} \tag{2.19}$$

2.5.1 Approaches to Adjust Pearson's χ^2

The rationale behind these approaches is to directly adjust the standard χ^2 test for the clustering of responses within the intact units. These approaches are intuitively attractive since they yield the standard Pearson χ^2 statistic if the estimated intraclass correlation is 0.

2.5.1.1 Donner and Donald's Adjustment

Donner (1989) and Donner and Donald (1987) discussed an adjustment that depends on clustering correction factors computed separately in each treatment group. The resulting statistic is given by

$$\chi_A^2 = \sum_{i=1}^{2} \frac{(Y_i - N_i\hat{P})^2}{N_i C_i \hat{P}(1 - \hat{P})} \tag{2.20}$$

where

$$C_i = 1 + (\bar{n}_{ai} - 1)\hat{\rho} \tag{2.21}$$

is an estimate of the design effect (or "clustering effect") in group $i(=1,2)$. Note that in some situations one may assume that $C_1 = C_2$, that is, estimates of population design effects are homogeneous across treatment groups. This assumption will hold under H_0 provided that the clusters are randomly assigned to treatment groups, but may not hold for observational comparisons, particularly if the mean cluster sizes in the two comparison populations are quite different (Donner et al., 1994). When $\hat{\rho} = 0$, χ_A^2 reduces to the standard Pearson chi-square χ_P^2.

2.5.1.2 Procedures Based on Ratio Estimate Theory

Rao and Scott (1992) proposed a method for testing H_0 that regards the observed response rates $\hat{P}_i$ as ratios rather than proportions. The estimated design effects in each group are computed as

$$d_i = \frac{\hat{V}_R(\hat{P}_i)}{\hat{V}_B(\hat{P}_i)}$$

where $\hat{V}_B(\hat{P}_i) = \hat{P}_i(1 - \hat{P}_i)/N_i$ is the estimated binomial variance and $\hat{V}_R(\hat{P}_i)$ is the estimated ratio variance (see Cochran, 1977) given by

$$\hat{V}_R(\hat{P}_i) = \frac{1}{k_i(k_1 - 1)N_i^2} \sum_{j=1}^{k_i} (y_{ij} - n_{ij}\hat{P}_i)^2 = v_i$$

The design effect d_i is used to compute the effective sample size in each group, $\tilde{N}_i = N_i/d_i$, the effective number of successes, $\tilde{y}_i = y_i/d_i$, and the effective overall response rate, $\tilde{P} = \sum_{i=1}^{2} \tilde{y}_i / \sum_{i=1}^{2} \tilde{N}_i$.

The test statistic that accounts for the design effect is

$$\chi_{RS}^2 = \sum_{i=1}^{2} \frac{(\tilde{y}_i - \tilde{N}_i\tilde{P})^2}{\tilde{N}_i\tilde{P}(1 - \tilde{P})} \tag{2.22}$$

The statistic χ_{RS}^2 does not explicitly involve the concept of within-cluster correlation and does not make any assumptions on the nature of clustering.

In particular, it does not assume the homogeneity of design effects. Therefore, the approach is applicable to nonexperimental trials. Donner et al. (1994) noted, however, that for trials involving random allocation of clusters to treatment groups, the assumption of homogeneous design effect is guaranteed at least under H_0. Donner et al. (1994) showed through extensive Monte-Carlo studies that χ_A^2 is valid in studies having as few as 10 clusters per group, and the number of clusters per group required to ensure the validity of χ_{RS}^2 may be substantially more.

2.5.1.2.1 Confidence Interval Construction

When the effect of intervention is measured by the risk difference $\hat{\delta} = \hat{P}_1 - \hat{P}_2$, one may construct an approximate two-sided $(1 - \alpha)$ 100% confidence interval on $P_1 - P_2$. The standard error of $\hat{\delta}$ is consistently estimated by

$$\hat{V}(\hat{\delta}) = \left[\frac{C_1 \hat{P}_1 (1 - \hat{P}_1)}{N_1} + \frac{C_2 \hat{P}_2 (1 - \hat{P}_1)}{N_2} \right]$$

where $C_j (j = 1, 2)$ is given by Equation 2.21.

The proposed confidence interval on δ, the true risk difference, is therefore

$$(\hat{P}_1 - \hat{P}_2) \pm z_{\alpha/2} \sqrt{\hat{V}(\hat{\delta})}$$

where $z_{\alpha/2}$ is the $(1 - \alpha)$ 100% two-sided critical value of the standard normal distribution.

Example 2.4 (Continued)

The summary statistics of Weil's data are

	Control	Treatment	Total
Y	142	112	254
N	158	147	305

Here, $\hat{P}_1 = 0.899$, $\hat{P}_2 = 0.760$, $\hat{P} = 0.83$, $\chi_P^2 = \frac{158(0.899 - 0.83)^2 + 147(0.760 - 0.83)^2}{(0.83)(0.17)} = 10.24$, and p-value $= 0.001$, indicating a significant difference in mortality between the two groups.

Now, when we adjust for clustering, the estimated ICC is $\hat{\rho} = 0.25$, $\bar{n}_{a1} = 10.8$, $\bar{n}_{a2} = 8.92$ so that $C_1 = 3.45$ and $C_2 = 3.20$. The adjusted χ^2 statistic is

$$\chi_A^2 = \frac{(142 - 158(0.83))^2}{(158)(3.45)(0.83)(0.17)} + \frac{(112 - 147(0.83))^2}{(147)(3.2)(0.83)(0.17)} = 3.043$$

and the p-value $= 0.081$.

This indicates that the difference in mortality between the two groups is not significant at $\alpha = 5\%$ and shows how failure to take into account cluster effects can lead to spurious statistical inference.

Further, $\hat{\delta} = 0.899 - 0.760 = 0.139$ with an estimated standard error of 0.042, so that the unadjusted 95% confidence limits are (0.059, 219).

However, when clustering is adjusted for, the estimated standard error is 0.076 and the confidence interval is $(-0.010, 0.288)$, which is much wider than when the clustering is ignored.

The following SAS code reads in the grouped data, generates the ungrouped data, computes the unadjusted χ^2 test, and runs the linear model to produce statistics for ICC.

```
* Grouped Data;
data weil;
input group $ litter n dead @@;
alive = n-dead;
cards;
c 1 13 13 c 2 12 12 c 3 9 9 c 4 9 9
c 5 8 8 c 6 8 8 c 7 13 12 c 8 12 11
c 9 10 9 c 10 10 9 c 11 9 8 c 12 13 11
c 13 5 4 c 14 7 5 c 15 10 7 c 16 10 7
t 17 12 12 t 18 11 11 t 19 10 10 t 20 9 9
t 21 11 10 t 22 11 9 t 23 11 9 t 24 9 8
t 25 9 8 t 26 5 4 t 27 9 7 t 28 7 4
t 29 10 5 t 30 6 3 t 31 10 3 t 32 7 0
;

* Ungrouped Data;
data new; set weil;
do i=1 to dead; y=1; output; end;
do i=1 to alive; y=0; output; end;

proc freq data=new;
tables group*y /nocol nopercent chisq;
run;

* Producing an overall estimate of ICC;
proc glm data=new;
class litter;
model y=litter;
run;
```

The SAS output is not shown.

The following R code reads in the grouped data, ungroups it to run ANOVA to get statistics for each group for ICC, and then converts back into the grouped data format (shown as a technique only) to compute Rao–Scott and Donner adjusted χ^2 tests.

```
# Reading the grouped Weil(1970)data
weiln <- data.frame(group = c(rep("c",16),rep("t",16)),
litter=1:32,
n=c(13,12,9,9,8,8,13,12,10,10,9,13,5,7,10,10,12,11,10,9,11,11,11,9,9,5,9,7,10,6,
10,7),
dead=c(13,12,9,9,8,8,12,11,9,9,8,11,4,5,7,7,12,11,10,9,10,9, 9,8,8,4,7,4, 5,3,3,0))
```

```
# Un-grouping the data
y1 <- data.frame(lapply(weiln, function(x) rep(x,weiln$dead)),
y=1)[,c(1,2,5)]
y0 <- data.frame(lapply(weiln, function(x) rep(x, weiln$n-weiln$dead)),
y = 0)[,c(1,2,5)]
weil <- rbind(y1,y0)
```

```
# Fiting linear model to get statistics by group for ICC
by(weil, weil[,1], function(x) anova(lm(y ~ factor(litter), data=x)))
```

```
# Convering back to grouped data – shown only as a technique
weiln <- data.frame(cbind(aggregate(weil[,3], weil[,1:2], length),
aggregate(weil[,3], weil[,1:2], sum)[,3]))
names(weiln) <-c("group","litter","n", "dead")
```

```
# Computing Rao-Scott Chi-square test adjusted for clusters (litter)
raoscott(cbind(dead, n - dead) ~ group, data = weiln)
# Computing Donner Chi-square test adjusted for clusters (litter)
donner(cbind(dead, n - dead) ~ group, data = weiln)
```

The output from Rao–Scott and Donner methods is shown below.

Test of proportion homogeneity (Rao and Scott, 1992)

- - - - - - - - - - - - - - - - - - -

raoscott(formula = cbind(dead, n - dead) ~ group, data = weiln)
N = 32 clusters, n = 305 subjects, y = 254 cases, I = 2 groups.

Data and design effects:
group N n y p vbin vratio deff
1   c 16 158 142 0.8987 0.000576 0.000710 1.232
2   t 16 147 112 0.7619 0.001234 0.004553 3.689

Adjusted chi-squared test:
X2 = 4.9, df = 1, P(> X2) = 0.0266

Test of proportion homogeneity (Donner, 1989)

- - - - - - - - - - - - - - - - - - -

donner(formula = cbind(dead, n - dead) ~ group, data = weiln)
N = 32 clusters, n = 305 subjects, y = 254 cases, I = 2 groups.

Data and correction factors:
group N n y p C
1   c 16 158 142 0.8987 3.181
2   t 16 147 112 0.7619 3.000

Intracluster correlation (anova estimate): 0.2326
Adjusted chi-squared test:
X2 = 3.3, df = 1, P(> X2) = 0.0685

2.5.1.3   *Adjusted χ^2 for Studies Involving More than Two Groups*

Suppose that it is of interest to compare H groups and each group has k_h clusters $(h = 1, 2, \ldots, H)$. Denote the number of subjects belonging to cluster i in group h by m_{hi}. The null hypothesis of interest may be specified as H_0: $P_1 = P_2 = \cdots = P_H = P$, where P_h is the probability that the outcome on a randomly selected subject group h is a success.

Let y_{hi} denote the number of successes for cluster i in group h. Then the total number of observations in the hth group is given by $M_h = \sum_{i=1}^{k_h} m_{hi}$, and the total number of successes by $y_h = \sum_{i=1}^{k_h} m_{hi}$.

We denote the number of clusters in the study by $k = \sum_{h=1}^{H} k_h$.

Let $\hat{P} = \sum_{h=1}^{H} y_h / \sum_{h=1}^{H} M_h$ denote the overall success rate in the sample, and $\hat{Q} = 1 - \hat{P}$. If there is no within-cluster effect, H_0 may be tested by the standard Pearson χ^2 statistic with $H - 1$ degrees of freedom. Donner et al. (1994) showed that this statistic may be written as

$$\chi^2 = \sum_{h=1}^{H} \chi_h^2$$

where

$$\chi_h^2 = \frac{\left(y_h - M_h\hat{P}\right)^2}{M_h\hat{P}} + \frac{\left(M_h - y_h - M_h\hat{Q}\right)^2}{M_h}$$

In the presence of clustering, χ^2 is no longer valid but may be adjusted to account for the within-cluster correlation effect. To construct this adjusted statistic, say χ_A^2, let $\hat{P}_{hi}$ denote the proportion of successes in cluster i in group h $(i = 1, 2, \ldots, k_h, h = 1, 2, \ldots, H)$, $\hat{P}_h = y_h / M_h$ the overall success rate in group h, and $M = \sum_h \sum_i m_{hi}$ the total number of observations in the sample. Then, the mean square error among clusters within groups is $\mathrm{MSB} = \sum_h \sum_i m_{hi}(\hat{P}_{hi} - \hat{P}_h)^2 / (k - H)$, and the mean square error within the cluster is $\mathrm{MSW} = \sum_h \sum_i y_{hi}(1 - \hat{P}_{hi}) / (M - k)$.

The clustering effect is measured by the ICC, which is estimated by

$$\hat{\rho} = \frac{\mathrm{MSB} - \mathrm{MSW}}{\mathrm{MSB} + (m_0 - 1)\mathrm{MSW}}$$

where $m_0 = \left[M - \sum_h \sum_i \frac{m_{hi}^2}{m_h}\right] / (k - H)$.

According to Donner (1992), the adjusted χ^2 statistic may now be computed as

$$\chi_A^2 = \sum_{h=1}^{H} (\chi_h^2/C_h)$$

where

$$C_h = \frac{\sum_{i=1}^{kh} m_{hi} C_{hi}}{\sum_{i=1}^{kh} m_{hi}} \quad \text{and} \quad C_{hi} = 1 + (m_{hi} - 1)\hat{\rho}$$

An approximate test of H_0 is obtained by referring χ_A^2 to tables of χ^2 distribution with $H - 1$ degrees of freedom.

Example 2.5   A Hypothetical Drug Trial

The data are the result of a drug trial aimed at comparing the effect of four antibiotics against "shipping fever" in calves. Calves arrive in trucks at the feedlot and are checked upon arrival for signs of the disease. Animals that are confirmed as cases (from the same truck) are randomized as a group to one of the four treatment regimes. The following table (Table 2.15) gives the number of treated animals within a 2-week period and the number of deaths at the end of the 2 weeks.

TABLE 2.15

Hypothetical Drug Trial to Data

Drug 1	Treated animals	30	25	25	32	12	10	10
	Deaths	3	0	4	10	0	0	1
Drug 2	Treated animals	30	30	15	15	20	19	
	Deaths	1	1	1	1	4	0	
Drug 3	Treated animals	30	35	30	10	25		
	Deaths	5	7	9	1	2		
Drug 4	Treated animals	40	10	25	20	19	25	
	Deaths	10	1	1	2	1	2	

We would like to test the hypothesis that the mortality rates are the same for all treatments. Let p_i denote the mortality rate of the ith treatment. Hence, the null hypothesis would be $H_0: p_1 = p_2 = \cdots = p_I$.

Since $\hat{p}_i = \sum_{i=1}^{I} y_i / \sum_{i=1}^{I} n_i$, where $n_1 = 144$, $n_2 = 129$, $n_3 = 130$, $n_4 = 139$, and $\hat{p}(1 - \hat{p}) = 0.1236 (0.8764) = 0.1083$, then the uncorrected χ^2 is given by

$$\chi^2 = 0.002606 + 4.520 + 4.47 + 0.00217 = 8.995$$

Comparing this to a χ_3^2 value of 7.81, the null hypothesis is rejected. The p-value is 0.029. This implies that there is a significant difference in the

proportions of dead animals for the four different antibiotics. To estimate
the intracluster correlation, the ANOVA results obtained from SAS are
summarized in the following table:

Treatment	SSB	DF	SSW	DF	N_i
1	1.915	6	13.835	137	144
2	0.504	5	7.00	123	129
3	0.763	4	18.807	125	130
4	0.974	5	13.947	133	139

MSB $= 0.208$ and MSW $= 0.103$, $n_0 = 21.934$, and thus $\hat{\rho} = 0.044$.

Since $\bar{n}_{a1} = 24.43$, $\bar{n}_{a2} = 23.34$, $\bar{n}_{a3} = 28.85$, and $\bar{n}_{a4} = 26.708$, then $C_1 = 2.023$, $C_2 = 1.98$, $C_3 = 2.22$, and $C_4 = 2.13$.

To facilitate the computations, we summarize the results as follows:

Treatment	C_i	$\hat{P}_i$	N_i	Components of χ_A^2 of Equation 2.2
1	2.023	0.13	144	0.0013
2	1.98	0.06	129	2.28
3	2.22	0.18	130	2.008
4	2.13	0.12	139	0.001

Hence $\chi_D^2 = 4.29$, which indicates that there is no significant difference
between the mortality rates.

Rao and Scott's method

The computations are summarized as follows:

Drug 1: $\hat{P}_1 = \dfrac{18}{144} = 0.125$

Cluster	y_{1j}	n_{1j}	$(y_{1j} - n_{1j}\hat{P}_i)$
1	3	30	0.563
2	0	25	9.766
3	4	25	0.766
4	10	32	36.00
5	0	12	2.25
6	0	10	1.563
7	1	10	0.063
Total	18	144	50.969

$v_1 = 0.003, d_1 = 3.775$

$\tilde{Y}_1 = 4.768, \tilde{N}_1 = 38.141$

Drug 2: $\hat{P}_2 = \dfrac{8}{129} = 0.062$

Cluster	y_{2j}	n_{2j}	$(y_{2j} - n_{2j}\hat{P}_i)$
1	1	30	0.74
2	1	30	0.74
3	1	15	0.005
4	1	15	0.005
5	4	20	7.616
6	0	19	1.388
Total	8	129	10.495

$v_2 = 0.0008, d_2 = 1.678$

$\tilde{Y}_2 = 4.767, \tilde{N}_2 = 76.863$

Drug 3: $\hat{P}_3 = \dfrac{24}{130} = 0.184$

Cluster	y_{3j}	n_{3j}	$(y_{3j} - n_{3j}\hat{P}_i)$
1	5	30	0.27
2	7	35	0.31
3	9	30	12.11
4	1	10	0.716
5	2	25	6.76
Total	24	130	20.17

$v_3 = 0.0015, d_3 = 1.285$

$\tilde{Y}_3 = 18.676, \tilde{N}_3 = 101.161$

Drug 4: $\hat{P}_4 = \dfrac{17}{139} = 0.122$

Cluster	y_{4j}	n_{4j}	$(y_{4j} - n_{4j}\hat{P}_i)$
1	10	40	26.09
2	7	35	0.05
3	9	30	4.234
4	1	10	0.198
5	2	25	1.752
6	2	25	1.118
Total	17	139	33.442

$v_4 = 0.0021, d_4 = 2.69$

$\tilde{Y}_4 = 6.32, \tilde{N}_4 = 51.68$

Hence, $\chi^2_{RS} = 5.883$, which again does not exceed the $\chi^2_{3,0.05}$ value of 7.81, so we have no reason to reject the null hypothesis. This implies that there is no significant difference between the mortality rates.

From this example, we can see the importance of accounting for intracluster correlations, as the resulting conclusion about the equality of the proportions is different when the correlation is taken into account.

The following SAS program reads the grouped data, generates the ungrouped data, and runs the linear models to compute statistics for ICC for each drug level.

```
* Grouped Data;
data drug;
input drug truck n dead @@;
alive = n-dead;
cards;
1 1 30 3 1 2 25 0 1 3 25 4 1 4 32 10
1 5 12 0 1 6 10 0 1 7 10 1 2 8 30 1
2 9 30 1 2 10 15 1 2 11 15 1 2 12 20 4
2 13 19 0 3 14 30 5 3 15 35 7 3 16 30 9
3 17 10 1 3 18 25 2 4 19 40 10 4 20 10 1
4 21 25 1 4 22 20 2 4 23 19 1 4 24 25 2
;

* Un-grouped Data;
data new; set drug;
do i=1 to dead; y=1; output; end;
do i=1 to alive; y=0; output; end;

* Producing statistics to compute ICC for each drug level;
proc glm data=new;
class truck;
model y = truck;
by drug;
run; quit;
```

The SAS output is not shown.

The following R code reads in the grouped data, ungroups it to run ANOVA to get statistics for each drug level for ICC, and then uses the grouped data to compute Rao–Scott and Donner adjusted χ^2 tests.

```
# Reading the grouped 'drug' data
drugn <- data.frame(drug=c(rep(1,7),rep(2,6),rep(3,5),rep(4,6)),
truck=1:24,
n=c(30,25,25,32,12,10,10,30,30,15,15,20,19,30,35,30,10,25,40,10,25,20,19,25),
dead=c(3,0,4,10,0,0,1,1,1,1,1,4,0,5,7,9,1,2,10,1,1,2,1,2))

# Un-grouping the data
y1 <- data.frame(lapply(drugn, function(x) rep(x,drugn$dead)),
    y=1)[,c(1,2,5)]
```

```
y0 <- data.frame(lapply(drugn, function(x) rep(x, drugn$n-drugn$dead)),
y = 0)[,c(1,2,5)]
drug <- rbind(y1,y0)

# Fiting linear model to get statistics by group for ICC
by(drug, drug[,1], function(x) anova(lm(y ~ factor(truck), data=x)))
# Computing Rao-Scott Chi-square test adjusted for clusters (litter)
raoscott(cbind(dead, n - dead) ~ drug, data = drugn)
# Computing Donner Chi-square test adjusted for clusters (litter)
donner(cbind(dead, n - dead) ~ drug, data = drugn)
```

The output from Rao–Scott and Donner methods is shown below.

Test of proportion homogeneity (Rao and Scott, 1992)
- -
raoscott(formula = cbind(dead, n - dead) ~ drug, data = drugn)
N = 24 clusters, n = 542 subjects, y = 67 cases, I = 4 groups.

Data and design effects:

	drug	N	n	y	p	vbin	vratio	deff
1	1	7	144	18	0.12500	0.0007595	0.0028676	3.775
2	2	6	129	8	0.06202	0.0004509	0.0007568	1.678
3	3	5	130	24	0.18462	0.0011579	0.0014880	1.285
4	4	6	139	17	0.12230	0.0007723	0.0020771	2.690

Adjusted chi-squared test:
$X2 = 5.9$, $df = 3$, $P(> X2) = 0.1174$

Test of proportion homogeneity (Donner, 1989)
- -
donner(formula = cbind(dead, n - dead) ~ drug, data = drugn)
N = 24 clusters, n = 542 subjects, y = 67 cases, I = 4 groups.

Data and correction factors:

	drug	N	n	y	p	C
1	1	7	144	18	0.12500	2.030
2	2	6	129	8	0.06202	1.982
3	3	5	130	24	0.18462	2.224
4	4	6	139	17	0.12230	2.129

Intracluster correlation (anova estimate): 0.0439

Adjusted chi-squared test:
$X2 = 4.3$, $df = 3$, $P(> X2) = 0.2318$

2.5.2 Inference on the Common Odds Ratio

Consider a series of 2×2 tables wherein the notation has been changed to accommodate multiple tables, groups, and clusters. Let n_{ijt} be the size of the

tth cluster in the jth group ($j=1$ for *exposed* and $j=2$ for *unexposed*) from the ith table, and k_{ij} the number of clusters in the jth group from the ith table. To further clarify this altered notation, Tables 2.16 and 2.17 describes the data layout for the ith stratum.

TABLE 2.16

Stratum		Cluster			
		1	2	...	k_{ij}
Exposed (E^+)	Cluster size	n_{i11}	n_{i12}	...	$n_{i1k_{ij}}$
$j=1$	Number of deaths	y_{i11}	y_{i12}	...	$y_{i1k_{ij}}$
Unexposed (E^-)	Cluster size	n_{i21}	n_{i22}	...	$n_{i2k_{ij}}$
$j=2$	Number of deaths	y_{i21}	y_{i22}	...	$y_{i2k_{ij}}$

TABLE 2.17

		D^+	D^-	
$j=1$	E^+	y_{i1}	$y_{i1}-n_{i1}$	n_{i1}
$j=2$	E^-	y_{i2}	$y_{i2}-n_{i2}$	n_{i2}

where $y_{ij}=\sum_{t=1}^{k_{ij}}y_{ijt}$ and $n_{ij}=\sum_{t=1}^{k_{ij}}n_{ijt}$ ($j=1,2;i=1,2,\ldots,k$).

Now, because the sampling units are clusters of individuals, the χ^2_{mh} statistic used to test H_0: $\psi=1$ would not be appropriate. To adjust this statistic for the clustering effect, we introduce two procedures by Donald and Donner (1987) and by Rao and Scott (1992).

2.5.2.1 Donald and Donner's Adjustment

Because we have $2k$ rows in Table 2.16, an intraclass correlation ρ is first estimated from each row. Let $\hat{\rho}_{ij}$ be the estimate of ρ_{ij} from the jth row in the ith table. Under a common correlation assumption, it is reasonable to construct an overall estimate of ρ as

$$\hat{\rho}_A = \frac{1}{2k}\sum_{i=1}^{k}\sum_{j=1}^{2}\hat{\rho}_{ij}$$

Let $\hat{D}_{ijt}=1+(n_{ijt}-1)\hat{\rho}_A$ be the correction factor for each cluster and B_{ij} the weighted average of such correction factors where the weights are the cluster sizes themselves. Therefore, we write

$$B_{ij}=\frac{\sum_{t=1}^{k_{ij}}n_{ijt}\hat{D}_{ijt}}{\sum_{t=1}^{k_{ij}}n_{ijt}}$$

Donald and Donner (1987) suggested that the Mantel–Haenszel test statistic on $H_0: \psi = 1$, adjusted for the clustering effect, is given by

$$\chi^2_{mhc} = \frac{\left[\sum_{i=1}^{k} \dfrac{y_{i1}(n_{i2} - y_{i2}) - y_{i2}(n_{i1} - y_{i1})}{n_{i1}B_{i1} + n_{i2}B_{i2}} \right]^2}{\sum_{i=1}^{k} \dfrac{n_{i1}n_{i2}y_{.i}(n_{i.} - y_{.i})}{(n_{i1}B_{i1} + n_{i2}B_{i2})n_i^2}}$$

Since cluster sampling affects the variance of the estimated parameters, the variance $\hat{V}_{mh}$ of $\hat{\psi}_{mh}$ is no longer valid. Donald and Donner defined the cluster variant $\hat{b}_i^*$ of the $\hat{b}_i$ contained in Hauck's formula 2.18 as

$$\hat{b}_i^* = \frac{B_{i1}}{n_{i1}\hat{P}_{i1}\hat{q}_{i1}} + \frac{B_{i2}}{n_{i2}\hat{P}_{i2}\hat{q}_{i2}}$$

The corrected variance $\hat{V}_{mhc}$ is

$$\hat{V}_{mhc} = \frac{\hat{\psi}_{mh}^2 \sum_{i=1}^{k} \hat{w}_i^2 \hat{b}_i^*}{\left(\sum_{i=1}^{k} \hat{w}_i \right)^2}$$

Hence a $(1 - \alpha)\,100\%$ confidence limits on ψ_{mh} after adjusting for clustering is $\hat{\psi}_{mh} \pm Z_{\alpha/2}\sqrt{\hat{V}_{mhc}}$.

2.5.2.2 Rao and Scott's Adjustment

This adjustment requires the computation of the variance inflation factors d_{ij} using the cluster-level data (y_{ijt}, n_{ijt}), where $t = 1, 2, \ldots, k_{ij}$. The inflation factor is computed in two steps. First,

$$v_{ij} = \frac{k_{ij}}{(k_{ij} - 1)n_{ij}^2} \sum_{t=1}^{k_{ij}} \left(y_{ijt} - n_{ijt}\hat{p}_{ij} \right)^2$$

where

$$\hat{P}_{ij} = \frac{y_{ij}}{n_{ij}}$$

and then

$$d_{ij} = \frac{n_{ij}v_{ij}}{\hat{p}_{ij}\hat{q}_{ij}}$$

An asymptotically (that is for large k_{ij} for each i and j) valid test of $H_0: \psi = 1$ is obtained by replacing (y_{ij}, n_{ij}) by $(\tilde{y}_{ij}, \tilde{n}_{ij})$, where $\tilde{y}_{ij} = y_{ij}/d_{ij}$ and $\tilde{n}_{ij} = n_{ij}/d_{ij}$.

To construct an asymptotic confidence interval on ψ_{mh}, (y_{ij}, n_{ij}) is replaced by $(\tilde{y}_{ij}, \tilde{n}_{ij})$ in $\hat{\psi}_{mh}$ to get

$$\tilde{\psi}_{mhc} = \frac{\sum_{i=1}^{k} \dfrac{\tilde{y}_{i1}(\tilde{n}_{i2} - \tilde{y}_{i2})}{(\tilde{n}_{i1} + \tilde{n}_{i2})}}{\sum_{i=1}^{k} \dfrac{\tilde{y}_{i2}(\tilde{n}_{i1} - \tilde{y}_{i1})}{(\tilde{n}_{i1} + \tilde{n}_{i2})}}$$

as the clustered adjusted point estimator of ψ_{mh}. Similarly, Hauck's variance estimator for $\tilde{\psi}_{mhc}$ becomes

$$\tilde{V}_{mhc} = \frac{\tilde{\psi}_{mhc}^2 \left(\sum_{i=1}^{k} \tilde{w}_i^2 \tilde{b}_i \right)}{\left(\sum_{i=1}^{k} \tilde{w}_i \right)^2}$$

where

$$\tilde{w}_i = \left(\tilde{n}_{i1}^{-1} + \tilde{n}_{i2}^{-1} \right)^{-1} \tilde{p}_{i2} \left(1 - \tilde{p}_{i1} \right)$$

$$\tilde{b}_i = \frac{d_{i1}}{n_{i1}\tilde{p}_{i1}(1 - \tilde{p}_{i1})} + \frac{d_{i2}}{n_{i2}\tilde{p}_{i2}(1 - \tilde{p}_{i2})}$$

and

$$\tilde{p}_{ij} = \frac{\tilde{y}_{ij}}{\tilde{n}_{ij}} \quad j = 1, 2$$

Example 2.6

The following data are the result of a case–control study to investigate the association between bovine leukemia virus (BLV) infection and bovine immunodeficiency virus (BIV) infection. Each BLV$^+$ cow was matched on sex and age (within 2 years) with a BLV$^-$ cow from a different herd. The pedigree relatives of a BLV$^+$ cow constituted clusters of BIV$^+$ or BIV$^-$, while the pedigree relatives of a BLV$^-$ cow constituted clusters of BIV$^+$ or BIV$^-$ (Table 2.18).

A region-stratified (unmatched) analysis is conducted to test the above hypothesis using

1. Mantel–Haenszel one degree of freedom χ^2 test on the significance of the common odds ratio and a 95% confidence interval using Hauck's variance formula.
2. Adjusted χ^2 test and the variance expression for clustering using Donald and Donner's procedure and Rao and Scott's procedure.

TABLE 2.18

Case–Control Study Results for Investigation of Association between BLV Infection and BIV Infection

Region 1				Region 2			
BLV+ cows		Controls		BLV+ cows		Controls	
BIV+	BIV−	BIV+	BIV−	BIV+	BIV−	BIV+	BIV−
1	4	0	4	7	1	0	2
1	5	0	4	6	1	0	0
1	2	0	3	0	0	1	6
2	4	0	2	1	1	0	6
0	1	0	4	0	3	0	2
2	0	0	7	0	1	1	0
1	1	0	3	1	1	1	0
1	2	1	1				
2	1	2	5				
3	0	0	3				
1	1	1	2				
2	4	0	6				
1	1	0	4				

From Table 2.18 we construct the following two 2 × 2 tables

	Region 1		Region 2	
	BLV+	BLV−	BLV+	BLV−
BLV+	18	26	15	8
BLV−	4	48	3	16

The Mantel–Haenszel common odds ratio is given by

$$\hat{\psi}_{MH} = \frac{\dfrac{(18)(48)}{96} + \dfrac{(15)(16)}{42}}{\dfrac{(4)(26)}{96} + \dfrac{(3)(8)}{42}} = 8.89$$

and Hauck's variance is 17.85.

Now, the one degree of freedom chi-squared test of the common odds ratio will be shown using three methods:

1. Uncorrected
2. Donald and Donner's adjustment
3. Rao and Scott's adjustment

Uncorrected chi-squared test of common odds ratio

H_0: No association between BIV and BLV status in pedigree.

$$\chi^2 = \frac{\left(|33 - 19.94| - \frac{1}{2}\right)^2}{6.86} = 24.863$$

Thus, since 24.863 exceeds the $\chi^2_{(1,0.05)}$ value of 3.84, the null hypothesis is rejected, implying that there is a strong association between BIV and BLV status.

Donald and Donner's adjustment

H_0: No association between BIV and BLV status in pedigree.

The χ^2_{mhc} for Donald and Donner is

$$\chi^2_{mhc} = \frac{\left[\sum_{i=1}^{k} \frac{y_{i1}(n_{i2} - y_{i2}) - y_{i2}(n_{i1} - y_{i1})}{n_{i1}B_{i1} + n_{i2}B_{i2}}\right]^2}{\sum_{i=1}^{k} \frac{n_{i1}n_{i2}y_{.i}(n_{i.} - y_{.i})}{(n_{i1}B_{i1} + n_{i2}B_{i2})n_i^2}}$$

The estimated common intraclass correlation is given by

$$\hat{\rho}_A = \frac{1}{2k} \sum \sum \hat{\rho}_{ij} = \frac{1}{2(2)}(-0.0186 + 0.08655 + 0.5920 + 0.3786) = 0.26$$

Now, the correction factor for each cluster is

$$\hat{D}_{ijt} = 1 + (n_{ijt} - 1)\hat{\rho}_A$$

and the weighted average of the correction factors is

$$B_{ij} = \frac{\sum n_{ijt}\hat{D}_{ijt}}{\sum n_{ijt}}$$

So that

$$B_{11} = \text{Region 1 BLV}^- = 1.870026 \quad B_{12} = \text{Region 1 BLV}^+ = 1.768454$$

$$B_{21} = \text{Region 2 BLV}^- = 1.952450 \quad B_{22} = \text{Region 2 BLV}^+ = 2.047695$$

and the χ^2_{mhc} using Donald and Donner's adjustment is

$$\chi^2_{mhc} = \left[\frac{\dfrac{18(52-4)-4(44-18)}{44(1.7685)+52(1.87)} + \dfrac{15(19-3)-3(23-15)}{23(2.048)+19(1.952)}}{\dfrac{52(44)(22)(96-22)}{(96)(96)(44(1.7685)+52(1.87))} + \dfrac{23(19)(18)(42-18)}{(42)(42)(23(2.048)+19(1.952))}}\right]^2$$

$$= 13.33$$

Because 13.33 is larger than the $\chi^2_{(1,0.05)}$ value of 3.84, the null hypothesis is rejected, implying that when we adjust for the intracluster correlation, there is a significant association between the BLV and the BIV status.

The value of the variance is now

$$\hat{V}_{mhc} = \frac{\hat{\psi}^2_{mh} \sum_{i=1}^{k} \hat{w}_i^2 \hat{b}_i^*}{\left(\sum_{i=1}^{k} \hat{w}_i\right)^2}$$

where

$$\hat{b}_i^* = \frac{B_{i1}}{n_{i1}\hat{P}_{i1}\hat{q}_{i1}} + \frac{B_{i2}}{n_{i2}\hat{P}_{i2}\hat{q}_{i2}}$$

$$\hat{w}_i = \left(\frac{1}{n_{i1}} + \frac{1}{n_{i2}}\right)^{-1} \hat{p}_{i2}q_{i1}$$

$$\hat{q}_{ij} = 1 - p_{ij}, \quad j = 1,2$$

The results of these computations show that $\hat{w}_1 = 1.085$, $\hat{w}_2 = 0.572$, $\hat{b}_1^* = 0.673$, and $\hat{b}_2^* = 1.165$. The variance is equal to 33.791.

Rao and Scott's Adjustment
The null hypothesis of no association between BIV and BLV status is tested using the following steps. The χ^2 is adjusted by the variance inflation factor, d_{ij}. First, we compute

$$v_{ij} = \frac{k_{ij}}{(k_{ij}-1)n_{ij}^2} \sum_{t=1}^{k_{ij}} (y_{ijt} - n_{ijt}\hat{p}_{ij})^2$$

where $\hat{p}_{ij} = y_{ij}/n_{ij}$.

The inflation factor d_{ij} is calculated using

$$d_{ij} = \frac{n_{ij}v_{ij}}{\hat{p}_{ij}\hat{q}_{ij}} \quad \tilde{y}_{ij} = \frac{y_{ij}}{d_{ij}} \quad \tilde{n}_{ij} = \frac{n_{ij}}{d_{ij}}$$

Here, $d_{11} = 0.93$, $d_{12} = 1.32$, $d_{21} = 2.23$, and $d_{22} = 1.70$. Calculation of the adjusted χ^2 is therefore given by $\chi^2_{mhc} = 18.69$.

Once again we reject the null hypothesis, which means that there is a significant association between the BLV and the BIV status. With the Rao and Scott adjustment, the variance estimate is now

$$\tilde{V}_{mhc} = \frac{\tilde{\psi}^2_{mhc} \left(\sum_{i=1}^{k} \tilde{w}_i^2 \tilde{b}_i\right)}{\left(\sum_{i=1}^{k} \tilde{w}_i\right)^2} = 29.851$$

The following SAS program sets up the data, computes the Mantel–Haenszel common odds ratio, and tests for the equality of the odds ratio across the

strata. The SAS PROC GLM produces the ANOVA results for four combinations of region and BLV status from where the overall common intracluster
correlation and adjusted tests of the significance of the common odds ratio
may be computed. The SAS output is not shown.

```
data virus;
input region pedigree BLV$ BIV count @@;
cards;
1 1 y 1 1 1 1 y 0 4 1 2 y 1 1 1 2 y 0 5
1 3 y 1 1 1 3 y 0 2 1 4 y 1 2 1 4 y 0 4
1 5 y 1 0 1 5 y 0 1 1 6 y 1 2 1 6 y 0 0
1 7 y 1 1 1 7 y 0 1 1 8 y 1 1 1 8 y 0 2
1 9 y 1 2 1 9 y 0 1 1 10 y 1 3 1 10 y 0 0
1 11 y 1 1 1 11 y 0 1 1 12 y 1 2 1 12 y 0 4
1 13 y 1 1 1 13 y 0 1 1 14 n 1 0 1 14 n 0 4
1 15 n 1 0 1 15 n 0 4 1 16 n 1 0 1 16 n 0 3
1 17 n 1 0 1 17 n 0 2 1 18 n 1 0 1 18 n 0 4
1 19 n 1 0 1 19 n 0 7 1 20 n 1 0 1 20 n 0 3
1 21 n 1 1 1 21 n 0 1 1 22 n 1 2 1 22 n 0 5
1 23 n 1 0 1 23 n 0 3 1 24 n 1 1 1 24 n 0 2
1 25 n 1 0 1 25 n 0 6 1 26 n 1 0 1 26 n 0 4
2 27 y 1 7 2 27 y 0 1 2 28 y 1 6 2 28 y 0 1
2 29 y 1 0 2 29 y 0 0 2 30 y 1 1 2 30 y 0 1
2 31 y 1 0 2 31 y 0 3 2 32 y 1 0 2 32 y 0 1
2 33 y 1 1 2 33 y 0 1 2 34 n 1 0 2 34 n 0 2
2 35 n 1 0 2 35 n 0 0 2 36 n 1 1 2 36 n 0 6
2 37 n 1 0 2 37 n 0 6 2 38 n 1 0 2 38 n 0 2
2 39 n 1 1 2 39 n 0 0 2 40 n 1 1 2 40 n 0 0
;

proc format;
value $blvf y='BLV+'
    n='BLV-';
 value bivf 1='BIV+'
    0='BIV-';

* Odds ratios of the two regions and the common odds ratio;
proc freq data=virus order=formatted;
    weight count;
    tables region*blv*biv / norow nocol nopercent measures cmh noprint;
format blv $blvf. biv bivf.; run;

* Computing the intraclass correlations;
proc sort data=virus; by region blv;

proc glm; by region blv;
    class pedigree;
```

```
    freq count;
    model biv = pedigree;
  run; quit;
```

The following R code reads the data in grouped form, ungroups it to run ANOVA to get statistics for each drug level to compute overall ICC, and then uses the grouped data to compute Rao–Scott and Donner adjusted χ^2 tests.

```
# Reading the virus data in the grouped (y/n) form
virusn <- data.frame(region=c(rep(1,26),rep(2,12)),
blv=c(rep("y",13),rep("n",13),rep("y",6),rep("n",6)),
pedigree=1:38,
n =c(5,6,3,6,1,2,2,3,3,3,2,6,2,4,4,3,2,4,7,3,2,7,3,3,6,4,8,7,2,3,1,2,2,7,6,2,1,1),
biv =c(1,1,1,2,0,2,1,1,2,3,1,2,1,0,0,0,0,0,0,0,1,2,0,1,0,0,7,6,1,0,0,1,0,1,0,0,1,1))
```

```
# Un-grouping the data
y1 <- data.frame(lapply(virusn, function(x) rep(x,virusn$biv)), y=1)
[,c(1:3,6)]
y0 <- data.frame(lapply(virusn, function(x) rep(x, virusn$n-virusn$biv)),
y = 0)[,c(1:3,6)]
virus <- rbind(y1,y0)
```

```
# Fitting linear models by clusters (pedigree) to get statistics for ICC
by(virus, virus[,c(1,2)], function(x) anova(lm(y ~ factor(pedigree),
data=x)))
```

2.6 Sample Size Requirements for Clustered Binary Data

2.6.1 Paired Sample Design

The determination of the sample size in a study that aims at testing for difference in proportions is an important issue. For the matched-pair design where McNemar test is used, Miettenen (1968) and Conner (1987) obtained several approximations to sample size. Specifically, the basic model used by both authors is represented in Table 2.19.

TABLE 2.19

Paired Dichotomous Data

		Y_2		
		1	0	
Y_1	1	P_{11}	P_{10}	P_1
	0	P_{01}	P_{00}	$1 - P_1$
		P_2	$1 - P_2$	1

where P_{ij} is the probability that a matched pair has response $Y_1 = i$ and $Y_2 = j$, $(i, j = 0, 1)$. Also $P_1 = P_{11} + P_{10}$, $P_2 = P_{11} + P_{01}$, and $\eta = P_{10} + P_{01}$ is the probability that the response of a case and its matched control disagrees. Formally, we need to determine the number of pairs n, necessary to have power $1 - \beta$ of detecting a difference $\delta = P_1 - P_2 > 0$ when a one-sided test of size α is to be used. By an argument similar to that of Snedecor and Cochran (1981), Conner showed that

$$n = \frac{\left[Z_\alpha n^{1/2} + Z_\beta (\eta - \delta^2)^{1/2} \right]^2}{\delta^2}$$

where Z_α and Z_β are the percentiles of the standard normal distribution as defined in Chapter 1.

Note that the above equation requires η to be known for the sample size to be determined. Since one can write $\eta = P_{10} + P_{01} = P_1 + P_2 - 2P_2 \Pr(Y_1 = 1 | Y_2 = 1)$, then η is minimum when the conditional probability $P_{1|1} = \Pr(Y_1 = 1 | Y_2 = 1)$ is maximum, and η is maximum when $P_{1|1}$ is minimum. Because $P_{1|1} = P_{11}/P_2$, it is maximized or minimized when P_{11} is maximized or minimized. Clearly, the issue of providing a plausible value for η is quite complicated. However, Connor (1987) argued that sample size formula for the independent outcome situation provides a conservative estimate of the sample size. This is given by

$$n' = \frac{(Z_\alpha \sigma_0 + Z_\beta \sigma_A)^2}{\delta^2}$$

where $\sigma_0^2 = 2 P_1 (1 - P_1)$ and $\sigma_A^2 = P_1(1 - P_1) + (P_1 - \delta)(1 - P_1 + \delta)$.

2.6.2 Comparative Studies for Cluster Sizes Greater than or Equal to 2

Recall that for continuous responses, the introduction of the parameter ρ allows the formalization of the within-cluster dependence. In the case of a dichotomous response, an analogue to ρ has been developed, as seen in the previous sections. Donner (1981) developed sample size expression required for testing $H_0: P_1 = P_2$, where P_1 and P_2 are the underlying success probabilities, given by

$$N' = \frac{(Z_\alpha + Z_\beta)^2 \sigma_d^2 (1 + (n - 1)\rho)}{\delta^2}$$

where n as usual is the cluster size, $N' = nk$ and $\sigma_d^2 = P_1(1 - P_1) + P_2(1 - P_2)$. In case the exact cluster size n is not known, it should be replaced by the largest expected cluster size.

Example 2.7

Consider a study in which the outcome of interest is hypertension status and the unit of randomization is a spouse pair. Previous studies estimated the within-pair correlation by $\hat{\rho} = 0.25$. Suppose the epidemiologist would like a 90% probability at $\alpha = 0.05$ (two-tailed) of detecting a significant difference between two ethnic groups (e.g., white versus black), where it is believed that the percentage of hypertension among the white is 15% and among the black 20%. Using the above expression we have

$$N' = \frac{(1.96 + 1.28)^2[(0.15)(0.85) + (0.20)(0.80)][1 + 0.25]}{(0.5)^2}$$

$$= 1509$$

Thus, the study must be designed to allocate $1509/2 \approx 755$ couples from each group. If no clustering effect was present ($\rho = 0$), $N' = 1207$, and hence 604 would be required in each group to provide the same statistical power.

2.7 Discussion

An extensive literature has been developed on the methodological issues that arise when the risk of disease is compared across treatment groups when the sampling units are clusters of individuals. The presence of the so-called "cluster effects" invalidates the standard Pearson's χ^2 test of homogeneity and makes the reported confidence interval on the common odds ratio unrealistically narrow. In the previous section, we introduced the most commonly used techniques of adjusting clustering effects. It is debatable as to which technique is most appropriate.

Extensive simulation studies conducted by Ahn and Odom-Maryon (1995) and Donner et al. (1994) showed that each approach has its advantages. Ahn and Odom-Maryon preferred Rao and Scott's adjustment on the length of the confidence interval of the Mantel–Haenszel common odds ratio. The reason was that the ANOVA estimator of the intraclass correlation ρ, needed for Donner's adjustment, is positively biased, and hence the confidence interval would be spuriously wide when $\rho = 0$. On the other hand, Donner et al.'s (1994) simulations showed that the adjustment to Pearson's χ^2 test of homogeneity based on the pooled estimate of the intraclass correlations performs better than methods that separately estimate design effects from each group. The reason was that under randomization, the assumption of a common population design effect is more likely to hold, at least under the null hypothesis. They also stressed the need for more research in this area, to investigate the finite-sample properties of methods that do not require the assumption of a common design effect.

The A-Cluster 2.1 software by the World Health Organization (2000) has implemented the analysis of cluster-randomized trials with continuous as well as the binary outcomes discussed in this chapter. The program incorporates the analysis of data and the estimation of sample size for parallel group, matched pair, and the stratified designs using Donald and Donner (1987) and Rao and Scott (1992) adjustments for clustering to the usual χ^2 test statistics.

Exercises

2.1 The following table summarizes the results of a case–control study. The main objective of the study was to investigate risk factors associated with the incidence of tick-borne diseases in "small-holder" dairy farms in one of the northern districts near Nairobi, Kenya. A case farm is a farm where animals are sprayed regularly, while a control farm is a farm where animals are not sprayed at all. The following table gives the distribution of the number of farms classified by size (i.e., number of animals on the farm) and the number of animals confirmed to have a tick-borne disease.

   (a) For the case and the control farms, test separately whether the number of sick animals follows a binomial distribution.
   (b) Is the rate of infection in control farms different from the case farms?

State your hypotheses and assumptions. Explain each step in the analyses and write your conclusions clearly.

Number of Sick Animals	Herd Size 1 ca	ct	2 ca	ct	3 ca	ct	4 ca	ct
0	10	2	20	2	10	1	5	1
1	8	1	10	2	5	0	1	1
2			2	10	0	4	0	2
3					0	4	0	5
4							0	5

ca: case and ct: control.

2.2 The data in the following table are from a study on the teratogenic effects of certain chemical (tetrabromodibenzo-*p*-dioxin or TBDD) in C57BL/6N mice. The responses are the proportions Y/n of cleft palate incidence in each litter for pregnant dams treated on gestation day 10 and examined on gestation day 18.

Dose	Y_{ij}	n_{ij}	Dose	Y_{ij}	n_{ij}	Dose	Y_{ij}	n_{ij}	Dose	Y_{ij}	n_{ij}
3	0	7	6	0	8	24	0	9	96	6	7
3	0	11	6	0	9	24	0	9	96	7	7
3	0	10	6	0	9	24	0	7	96	3	3
3	0	9	6	0	10	24	0	9	96	9	9
3	0	10	6	0	8	24	0	5	96	10	10
3	0	8	6	0	8	24	0	9	96	2	3
3	0	7	6	0	10	24	0	8	96	7	8
3	0	10	12	0	3	24	1	9	96	1	3
3	0	9	12	0	9	24	0	11	96	9	9
3	0	10	12	0	7	24	0	6	96	8	9
3	0	2	12	0	8	24	0	9	96	8	8
3	0	9	12	0	9	24	0	9	192	6	6
3	0	9	12	0	5	24	0	8	192	9	9
3	0	10	12	0	6	24	0	6	192	4	4
3	0	9	12	0	8	24	0	9	192	6	6
6	0	11	12	0	8	48	3	5	192	7	7
6	0	6	12	0	9	48	2	9	192	10	10
6	0	3	12	0	10	48	0	8	192	7	7
6	0	7	12	0	6	48	0	8	192	5	5
6	0	3	12	0	8	48	0	10	192	9	9
6	0	9	12	0	9	48	0	5	192	4	4
6	0	10	12	0	10	48	0	8	192	7	7
6	0	9	12	0	9	48	0	3	192	8	8
6	0	3	12	0	7	48	4	9	192	9	9
6	0	9	24	0	8	48	0	9	192	10	10
6	0	11	24	0	11	48	0	8			

(a) Is there a significant difference between dose levels on the incidence of cleft palate?

(b) Test the above hypothesis by accounting for the dose structure in a logistic regression model (take $X = \log_{10}$ (dose) as a covariate).

What do you conclude?

2.3 Run the SAS and R programs given in Example 2.6 to compute the common odds ratio and test the significance of the common odds ratio using unadjusted and adjusted χ^2 tests and verify the calculations in the example.

2.4 An investigator is interested in comparing prevalence of mastitis in four breeds of dairy cattle. He selects herds of the four breeds (exactly one breed in each herd) to obtain the following data. The table shows herd size, followed by the number of cases in brackets.

Breed 1	30(10)	47(2)	48(2)	24(0)
Breed 2	21(0)	31(0)	46(11)	
Breed 3	10(5)	43(20)	32(9)	43(0)	37(22)
Breed 4	17(1)	35(10)	41(3)	

Verify the following results:

Pooled prevalence $\hat{p} = 0.188$, mean herd size $m = 33.667$.

The usual χ^2 ignoring herds is

$$\sum \frac{(\text{observed} - \text{expected})^2}{\text{expected}} = 37.926$$

Compare the χ^2 tables with three degrees of freedom. Verify that the p-value is <0.001.

To account for clustering, we need to calculate the intracluster correlation coefficient. Write a SAS program to calculate the following quantities needed to evaluate the pooled intraclass correlation. For each breed, calculate SSB and SSW and verify the following results.

Breed	SSB	SSW	Number of Herds (n_h)
1	2.186	10.498	4
2	1.396	8.370	3
3	8.409	28.585	5
4	1.028	10.865	3

$$\text{MSB} = \frac{\sum \text{SSB}}{\sum (n_h - 1)} \qquad \text{MSW} = \frac{\sum \text{SSW}}{N - \sum n_h}$$

where N is the total number of animals. Show that $\text{MSB} = 1.184$, $\text{MSW} = 0.119$, and hence $\hat{\rho} = \frac{\text{MSB} - \text{MSW}}{\text{MSB} + (M-1)\text{MSW}} = 0.210$, correction factor $C = 1 + (m - 1)$ $\hat{\rho} = 7.857$, and corrected χ^2 is $37.926/7.857 = 4.827$.

What is the number of appropriate degrees of freedom associated with the above corrected χ^2 value?

2.5   This exercise is an illustration on the use of stratified analysis when the randomization unit is a cluster (litter). Use the χ^2 test to compare between the two treatments with respect to death rate.

Stratum I	Treatment I	Litter size	15	13	12	15	10	9	$\hat{p} = 0.122$
		Mortality	2	0	2	5	0	0	
	Treatment II	Litter size	16	15	13	13	11	12	$\hat{p} = 0.063$
		Mortality	1	0	1	0	3	0	
Stratum II	Treatment I	Litter size	14	16	15	9	14		$\hat{p} = 0.122$
		Mortality	4	5	3	0	3		
	Treatment II	Litter size	16	7	12	15	11		$\hat{p} = 0.122$
		Mortality	4	0	0	3	0		

	Stratum I			Stratum II		
	$D(x)$	$A(y)$	Total	$D(x)$	$A(y)$	Total
Treatment I	9	65	$74 = n_{11}$	15	53	$68 = n_{21}$
Treatment II	5	75	$80 = n_{12}$	7	54	$61 = n_{22}$
Total	$14 = x_1$	$140 = y_1$	$154 = n_1$	$22 = x_2$	$107 = y_2$	$129 = n_2$

If the odds ratio ψ is assumed to be the same in both strata, the Mantel–Haenszel procedure tests the hypothesis $\psi = 1$. (When $\psi = 1$, the relative risk is 1.)

$$\chi^2_{MH} = \frac{\left(\sum_t \dfrac{x_{1t}y_{2t} - x_{2t}y_{1t}}{n_t} \right)^2}{\sum_t \dfrac{n_{1t}n_{2t}x_t y_t}{(n_t - 1)n_t^2}}$$

Show that $\chi^2_{MH} = 414$. What is the p-value associated with the test?

To account for clustering, compute SSB and SSW for each of the four treatment groups (rows) using PROC GLM in SAS. Verify the following results:

	SSB	SSW	Litters
Stratum 1, Row 1	1.172	6.733	6
Stratum 1, Row 2	0.645	4.042	6
Stratum 2, Row 1	0.639	11.052	5
Stratum 2, Row 2	0.792	5.400	5

$$\text{MSB} = \frac{\sum \text{SSB}}{\sum (n_h - 1)} = 0.181 \quad \text{MSW} = \frac{\sum \text{SSW}}{N - \sum n_h} = 0.104$$

$$\hat{\rho} = \frac{\text{MSB} - \text{MSW}}{\text{MSB} + (m - 1)\text{MSW}} = 0.054$$

Compute the correction factor for each cluster size, m

$$c_m = 1 + (m - 1)(0.054)$$

and for each row compute the weighted mean, B_{jt}.
For example, $B_{11} = \dfrac{15C_{15} + 13C_{13} + \cdots + 9C_9}{15 + 13 + \cdots + 9} = 1.633.$

Show that the corrected Mantel–Haenszel χ^2 statistic is as given below:

$$
\chi^2_{MH} = \frac{\left(\sum_t \dfrac{x_{1t}y_{2t} - x_{2t}y_{1t}}{n_{1t}B_{1t} + n_{2t}B_{2t}} \right)^2}{\sum_t \dfrac{n_{1t}n_{2t}x_t y_t}{(n_{1t}B_{1t} + n_{2t}B_{2t})n_t^2}}
$$

$$
= \frac{(1.373 + 2.03)^2}{3.198 + 4.548}
$$

$$
= 2.489
$$

2.6   Analyze the smoking cessation data of Chapter 1 to compare the two proportions of correlated responses. Consider each school a cluster.

2.7   Run the SAS and R programs given in Example 2.6, analyze Weil's data, and verify the results reported in the example.

3

Modeling Binary Outcome Data

CONTENTS

3.1 Introduction

In many research problems, it is of interest to study the effects that some variables exert on others. One sensible way to describe this relationship is to relate the variables by some sort of mathematical equation. In most applications, statistical models are mostly mathematical equations constructed to approximately relate the response (dependent) variables to a group of predictor (independent) variables.

When the response variable, denoted by y, is continuous and believed to depend linearly on k variables $x_1, x_2, \ldots, x_k$ through unknown parameters $\beta_0, \beta_1, \ldots, \beta_k$, then this linear (where "linear" is used to indicate linearity in the unknown parameters) relationship is given as

$$y_i = \sum_{j=0}^{k} \beta_j x_{ji} + \varepsilon_i \tag{3.1}$$

where $x_{0i} = 1$ for all $i = 1, 2, \ldots, n$.

The term ε_i is the unobservable random error representing the residual variation and is assumed to be independent of the systematic component $\sum_{j=0}^{k} \beta_j x_{ji}$. It is also assumed that $E(\varepsilon_i) = 0$ and $V(\varepsilon_i) = \sigma^2$; hence, $E(y_i) = \sum_{j=0}^{k} \beta_j x_{ji}$ and $V(y_i) = \sigma^2$.

To fit the model 3.1 to the data (y_i, x_i), one has to estimate the parameters $\beta_0, \beta_1, \ldots, \beta_k$. The most commonly used methods of estimation are (i) the method of least squares and (ii) the method of maximum likelihood.

Applications of these methods of estimation to the linear regression model 3.1 are extensively discussed in Mosteller and Tukey (1977), Draper and Smith (1981), and many other sources. It should be noted that no assumptions are needed on the distribution of the response variable y (except the independence of $(y_1, y_2, \ldots, y_n)$ to estimate the parameters by the method of least squares. However, the maximum likelihood requires that the sample $y = (y_1, y_2, \ldots, y_n)$ be randomly drawn from a distribution where the specified structure of that distribution in most applications is

$$N \left(\sum_{j=0}^{k} \beta_j x_{ji}, \sigma^2 \right)$$

The least squares estimates of the regression parameters will then coincide with those obtained by the method of maximum likelihood. Another remark that should be made here is that there is nothing in the theory of least squares that restricts the distribution of the response variable to be continuous, discrete, or of bounded range. For example, suppose that we would like to model the proportion $\hat{p}_i = \frac{y_i}{n_i}$ $(i = 1, 2, \ldots, m)$ of individuals suffering from some respiratory illness, observed over several geographical regions, as a function of k covariates, where $y_i = \sum_{j=1}^{n_i} y_{ij}$, in which $y_{ij} = 1(0)$ if disease is present (absent). We further assume, conditional on the observed covariates, that y_i is binomially distributed with mean p_i. That is, we assume the relationship between $E(y_i | x_{ji}) = p_i$ and the covariates to be

$$p_i = \sum_{j=0}^{k} \beta_j x_{ji} \tag{3.2}$$

The least squares estimates are obtained by minimizing

$$s^2 = \sum_{i=1}^{n} \left(\hat{p}_i - \sum_{j=0}^{k} \beta_j x_{ji} \right)^2$$

Several problems are encountered when the least squares method is used to fit model 3.2. One of the assumptions of the method of least squares is the homogeneity of variance, that is, $V(y_i) = \sigma^2$, i.e., the variance does not vary from one observation to another. For binary data, y_i follows a binomial distribution with mean $n_i p_i$ and variance $n_i p_i (1 - p_i)$ so that

$$V(\hat{p}_i) = \frac{p_i(1 - p_i)}{n_i}$$

As proposed by Cox and Snell (1989), one can deal with the variance heterogeneity by applying the method of weighted least squares using the reciprocal variance as a weight. The weighted least squares estimates are thus obtained by minimizing

$$s_w^2 = \sum_{i=1}^{n} w_i \left(\hat{p}_i - \sum_{j=0}^{k} \beta_j x_{ji} \right)^2 \tag{3.3}$$

where $w_i = [V(\hat{p}_i)]^{-1}$ depends on p_i, which in turn depends on the unknown parameters $\beta_0, \beta_1, \ldots, \beta_k$ through the relationship 3.2. The model 3.2 can be fitted quite easily using PROC REG in SAS together with the WEIGHT statement, where $\hat{w}_i$ are the specified weights. Note that $0 \le p_i \le 1$ and the estimates $\hat{\beta}_0, \hat{\beta}_1, \ldots, \hat{\beta}_k$ of the regression parameters are not constrained. That is, they are permitted to attain any value in the interval $(-\infty, \infty)$. Since the fitted values are obtained by substituting $\hat{\beta}_0, \hat{\beta}_1, \ldots, \hat{\beta}_k$ in Equation 3.2,

$$\hat{p}_i = \sum_{j=0}^{k} \hat{\beta}_j x_{ji}$$

Thus, there is no guarantee that the fitted values should fall in the interval [0,1].

To overcome the difficulties of using the method of least squares to fit a model where the response variable has a restricted range, it is suggested that a suitable transformation be employed so that the fitted values of the transformed parameter vary over the interval $(-\infty, \infty)$.

This chapter is devoted to the analysis of binomially distributed data where the binary responses are independent, with special attention given to situations where the binary responses are obtained from clusters and hence cannot be assumed to be independent. The chapter is organized as follows: In

Section 3.2 we introduce the logistic transformation and establish the relationship between the regression coefficient and the odds ratio parameter. Model-building strategies are discussed in Sections 3.3 and 3.4, and measures of goodness of fit are introduced in Section 3.5. Approaches to modeling correlated binary data are discussed in Section 3.3. In this section, population average and cluster-specific models are investigated with examples.

3.2   The Logistic Regression Model

Let us consider the following example that may help the reader understand the motives of the logistic transformation. Suppose that we have a binary variable y that takes the value 1 if a sampled subject is diseased, and 0 otherwise. Let $P(D) = P[y = 1] = \pi$ and $P(\overline{D}) = P[y = 0] = 1 - \pi$. Moreover, suppose that X is a risk factor that has normal distribution with mean μ_1 and variance σ^2 in the population of diseased, that is

$$X|D = N(\mu_1, \sigma^2)$$

Meaning that, given the information that the individual is diseased, the conditional distribution of X is $N(\mu_1, \sigma^2)$. Hence

$$f(X|D) = \frac{1}{\sigma\sqrt{2\pi}} \exp\left[-\frac{(x - \mu_1)^2}{2\sigma^2}\right]$$

In a similar manner, we assume that the distribution of the risk factor X in the population of nondiseased has a mean μ_2 and variance σ^2. That is

$$f(X|\overline{D}) = \frac{1}{\sigma\sqrt{2\pi}} \exp\left[-\frac{(x - \mu_2)^2}{2\sigma^2}\right]$$

Since $p = P[y = 1|X = x] = \dfrac{p(y = 1, X = x)}{f(x)}$, then from Bayes' theorem

$$p = \frac{f(X|D)P(D)}{f(X|D)P(D) + f(X|\overline{D})P(\overline{D})}$$

$$= \frac{\dfrac{\pi}{\sigma\sqrt{2\pi}} \exp\left[-\dfrac{(x - \mu_1)^2}{2\sigma^2}\right]}{\dfrac{\pi}{\sigma\sqrt{2\pi}} \exp\left[-\dfrac{(x - \mu_1)^2}{2\sigma^2}\right] + \dfrac{1 - \pi}{\sigma\sqrt{2\pi}} \exp\left[-\dfrac{(x - \mu_2)^2}{2\sigma^2}\right]}$$

Therefore,

$$p = P[y = 1|X = x] = \frac{e^{\beta_0 + \beta_1 x}}{1 + e^{\beta_0 + \beta_1 x}} \tag{3.4}$$

In Equation 3.4 we have $\beta_0 = -\ln\left(\frac{1-\pi}{\pi}\right) - \frac{1}{2\sigma^2}(\mu_1 - \mu_2)(\mu_1 + \mu_2)$, $\beta_1 = \frac{\mu_1 - \mu_2}{\sigma^2}$, and

$$\ln\left(\frac{p}{1-p}\right) = \beta_0 + \beta_1 x \tag{3.5}$$

Therefore, the log-odds is a linear function of the explanatory variable x (here, the risk factor).

Remarks

The regression parameter β_1 has log-odds ratio interpretation in epidemiologic studies. To show this, suppose that the exposure variable has two levels (exposed, not exposed). Let us define a dummy variable x that takes the value 1 if the individual is exposed to the risk factor and 0 if not exposed.

From Equation 3.4 we have

$$P_{11} = P(y = 1|X = 1) = \frac{e^{\beta_0 + \beta_1}}{1 + e^{\beta_0 + \beta_1}}$$

$$P_{01} = P(y = 0|X = 1) = 1 - P_{11}$$

$$P_{10} = P(y = 1|X = 0) = \frac{e^{\beta_0}}{1 + e^{\beta_0}}$$

$$P_{00} = P(y = 0|X = 0) = 1 - P_{10}$$

The odds ratio is $\psi = \frac{P_{11}P_{00}}{P_{10}P_{01}} = e^{\beta_1}$, and it follows that $\ln(\psi) = \beta_1$.

The representation can be extended such that logit(p) is a function of more than just one explanatory variable.

Let $y_1, y_2, \ldots, y_n$ be a random sample of n successes out of $n_1, n_2, \ldots, n_n$ trials and let the corresponding probabilities of success be $p_1, p_2, \ldots, p_n$. If we wish to express the probability p_i as a function of the explanatory variables $x_{1i}, \ldots, x_{ki}$, then the generalization of Equation 3.5 is logit(p_i) = $\log\left(\frac{p_i}{1-p_i}\right) = \sum_{j=0}^{k} \beta_j x_{ji}$, $x_{0i} = 1$ for all $i = 1, 2, \ldots, n$.

We shall denote the linear function $\sum_{j=0}^{k} \beta_j x_{ji}$ by η_i, which is usually known as the *link function*.

Hence, $p_i = e^{\eta_i}/(1 + e^{\eta_i})$.

The binomially distributed random variable y_i, $i = 1, 2, \ldots, n$, has mean $\mu_i = n_i p_i$ and variance $n_i p_i q_i$. Fitting the model to the data is achieved by estimating the model parameters $\hat{\beta}_0, \hat{\beta}_1, \ldots, \hat{\beta}_k$.

The maximum likelihood method is used to estimate the parameters where the likelihood function is given by

$$L(\beta) = \prod_{i=1}^{n} \binom{n_i}{y_i} p_i^{y_i} q_i^{n_i - y_i}$$

$$= \prod_{i=1}^{n} \binom{n_i}{y_i} (e^{\eta_i})^{y_i} \left(\frac{1}{1 + e^{\eta_i}}\right)^{n_i}$$

The logarithm of the likelihood function is thus

$$l(\beta) = \sum_{i=1}^{n} [y_i \eta_i - n_i \ln(1 + e^{\eta_i})] \tag{3.6}$$

Differentiating $l(\beta)$ with respect to β_r, we have

$$\ell_r = \frac{\partial l(\beta)}{\partial \beta_r} = \sum_{i=1}^{n} [y_j x_{ri} - n_i x_{ri} e^{\eta_i} (1 + e^{\eta_i})^{-1}]$$

$$= \sum_{i=1}^{n} x_{ri}(y_i - n_i p_i) \quad r = 0, 1, 2, \ldots, k \tag{3.7}$$

The $k+1$ equations in Equation 3.7 can be solved numerically. The large-sample variance–covariance matrix of the maximum likelihood estimators is the inverse of Fisher's information matrix, I^{-1} (see Cox and Snell, 1989), where

$$I = -E(\ell_{rs}) = -E \left[\frac{\partial^2 l(\beta)}{\partial \beta_r \partial \beta_s} \right] = \sum_{i=1}^{n} n_i x_{ri} x_{si} p_i (1 - p_i)$$

The rth diagonal element in I^{-1} is $\hat{V}(\hat{\beta}_r) = V_{rr}$.

Once the parameters have been estimated, the predicted probabilities of success are given by

$$\hat{p}_i = \frac{e^{\hat{\eta}_i}}{1 + e^{\hat{\eta}_i}}$$

where $\hat{\eta}_i = \sum_{j=0}^{k} \hat{\beta}_j x_{ij}$.

The maximum likelihood-based $(1 - \alpha)100\%$ confidence interval on β_r is given approximately by $\hat{\beta}_r \pm z_{\alpha/2}(V_{rr})^{1/2}$. Wald's test on the null hypothesis $H_0: \beta_r = 0$ is given by referring $z = \hat{\beta}/(V_{rr})^{1/2}$ to the tables of standard normal distribution.

3.2.1 Coding Categorical Explanatory Variables and Interpretation of Coefficients

Recall that when Equation 3.4 is applied to the simple case of one independent variable that has two levels (exposed, not exposed), we defined a dummy variable X such that $X_i = 1$ if the ith individual is exposed, and $X_i = 0$ if the ith individual is not exposed.

Suppose that the exposure variable X has $m > 2$ categories. For example, X may be the strain or the breed of the animal, or it may be the ecological zone from which the sample is collected. Each of these variables (strain, breed, zone, etc.) is *qualitative* or a factor variable that can take a finite number of values known as the levels of the factor. To see how qualitative independent variables or factors are included in a logistic regression model, suppose that F is a factor with m distinct levels. There are various methods in which the indicator variables or the dummy variables can be defined. The choice of a particular method will depend on the goals of the analysis. One way to represent the m levels of the factor variable F is to define $m - 1$ dummy variables $f_1, f_2, \ldots, f_{m-1}$ such that the portion of the design matrix corresponding to these variables looks like Table 3.1.

TABLE 3.1

Dummy Variables for the Factor Variable F with m Levels

Level	f_1	f_2	$\ldots$	f_{m-1}
1	0	0		0
2	1	0	$\ldots$	0
3	0	1	$\ldots$	0
.	.	.	$\ldots$	.
.	.	.	$\ldots$	.
m	0	0	$\ldots$	1

Example 3.1

The following data are the results of a carcinogenic experiment. Different strains of rats have been injected with a carcinogen in their footpad. They were then put on a high-fat diet, and at the end of week 21 the number with tumors (y) was counted.

TABLE 3.2

Hypothetical Data: Counts of Rats with Tumors

	Strain 1	Strain 2	Strain 3	Strain 4
y_i	10	20	5	2
$n_i - y_i$	45	20	20	43
n_i	55	40	25	45
$\hat{\psi}$	4.780	21.500	5.375	

The last row of Table 3.2 gives the odds ratio for each strain level using strain 4 as the reference level. For example, for strain 1 the estimated odds ratio is

$$\hat{\psi}[\text{strain 1; strain 4}] = \frac{(10)(43)}{(45)(2)} = 4.780$$

Using strain 4 as a reference group we define the three dummy variables

$$X_j = \begin{cases} 1 & \text{if rat is from strain } j \ \ j = 1,2,3 \\ 0 & \text{otherwise} \end{cases}$$

The results of fitting the logistic regression model to the data in Table 3.2 are given in Table 3.3.

TABLE 3.3

Maximum Likelihood Analysis

Variable	Estimates	Standard Error	Wald χ^2	$\hat{\psi}$
Intercept	$\hat{\beta}_0 = -3.068$	0.723	17.990	
Strain 1	$\hat{\beta}_1 = 1.564$	0.803	3.790	4.780
Strain 2	$\hat{\beta}_2 = 3.068$	0.790	15.103	21.500
Strain 3	$\hat{\beta}_3 = 1.682$	0.879	3.658	5.375

Note that $\ln \hat{\psi}$ [strain 1; strain 4] $= \ln(4.78) = 1.56 = \hat{\beta}_1$. The standard error column shows the square roots of the diagonal elements of I^{-1}. Hence, as we mentioned earlier, the estimated parameters maintain their log-odds ratio interpretation even if we have more than one explanatory variable in the logistic regression function. One should also note that the estimated standard error of the odds ratio estimate from a univariate analysis is identical to the standard error of the corresponding parameter estimate obtained from the logistic regression analysis. For example

$$\text{SE}(\ln \hat{\psi}[\text{strain 3; strain 4}]) = \left(\frac{1}{5} + \frac{1}{20} + \frac{1}{2} + \frac{1}{43}\right)^{1/2} = 0.879$$

which is identical to $\text{SE}(\hat{\beta}_3)$ as shown in Table 3.3. Since the approximate $(1 - \alpha)100\%$ confidence limits for the parameter β_j are $\hat{\beta}_j \pm Z_{\alpha/2}\hat{\text{SE}}(\hat{\beta}_j)$, the limits for the corresponding odds ratio are obtained by taking the antilog transformation, giving the limits on the parameter β_j as $\exp[\hat{\beta}_j \pm Z_{\alpha/2}\hat{\text{SE}}(\hat{\beta}_j)]$.

3.2.2 Interaction and Confounding in Logistic Regression

In Example 3.1, we showed how the logistic regression model can be used to model the relationship between the proportion or the probability of developing tumors and the strain. Other variables could also be included in the model such as sex, the initial weight of each mouse, age, or other relevant variables. The main goal, of what then becomes a rather comprehensive model, is to adjust for the effect of all other variables and the effect of the differences in their distributions on the estimated odds ratios. It should be pointed out that the effectiveness of the adjustment (measured by the reduction in the bias of the estimated coefficient) depends on the appropriateness of the log-odds transformation and the assumption of constant slopes across the levels of a factor variable (Hosmer and Lemeshow, 1989). Departure from the constancy of slopes is explained by the existence of interaction. For example, if we have two factor variables, F_1 and F_2, where the response at a particular level of

F_1 varies over the levels of F_2, then F_1 and F_2 are said to interact. To model the interaction effect, one should include terms representing the main effects of the two factors as well as terms representing the two-factor interaction that is represented by a product of two dummy variables. Interaction is known to epidemiologists as "effect modification." Thus, a variable that interacts with a risk factor of exposure variable is termed an "effect modifier." To illustrate, suppose that factor F_1 has three levels (a_1, a_2, a_3), and factor F_2 has two levels (b_1, b_2). To model the main effects and their interactions, we first define the dummy variables.

$$A_i = \begin{cases} 1 & \text{if an observation belongs to the } i\text{th level of factor } F_1 (i = 1, 2) \\ 0 & \text{otherwise} \end{cases}$$

which means that a_3 is the referent group. Similarly, we define a dummy variable $B = 1$ if the individual belongs to the second level of factor F_2. Suppose that we have the following five data points (Table 3.4).

TABLE 3.4

Hypothetical Data of a Two-Factor Experiment

Observation	y	F_1	F_2
1	1	a_1	b_1
2	1	a_1	b_2
3	0	a_2	b_2
4	0	a_3	b_2
5	1	a_3	b_1

To model the interaction effect of F_1 and F_2, the data layout would be as in Table 3.5.

TABLE 3.5

Dummy Variables for Modeling Interaction of Two Factors

Observation	Y	A_1	A_2	B	A_1B	A_2B
1	1	1	0	0	0	0
2	1	1	0	1	1	0
3	0	0	1	1	0	1
4	0	0	0	1	0	0
5	1	0	0	0	0	0

Another important concept to epidemiologists is confounding. A confounder is a covariate that is associated with both the outcome variable (e.g., disease) and a risk factor. When both associations are detected, then the relationship between the risk factor and the outcome variable is said to be confounded.

Kleinbaum et al. (1988) recommended the following approach (which we extend to logistic regression) to detect confounding in the context of multiple linear regression. Suppose that we would like to describe the relationship between the outcome variable y and a risk factor x, adjusting for the effect of other covariates $x_1, x_2, \ldots, x_{k-1}$ (assuming no interactions are involved) so that

$$\eta = \beta_0 + \beta x + \beta_1 x_1 + \cdots + \beta_{k-1} x_{k-1}$$

Kleinbaum et al. argued that confounding is present if the estimated regression coefficient β of the risk factor x, ignoring the effects of $x_1, x_2, \ldots, x_{k-1}$, is meaningfully different from the estimate of β based on the linear combination that adjusts for the effect of $x_1, x_2, \ldots, x_{k-1}$.

Example 3.2

To determine the disease status of a herd with respect to listeriosis (a disease caused by bacterial infection), fecal samples are collected from selected animals, and a "group testing" technique is adopted to detect the agent responsible for the occurrence. One positive sample means that there is at least one affected animal in a herd, hence the entire herd is identified as a "case." In this example, we will consider possible risk factors, such as *herd size*, *type of feed*, and *level of mycotoxin in the feed*.

Herd sizes are defined as *small* (25–50), *medium* (50–150), and *large* (150–300). The two types of feed are *dry* and *not dry*; the three levels of mycotoxin are *low*, *medium*, and *high*. Table 3.6 indicates the levels of mycotoxin found in different farms and the associated disease occurrences.

TABLE 3.6

Occurrence of Listeriosis in Herds of Different Sizes Levels of Mycotoxin

Level of Mycotoxin	Type of Feed	Small		Medium		Large	
		Case	Control	Case	Control	Case	Control
Low	Dry	2	200	15	405	40	300
	Not dry	1	45	5	60	5	4
Medium	Dry	5	160	1	280	40	100
	Not dry	4	55	3	32	0	42
High	Dry	2	75	60	155	40	58
	Not dry	8	10	10	20	4	4

Before we analyze these data using multiple logistic regression, we should calculate some basic results. The study looks at the type of feed as the risk factor of primary interest. Suppose that we would like to look at the crude association between the occurrence of the disease (case/control) and the level of mycotoxin (low, medium, and high). Table 3.7 summarizes the relationship between the disease and the levels of mycotoxin, ignoring the effect of herd size and the type of feed.

TABLE 3.7

Disease Occurrence at Different Levels of Mycotoxin

Mycotoxin	Disease		
	D$^+$	D$^-$	$\hat{\psi}$
Low	68	1014	1.00
Medium	67	629	1.59
High	124	322	5.74

Note: "Low" is the referent level.

The estimated odds of disease for a farm with medium level of mycotoxin relative to a farm with low level is

$$\hat{\psi} = \frac{(1014)(67)}{(68)(629)} = 1.59$$

This suggests that herds with medium levels are about 1.5 times more likely to have diseased animals than herds with low levels. On the other hand, the likelihood of disease of a farm with high levels is about six times relative to a farm with low levels.

$$\hat{\psi} = \frac{(1014)(124)}{(322)(68)} = 5.74$$

Now we reorganize the data (Table 3.8) so as to look at the association between disease and the type of feed while adjusting for the herd size.

TABLE 3.8

Listeriosis Occurrence When Considering Herd Size and Type of Feed

Type of Feed	Herd Size					
	Small		Medium		Large	
	Case	Control	Case	Control	Case	Control
Dry	9	435	90	840	120	458
Not dry	13	110	18	112	9	10
n	567		1060		597	
$\hat{\psi}$	0.175		0.667		0.291	

When considering each herd size separately, we have the following results.

Small

	Case	Control	Total
Dry	9	435	444
Not dry	13	110	123
Total	22	545	567

$$\hat{\psi}_1 = \frac{990}{5655} = 0.175$$

$$\ln \hat{\psi}_1 = -1.743$$

$$\text{SE}(\ln \hat{\psi}_1) = \left(\frac{1}{9} + \frac{1}{435} + \frac{1}{13} + \frac{1}{110} \right)^{1/2}$$

$$= 0.446$$

Medium

	Case	Control	Total
Dry	90	840	930
Not dry	18	112	130
Total	108	952	1060

$$\hat{\psi}_2 = 0.667$$

$$\ln \hat{\psi}_2 = -0.405$$

$$\text{SE}(\ln \hat{\psi}_2) = 0.277$$

Large

	Case	Control	Total
Dry	120	458	578
Not dry	9	10	19
Total	129	468	597

$$\hat{\psi}_3 = 0.291$$

$$\ln \hat{\psi}_3 = -1.234$$

$$\text{SE}(\ln \hat{\psi}_3) = 0.471$$

The odds ratio of the association of feed type and diseased farm adjusting for the herd size is now computed using Woolf's method (1955) as

$$\ln \hat{\psi} = \frac{\sum \dfrac{\ln \hat{\psi}_j}{v(\ln \hat{\psi}_j)}}{\sum \dfrac{1}{v(\ln \hat{\psi}_j)}}$$

$$= \frac{\left(\dfrac{-1.743}{0.1991}\right) + \left(\dfrac{-0.405}{0.0767}\right) + \left(\dfrac{-1.234}{0.2216}\right)}{\left(\dfrac{1}{0.1991}\right) + \left(\dfrac{1}{0.0767}\right) + \left(\dfrac{1}{0.2216}\right)}$$

$$= -0.867$$

Thus, $\hat{\psi}_W = e^{-0.867} = 0.420$

The test for interaction using Woolf's χ^2 is obtained as follows:

$$V(\ln \hat{\psi}_W) = \frac{1}{\sum \dfrac{1}{V(\ln \hat{\psi}_j)}}$$

$$= 0.0443$$

$$\chi_w^2 = \sum \frac{1}{V(\ln \hat{\psi}_j)}(\ln \hat{\psi}_j - \ln \hat{\psi})^2$$

$$= \frac{(-1.74 + 0.867)^2}{0.1991} + \frac{(-0.405 + 0.867)^2}{0.0767} + \frac{(-1.234 + 0.867)^2}{0.2216}$$

$$= 7.22$$

Since χ_w^2 is greater than $\chi_{(0.05,2)}^2$, there is evidence of interaction between the herd size and the type of feed used on the farm. We investigate this further in the following section.

3.2.3 The Goodness of Fit and Model Comparisons

Measures of goodness of fit are statistical tools used to explore the extent to which the fitted responses obtained from the postulated model compare with the observed data. Clearly, the fit is good if there is a good agreement between the fitted and the observed data. The Pearson χ^2 and the likelihood ratio test (LRT) are the most commonly used measures of goodness of fit for categorical data. The following sections will give a brief discussion on how each of the χ^2 and the LRT criteria can be used as measures of goodness of fit of a logistic model.

3.2.3.1   *The Pearson χ^2 Statistic*

The Pearson χ^2 statistic is defined by

$$\chi^2 = \sum_{i=1}^{n} \frac{(y_i - n_i \hat{p}_i)^2}{n_i \hat{p}_i \hat{q}_i}$$

For the logistic regression model, $\hat{p}_i = \frac{e^{\hat{\eta}_i}}{1+e^{\hat{\eta}_i}}$, and $\hat{\eta}_i = \sum_{j=1}^{k} x_{ji}\hat{\beta}_j$ is the linear predictor, obtained by substituting the maximum likelihood estimator of β_j in η_i. The distribution of χ^2 is asymptotically that of a χ^2 with $(n-k-1)$ degrees of freedom (see Collett, 2003). Large values of χ^2 can be taken as evidence that the model does not adequately fit the data. Because the model parameters are estimated by the method of maximum likelihood, it is recommended that one uses the LRT statistic as a criterion for goodness of fit of the logistic regression model.

3.2.3.2   *The Likelihood Ratio Criterion (Deviance)*

Suppose that the model we would like to fit a model (called current model) with $k+1$ parameters, and that the log likelihood of this model given by Equation 3.6 is denoted by l_c. That is

$$l_c = \sum_{i=1}^{n} [y_i \ln p_i + (n_i - y_i) \ln(1 - p_i)]$$

Let $\hat{p}_i$ be the maximum likelihood estimator of p_i under the current model. Therefore, the maximized log-likelihood function under the current model is given by

$$\hat{l}_c = \sum_{i=1}^{n} [y_i \ln \hat{p}_i + (n_i - y_i) \ln(1 - \hat{p}_i)]$$

McCullagh and Nelder (1989) indicated that, to assess the goodness of fit of the current model, $\hat{l}_c$ should be compared with another log likelihood of a model where the fitted responses coincide with the observed responses. Such a model has as many parameters as the number of data points and is thus called the *full* or *saturated* model and is denoted by $\hat{l}_s$. Since, under the saturated model, the fitted p_i are the same as the observed proportions $\tilde{p}_i = y_i/n_i$, the maximized log-likelihood function under the saturated model is

$$\tilde{l}_s = \sum_{i=1}^{n} [y_i \ln \tilde{p}_i + (n_i - y_i) \ln(1 - \tilde{p}_i)]$$

The metric $D = -2(\hat{l}_c - \tilde{l}_s)$, which is called the *deviance*, was suggested by McCullagh and Nelder (1989) as a measure of goodness of fit of the current model.

As can be seen, the deviance is in fact the likelihood ratio criterion for comparing the current model with the saturated model. Now, since the two models are trivially nested, it is tempting to conclude from the large-sample likelihood theory that the deviance is distributed as a χ^2 with $(n - k - 1)$ degrees of freedom if the current model holds. However, from the standard theory leading to the χ^2 approximation for the null distribution of the likelihood ratio statistic, we find that if model A has p_A parameters and model B (nested in model A) has p_B parameters with $p_B < p_A$, then the likelihood ratio statistic that compares the two models has χ^2 distribution with degrees of freedom $p_B - p_A$ as $n \to \infty$ (with p_A and p_B both being fixed). If A is the saturated model, $p_A = n$, so the standard theory does not hold. In contrast to what has been reported in the literature, Firth (1991) pointed out that the deviance does not, in general, have an asymptotic χ^2 distribution in the limit as the number of data points increases. Consequently, the distribution of the deviance may be far from χ^2, even if n is large.

There are situations, however, when the distribution of the deviance can be reasonably approximated by a χ^2. The binomial model with large n_i is an example. In this situation, a binomial observation y_i may be considered a sufficient statistic for a sample of n_i independent binary observations, each with the same mean, so that $n_i \to \infty$ $(i = 1, 2, \ldots, n)$ plays the role in asymptotic computations as the usual assumption $n \to \infty$. In other words, the validity of the large-sample approximation to the distribution of the deviance, in logistic regression model fit, depends on the total number of individual binary observations $\sum n_i$ rather than on n, the actual number of data points y_i. Therefore, even if the number of binomial observations is small, the χ^2 approximation to the distribution of the deviance can be used as long as $\sum n_i$ is reasonably large.

More fundamental problems with the use of the deviance for measuring goodness of fit arise in the important special case of binary data, where $n_i = 1$ $(i = 1, 2, \ldots, n)$. The likelihood function for this case is

$$L(\beta) = \prod_{i=1}^{n} p_i^{y_i} (1 - p_i)^{1 - y_i}$$

For the saturated model $\hat{p}_i = y_i$ and

$$\hat{l}_c = \sum_{i=1}^{n} [y_i \ln \hat{p}_i + (1 - y_i) \ln(1 - \hat{p}_i)]$$

Now, since $y_i = 0$ or 1, $\ln y_i = (1 - y_i) \ln(1 - y_i) = 0$, the deviance is

$$D = -2 \sum_i \left\{ y_i \ln\left(\frac{\hat{p}_i}{1 - \hat{p}_i}\right) + \ln(1 - \hat{p}_i) \right\} \tag{3.8}$$

We now show that D depends only on the fitted value $\hat{p}_i$ and so is uninformative about the goodness of fit of the model. To see this, using Equation 3.7

where $n_i = 1$, we have

$$\frac{\partial l(\beta)}{\partial \beta_r} = \sum_i x_{ri}(y_i - \hat{p}_i) = 0 \tag{3.9}$$

Multiplying both sides of Equation 3.9 by $\hat{\beta}_r$ and summing over r

$$\sum (y_i - \hat{p}_i)\sum_r \beta_r x_{ri} = 0$$

$$= \sum (y_i - \hat{p}_i)\ln\left(\frac{\hat{p}_i}{1 - \hat{p}_i}\right)$$

from which

$$\sum y_i \ln\left(\frac{\hat{p}_i}{1 - \hat{p}_i}\right) = \sum \hat{p}_i \ln\left(\frac{\hat{p}_i}{1 - \hat{p}_i}\right) \tag{3.10}$$

Substituting Equation 3.10 into 3.8 we get

$$D = -2\sum_i \left\{\hat{p}_i \ln\left(\frac{\hat{p}_i}{1 - \hat{p}_i}\right) + \ln(1 - \hat{p}_i)\right\}$$

Therefore, D is completely determined by $\hat{p}_i$ and hence useless as a measure of goodness of fit of the current model. However, in situations where model A is nested in another model B, the difference in deviance of the two models can be used to test the importance of those additional parameters in model B.

Pearson's $\chi^2 = \sum_{i=1}^{n} \frac{(y_i - \hat{p}_i)^2}{\hat{p}_i \hat{q}_i}$ encounters similar difficulties. It can be verified that, for binary data ($n_i = 1$ for all i), χ^2 always takes the value n and is therefore completely uninformative. Moreover, the χ^2 statistic, unlike the difference in deviance, cannot be used to judge the importance of additional parameters in a model that contains the parameters of another model.

We now explain how the difference in deviance can be used to compare models. Suppose that we have two models with the following link functions:

Model	Link (η)
A	$\sum_{j=0}^{p_1} \beta_j x_{ji}$
B	$\sum_{j=0}^{p_1+p_2} \beta_j x_{ji}$

Model A contains $p_1 + 1$ parameters and is therefore nested in model B, which contains $p_1 + p_2 + 1$ parameters. The deviance under model A denoted by D_A carries $(n - p_1 - 1)$ degrees of freedom, while that of model B denoted by D_B carries $(n - p_1 - p_2 - 1)$ degrees of freedom. The difference $D_A - D_B$ has an approximate χ^2 distribution with $(n - p_1 - 1) - (n - p_1 - p_2 - 1) = p_2$ degrees of freedom. This χ^2 approximation to the difference between two deviances can be used to assess the combined effect of the p_2 covariates in model B on the response variable y. The model comparison based on the difference between deviances is equivalent to the analysis based on the LRT. In the following example, we illustrate how to compare models using the LRT.

Example 3.2 (Continued)

Here, we apply the concept of difference between deviances or LRT to test for the significance of the added variables. First, we fit two logistic regression models, one with main effects (A) and another with main effects and interactions (B).

The following SAS program sets up the data and runs the models.

```
data toxin;
input toxin $ feed $ hsize $ case count @@;
cards;
low dry small 1 2 low dry small 0 200 low wet small 1 1
low wet small 0 45 med dry small 1 5 med dry small 0 160
med wet small 1 4 med wet small 0 55 high dry small 1 2
high dry small 0 75 high wet small 1 8 high wet small 0 10
low dry medium 1 15 low dry medium 0 405 low wet medium 1 5
low wet medium 0 60 med dry medium 1 15 med dry medium 0 280
med wet medium 1 3 med wet medium 0 32 high dry medium 1 60
high dry medium 0 155 high wet medium 1 10 high wet medium 0 20
low dry large 1 40 low dry large 0 300 low wet large 1 5
low wet large 0 4 med dry large 1 40 med dry large 0 100
med wet large 1 0 med wet large 0 2 high dry large 1 40
high dry large 0 58 high wet large 1 4 high wet large 0 4
;

* Model with main effects only;
proc logistic descending data=toxin;
weight count;
class toxin (ref='low') feed (ref='dry') hsize (ref='small')/ param=ref;
model case= toxin feed hsize;
run;

*Model with main effects and mycotoxin by feed type interaction;
proc logistic descending data=toxin;
weight count;
class toxin (ref='low') feed (ref='dry') hsize (ref='small')/ param=ref;
model case= toxin feed hsize toxin*feed;
run;
```

Selected SAS output from running the model A is displayed below:

Model Fit Statistics

Criterion	Intercept Only	Intercept and Covariates
AIC	1602.415	1362.475
SC	1603.970	1371.807
−2 Log L	1600.415	1350.475

Analysis of Maximum Likelihood Estimates

Parameter		DF	Estimate	Standard Error	Wald χ^2	$Pr > \chi^2$
Intercept		1	−4.3348	0.2684	260.8223	<0.0001
toxin	High	1	1.9898	0.1751	129.2018	<0.0001
toxin	Med	1	0.7288	0.1860	15.3544	<0.0001
feed	Wet	1	0.8637	0.2131	16.4325	<0.0001
hsize	Large	1	2.3400	0.2581	82.2175	<0.0001
hsize	Medium	1	1.0818	0.2487	18.9220	<0.0001

Odds Ratio Estimates

Effect	Point Estimate	95% Wald Confidence Limits	
toxin high versus low	7.314	5.190	10.308
toxin med versus low	2.073	1.439	2.984
feed wet versus dry	2.372	1.562	3.601
hsize large versus small	10.381	6.260	17.215
hsize medium versus small	2.950	1.812	4.803

Selected SAS output from running the model B is displayed below:

Model Fit Statistics

Criterion	Intercept Only	Intercept and Covariates
AIC	1602.415	1364.527
SC	1603.970	1376.970
−2 Log L	1600.415	1348.527

Analysis of Maximum Likelihood Estimates

Parameter			DF	Estimate	Standard Error	Wald χ^2	$\Pr > \chi^2$
intercept			1	−4.3456	0.2711	256.9229	<0.0001
toxin	High		1	2.0114	0.1906	111.3244	<0.0001
toxin	Med		1	0.8249	0.1995	17.0977	<0.0001
feed	Wet		1	1.1221	0.3604	9.6937	0.0018
hsize	Large		1	2.3128	0.2578	80.4674	<0.0001
hsize	Medium		1	1.0529	0.2491	17.8723	<0.0001
toxin*feed	High	wet	1	−0.1618	0.4749	0.1160	0.7334
toxin*feed	Med	wet	1	−0.7283	0.5527	1.7365	0.1876

One should realize that the parameter estimates of the main effects of model B are not much different from those of model A. Now, to test for the significance of the interaction terms using the deviance, we use the likelihood ratio. In the model without interaction, $-2 \log L = 1350.475$, and in the model with interaction, $-2 \log L = 1348.527$. Therefore, the value of the LRT statistic is $1350.475 - 1348.527 = 1.948$. Asymptotically, the deviance has a χ^2 distribution with degrees of freedom equal to $7 - 5 = 2$. Therefore, we do not have sufficient evidence to reject the null hypothesis of no interaction effect and conclude that the main effects model is adequate.

General Comments:

1. The main risk factor of interest in this study was the type of feed. Since the estimated coefficient of feed in model A is positive, then according to the way we coded that variable, dry feed seems to have sparing effect on the risk of listeriosis.

2. From model A, adjusting for herd size, the odds of a farm being a case with wet feed and high level of mycotoxin, relative to a farm with medium or low level of mycotoxin and dry feed, is $\exp(0.864 + 1.990) = 17.35$.

3. From the model with interaction, the same odds ratio estimate is $\exp(1.122 + 2.0114 - 0.1618) = 19.52$.

The difference, $19.52 - 17.35 = 2.17$, is the bias in the estimated odds ratio if the interaction effects were ignored. Note that epidemiologists are interested in measuring the magnitude of bias, in odds ratio estimate, due to omitted effects, even if these effects are not statistically significant.

To run these models in R, we need to enter the data first. The tabular data of Table 3.6 may be entered as follows:

```
toxin <- gl(3,2, 18, label = c("Low","Medium","High"))
feed <- gl(2,1, 18, label = c("Dry","Wet"))
```

```
hsize <- gl(3,6, 18, label = c("Small","Medium","Large"))
disease <- c(2,1,5,4,2,8,15,5,15,3,60,10,40,5,40,0,40,4)
nodisease <- c(200,45,160,55,75,10,405,60,280,32,155,20,300,4,100,2,58,4)
data.frame(toxin,feed,hsize,diseased,nodisease)
outcome <- cbind(disease,nodisease)
```

The following code will run the models A and B:

```
# Model A with main effects only
Logist_a <-glm(outcome~toxin+feed+hsize,family=binomial)
```

```
# Model B with interations
Logist_b<-glm(outcome~toxin+feed+hsize+toxin*feed,family=
binomial)
```

The output from model A is shown below:

Call:
glm(formula = outcome ~ toxin + feed + hsize, family = binomial)

Deviance Residuals:

Min	1Q	Median	3Q	Max
-2.2190	-1.2675	-0.2793	0.2844	2.5191

Coefficients:

	Estimate	Std. Error	z value	$Pr(>|z|)$	
(Intercept)	-4.3350	0.2684	-16.150	$< 2e-16$	***
toxinMedium	0.7288	0.1860	3.918	8.91e-05	***
toxinHigh	1.9898	0.1751	11.367	$< 2e-16$	***
feedWet	0.8637	0.2131	4.054	5.04e-05	***
hsizeMedium	1.0819	0.2487	4.350	1.36e-05	***
hsizeLarge	2.3401	0.2581	9.068	$< 2e-16$	***

—

Signif. codes: 0 '***' 0.001 '**' 0.01 '*' 0.05 '.' 0.1 ' ' 1
(Dispersion parameter for binomial family taken to be 1)

Null deviance: 284.66 on 17 degrees of freedom
Residual deviance: 34.72 on 12 degrees of freedom
AIC: 109.48

Number of Fisher Scoring iterations: 4

The "glm" function does not print the odds ratios and the confidence intervals. The odds ratio estimates and the 95% confidence intervals may, however, be easily computed, say for model A.

sum.coef<-summary(toxin_a)$coef

est<-exp(sum.coef[,1])
upper.ci<-exp(sum.coef[,1]+1.96*sum.coef[,2])
lower.ci<-exp(sum.coef[,1]-1.96*sum.coef[,2])

cbind(est,upper.ci,lower.ci)

The odds ratios and the 95% confidence intervals are

	est	lower.ci	upper.ci
(Intercept)	0.01310247	0.00774	0.02217
toxinMedium	2.07268339	1.4395	2.98443
toxinHigh	7.31432557	5.18993	10.30830
feedWet	2.37199521	1.56222	3.60153
hsizeMedium	2.95040995	4.80381	1.81209
hsizeLarge	10.38250307	6.26072	17.21790

Further, the "glm" would use the first level of a factorial explanatory variable as a reference. For some other level to be the reference, the order of the levels should be changed. For example, if large herd size is desired as a reference, then the following statement should be run before fitting the model.

(hsize <- relevel(hsize, ref="Large")

The best-fitting model may be realized using the step() function.

The above sections demonstrated fitting the logistic regression to binary data with several explanatory variables. A crucial assumption for the likelihood inference to be valid is the independence of the responses. This assumption may be valid if the individuals are randomly sampled. However, there are situations where sampling individuals may not be feasible. The remainder of this chapter will be devoted to discussions concerned with fitting regression models for binary data obtained from clusters of subjects.

3.3 Modeling Correlated Binary Outcome Data

3.3.1 Introduction

Data from clustered samples arise frequently in many statistical and epidemiologic investigations. We have already discussed in Chapters 1 and 2 that clustering may be as a result of observations that are repeatedly collected on the experimental units as in cohort studies, or may be due to sampling blocks of experimental units such as families, herds, and litters. The data of interest consist of a binary outcome variable y_{ij}, where $i = 1, 2, \ldots, k$ indexes the clusters and $j = 1, 2, \ldots, n_i$ indexes units within clusters. A distinguishing feature of such clustered data is that they tend to exhibit intracluster correlation. To obtain valid inference, the analysis of clustered data must account for the effect of this correlation within a regression model. Ignoring the clustering effect will affect the validity of statistical inference on the regression parameters β. The following section illustrates the diversity of the problems in which intracluster effect may be present through a number of examples.

Note that we shall investigate the problem of fitting regression models for clustered binary data, when the units are naturally aggregated. For example, the cluster may be a herd, a flock, a family, or a litter of pubs. However, there are special types of clusters of binary observations, such as longitudinal clustering that we deal with in Chapter 6. Correlated binary data from longitudinal studies where repeated measures of a binary outcome are gathered from independent samples of individuals need special modeling strategies, simply because the nature of the within-cluster (subject) correlation is different. Moreover, there are usually two types of covariates measured. The covariates of the first set are measured at the baseline and do not change during the course of the study. The covariates of the second set are measured at each time point. For longitudinal studies, we may be interested in how an individual's response changes over time, or more generally in the effect of change in covariates on the binary outcome.

The individual measurements within the cluster are called subunits of the cluster. Positive correlation among subunits is manifested by more homogeneous subunits and more variable cluster totals than would be expected with no correlation (i.e., simple Bernoulli sampling or binomial data). This effect is called extra-binomial variation or overdispersion. Ignoring this positive correlation in the analysis will result in statistical tests that overstate the significance of the differences seen among subunit responses. In Chapter 2, we focused on the analysis of correlated binary data from clinical and field trials. Here, we focus primarily on regression-type methods that can accommodate both continuous and categorical covariates.

Although modeling strategies for correlated binary data fall into several categories, in this chapter we shall focus on two models discussed briefly in Chapter 1:

- *Population average (PA) logistic regression models*: Model the marginal probabilities in terms of covariates, treating the correlation among cluster members as nuisance parameters. For these models, the "generalized estimating equations (GEE)" is the method of choice to account for the correlation when covariates are measured at both the cluster and the unit level.

- *Cluster-specific logistic regression models*: Allow the model for each cluster to differ by including cluster-specific parameters that can describe the correlation structure within the cluster. Since the number of such parameters grows along with the number of clusters, a popular approach is to consider these cluster-specific parameters as a random sample from some underlying distribution.

Once a modeling strategy has been chosen, there is also the issue of which method or methods can be used to fit the model. Because of the complexity of specifying a complete joint distribution for the set of correlated responses and the associated computational burdens, maximum likelihood estimation is not always feasible. However, pseudolikelihood and different types of approximations to the desired likelihoods have been used. We shall elaborate on this issue further in Chapter 4.

3.3.2 Population Average Models: The GEE Approach

The parameters of such models have a "population-averaged" interpretation in the sense that the effect of the covariates is averaged across clusters that form the population. Models and methods have been formulated that deal specifically with only the mean and within-cluster correlation.

An estimation approach that places the emphasis on estimating marginal mean parameters while treating the association parameters as nuisance is called the GEE approach for which software is readily available in SAS PROC (GENMOD). The marginal means are modeled via any generalized linear model (GLM), which includes the familiar linear regression and logistic regression models. For binary data, the logit (i.e., logistic regression), probit, or complementary log–log links are commonly used to relate the marginal mean to the linear combination of the covariates (i.e., the linear predictor $x'_{ij}\beta$).

If the analyst incorrectly assumed that all observations, both within and between clusters, were independent, maximum likelihood estimation of the β regression coefficients using standard software for GLMs would result in estimates, which were consistent, but not efficient. To obtain better efficiency, the association within clusters must be built into the estimation method. The GEE method provides a way to do this.

The introduction of GLM expanded the classical regression model by allowing the expected value of the response to be a nonlinear function of the linear predictor and the variance of the responses to depend on the expected value. The relationship between the variance and the expected value, however, is restricted to those found in exponential family distributions. The data distribution in GLM is completely specified, and thus maximum likelihood estimation is possible.

If the constraint that the marginal distributions have exponential family form is relaxed so that the variance can be an arbitrary function of the mean, then we obtain quasi-likelihood models (Wedderburn, 1974). For these models, which still make between- and within-cluster independence assumptions, a quasi-score equation is derived via a quasi-likelihood function.

The GEE approach extends quasi-likelihood models by including a within-cluster "working" correlation matrix in the quasi-score (estimating) equations. The analyst can specify a form of this within-cluster correlation matrix or allow it to be completely unspecified. For example, one could specify a common correlation for every pair of cluster members (which would be assumed the same in every cluster) called an "exchangeable" correlation structure or an autoregressive structure, where cluster members closer in time or space would be assumed to be more highly correlated than those further apart. These correlation structures will be dealt with in Chapter 6. This method allows unequal cluster sizes, but any missing data are assumed missing completely at random (MCAR) in the sense of Little and Rubin (1987).

The GEE method will produce consistent and asymptotically normal estimates of the β parameters under some general conditions and the correct specification of the mean, even if the working correlation structure is specified incorrectly. The stronger the within-cluster correlation and the closer the working correlation is to the true underlying correlation, the higher the gain in efficiency. The resulting estimates of correlation parameters are biased and less efficient. If they are considered nuisance parameters of no scientific interest, this lack of useful estimates is of little concern.

3.3.3   Cluster-Specific Models (Random Effects Models)

Cluster-specific models are differentiated from population average of marginal models by the inclusion of parameters, which are specific to cluster. A cluster-specific model includes covariates that are linearly related to the log odds of the marginal probability of a positive response. We might also expect the intercept and slope of the relationship to vary from cluster to cluster. A model with only one covariate would take a form similar to the mixed linear model discussed in Chapter 1. Recall that if the $\log [P_r(y_{ij} = 1|x_{ij})]$ is a linear function of one covariate x_{ij} such that

$$\text{logit}[\text{Pr}\,(y_{ij} = 1|x_{ij})] = \beta_{i1} + \beta_{i2}x_{ij} \qquad (3.11)$$

where β_{i1} and β_{i2} are the intercept and slope parameters for cluster i. Inference under this model is complicated by the fact that the number of parameters grows with the number of clusters. A popular approach to reducing the number of parameters in a cluster-specific model is to assume that the clusters are a random sample from some underlying population of clusters and that the parameter values for the clusters follow a distribution. A typical choice is the Gaussian distribution:

$$\begin{bmatrix} \beta_{i1} \\ \beta_{i2} \end{bmatrix} \sim N\left(\begin{bmatrix} \alpha_1 \\ \alpha_2 \end{bmatrix}, \Sigma \right)$$

where α_1 and α_2 are the mean intercept and slope values for the population of clusters, and Σ is a 2×2 covariance matrix. This assumed distribution on the parameters makes this cluster-specific model a random effect model. Models of this type are also commonly called mixed effects, hierarchical, or random coefficients models. If we define

$$\beta_{i1} = \alpha_1 + u_{i1} \quad \beta_{i2} = \alpha_2 + u_{i2}$$

then u_{i1} and u_{i2} are the deviations from the mean intercept and slope term for the ith cluster. We can rewrite the model for the ith cluster's response in terms of the mean intercept and slopes α_1 and α_2 (fixed effects), and the (unobserved) individual deviations as

$$\text{logit}[\Pr(y_{ij} = 1 | x_{ij})] = (\alpha_1 + u_{i1}) + (\alpha_2 + u_{i2})x_{ij}$$

where $\begin{bmatrix} u_{i1} \\ u_{i2} \end{bmatrix} \sim N(0, \sum)$.

In this formulation, the fixed effects α_1 and α_2 are interpreted as the typical parameter values for the population, while the random effects modify the average parameters to be specific to that cluster. Fitting the above model is done quite easily using the GLIMMIX/SAS macro as shown in this chapter.

The mixed effects model can be written in a more compact form as

$$\text{logit}(p_{ij}) = X_{ij}\beta + Z_{ij}\gamma_i \tag{3.12}$$

where β is a vector of fixed effects, γ_i a vector of random effects, X_{ij} and Z_{ij} are covariate vectors corresponding to the fixed effects and the random effects, respectively. In most applications, it is assumed that γ_i has a multivariate normal distribution with mean 0 and covariance matrix $\sum$, that is,

$$\gamma_i \sim \text{MVN}\left(0, \sum\right)$$

To estimate the model parameters, the method of maximum likelihood can be used. The likelihood function is given by

$$L(\beta, b_i) = \prod_{i=1}^{k}\prod_{j=1}^{n_i} p_{ij}^{y_{ij}}(1 - p_{ij})^{1-y_{ij}}$$

$$= \prod_{i=1}^{k}\prod_{j=1}^{n_i} \frac{[\exp(x_{ij}\beta + Z_{ij}\gamma_i)]^{y_{ij}}}{\exp(x_{ij}\beta + Z_{ij}\gamma_i)} \tag{3.13}$$

$$= \prod_{i=1}^{k} l(l_i)$$

The standard approach to dealing with a likelihood function that contains random variables is to integrate the likelihood function with respect to the distribution of these variables. After integrating out γ_i, the resulting function is called a "marginal likelihood," which depends on the fixed effects parameters and the parameters of the covariance matrix $\sum$. The maximum likelihood estimates of these parameters are those values that maximize the marginal likelihood function given as

$$L(\beta, D) = \prod_{i=1}^{k} \int l_i \frac{\exp\left(-\frac{1}{2} b_i D^{-1} b_i^T\right)}{(2\pi)^{k/2} |D|^{1/2}} \, db_i \tag{3.14}$$

The two problems associated with the direct maximization of the marginal likelihood (Equation 3.14) are:

1. Closed form expression for the integrals (Equation 3.14) is not available, so we cannot find exact maximum likelihood estimates.

2. The maximum likelihood estimator of the variance components does not take into account the loss in the degrees of freedom resulting from estimating fixed effects. This means that the maximum likelihood estimates of the variance components are biased in small samples. However, the GLIMMIX uses the restricted maximum likelihood (REML), which corrects for bias in the estimates of the variance components.

Models with random effects are expected to be more efficient than population average models, provided that we have correctly identified the correct distribution for the random component in the model. The random effects model can be extended to include more than one random component. For example, the health status (presence or absence of disease) of individuals in the same household, same counties, and in the same geographical area is often more similar than that of individuals from different households, counties, or regions. This may be due to common socioeconomic, environmental, and behavioral factors. The ability to quantify sources of unobserved heterogeneity in the health outcome of individuals is important for several reasons (see Katz et al., 1993). The within-household or counties or regional clustering of disease alters the effective sample size needed to provide accurate estimates of disease prevalence. Estimates of disease prevalence at each level of organization (household, county, region, etc.) can provide insight into the dynamics among the risk factors operating at each level. The ability to obtain separate estimates of the variance component for the random effect at each level of clustering may guide the policy makers as to which level of organization they should direct scarce health management dollars.

3.3.4   Interpretation of Regression Parameters

Since the two modeling approaches will often lead to different interpretations of the β parameters, an understanding of their differences is crucial. The choice of an appropriate model will be guided by how well the interpretations address the research question of interest.

Comparing the interpretations of β_k in the marginal model and as a fixed effects parameter in a cluster-specific model can be illustrated with the Miall and Oldham data discussed in Chapter 1. The family constitutes a cluster and siblings are the subunits of the cluster. The mother's hypertensive status ("Yes" if SBP is over or equal to 140 and "No" if SBP is under 140) was recorded at the beginning of the study. Thus, the mother's hypertensive status would be a cluster-level covariate and assumed not to change between subunits. Suppose that the siblings' SBP levels are similarly dichotomized, so that the response variable is binary.

Consider first a marginal model with an intercept, mother's hypertensive status, and age of the child at the time of measurement. If there were independence among the siblings' responses, the interpretation of the regression coefficient would be precisely that of a simple logistic regression model. In the marginal model, the dependence is recognized in the estimation methodology, but not in the model for the marginal mean. The parameter β for hypertension status represents the difference in the log odds ratio for diseased children with a hypertensive mother and those whose mother did not smoke at the baseline. Mathematically, this is the difference in the log odds of the mean risk between these two groups, where the mean is taken over all children (subunits), weighted by the working dependency structure used in the estimation method.

In a random effects model with fixed effects for the same covariates as listed above, plus a random effect for family (i.e., a random cluster effect), the interpretation is conditional on that random effect for the family. Within this family, the coefficient represents the magnitude of change in the log odds one would expect with sib's mother being diseased at baseline versus sib's mother being healthy at baseline. Since the model specifies that this coefficient is the same for all families, it is estimated by combining information from different families, such as averaging over all families according to the distribution of that random effect. Because the effect we are trying to measure is not observable, its estimation is heavily model based.

It should be noted that if there are no covariates measured on the individuals within the cluster, rather that the covariates are measured only at the cluster level, we can summarize the binary outcomes for a cluster as a binomial proportion. In this case, positive correlation between y_{ij} and y_{il} is then manifest as overdispersion or extrabinomial variation.

Before we illustrate through several examples how to model correlated binary data using the GEE and the mixed effects models, we remind the reader that when a regression model is fitted using the weighted least squares, we used the reciprocal of variance as the weights. If we inflate these variances with an appropriate inflation factor that accounts for the within-cluster correlation, we may use the "weighted" logistic regression to fit clustered binary data. Therefore, both the GEE and the weighted logistic regression would be population average models. Two methods of weighting will be used, the first utilizes Donner's adjustment and therefore is model based, and the second uses the inflation factor devised by Rao and Scott as shown in Chapter 2.

Example 3.3

This example will analyze experimental data taken from Paul (1982) on the number of live fetuses affected by treatment (control, low dose, and medium dose). The high dose was removed for the purpose of this example (Table 3.9).

TABLE 3.9

Data from Shell Toxicology Laboratory

Control		Low		Medium	
x^a	n^b	x	n	x	n
1	12	0	5	2	4
1	7	1	11	3	4
4	6	1	7	2	9
0	6	0	9	1	8
0	7	2	12	2	9
0	8	0	8	3	7
0	10	1	6	0	8
0	7	0	7	4	9
1	8	1	6	0	6
0	6	0	4	0	4
2	11	0	6	4	6
0	7	3	9	0	7
5	8	0	6	0	3
2	9	0	7	6	13
1	2	1	5	6	6
2	7	5	9	5	8
0	9	0	1	4	11
0	7	0	6	1	7
1	11	3	9	0	6
0	10			3	10
0	4			6	6
0	8				
0	10				
3	12				
2	8				
4	7				
0	8				

[a] Number of live fetuses affected by treatment.
[b] Total number of live fetuses.

To show how RS adjustment is used to correct for the effect of within-litter correlation in the framework of logistic regression, we first derive the inflation factor for each group. From Chapter 2, direct computations show that

Control $\hat{p}_1 = 0.135$, $v_1 = 0.00127$, $d_1 = 2.34$

Low $\hat{p}_2 = 0.135$, $v_2 = 0.0017$, $d_2 = 1.94$

Medium $\hat{p}_3 = 0.344$, $v_3 = 0.0036$, $d_3 = 2.41$

Moreover, the ANOVA estimator of the intralitter correlation needed to construct Donner's inflation factor is $\hat{\rho} = 0.261$. The following is the SAS program that can be used to analyze the data:

```
data dose;
input group $ y n @@;
if group='con' then do; x=-1; d=2.34; end;
if group='low' then do; x=0; d=1.94; end;
if group='med' then do; x= 1; d=2.41; end;
raoscott =1/d;
donner=1/(1+(n-1)*0.261);
litter=_n_;
cards;
con 1 12 con 1 7 con 4 6 con 0 6 con 0 7 con 0 8
con 0 10 con 0 7 con 1 8 con 0 6 con 2 11 con 0 7
con 5 8 con 2 9 con 1 2 con 2 7 con 0 9 con 0 7
con 1 11 con 0 10 con 0 4 con 0 8 con 0 10 con 3 12
con 2 8 con 4 7 con 0 8 low 0 5 low 1 11 low 1 7
low 0 9 low 2 12 low 0 8 low 1 6 low 0 7 low 1 6
low 0 4 low 0 6 low 3 9 low 0 6 low 0 7 low 1 5
low 5 9 low 0 1 low 0 6 low 3 9 med 2 4 med 3 4
med 2 9 med 1 8 med 2 9 med 3 7 med 0 8 med 4 9
med 0 6 med 0 4 med 4 6 med 0 7 med 0 3 med 6 13
med 6 6 med 5 8 med 4 11 med 1 7 med 0 6 med 3 10
med 6 6
;
* Model 1: Marginal Model: Logistic regression ignoring clustering;
proc logistic descending data=dose;
model y/n = x;


* Model 2: Marginal Model: Logistic regression accounting for
clustering using Rao-Scott's weights;
proc logistic descending data=dose;
model y/n = x;
weight raoscott;
run;


* Model 3: Marginal Model: Logistic regression accounting for
clustering using Donner's weights;
proc logistic descending data=dose;
model y/n =x;
weight donner;
run;
```

```
* Model 4: Cluster Specific GEE model with exchangeable
correlation structure;
proc genmod data=dose;
class litter;
model y/n = x / dist=bin link=logit;
repeated subject=litter /type=cs corrw;
run;


data new; set dose;
noty=n-y;
do i=1 to y; dead= 1; output; end;
do i=1 to noty; dead= 0; output; end;
run;


* Model 5: Cluster specific GLIMMIX model with exchangeable
correlation structure;
proc glimmix data=new;
class litter;
model dead =x/ solution dist=bin link=logit;
random intercept /subject=litter type=cs;
run;
```

Selected SAS output of fitting these models is given below.
Model 1: Marginal Model: Logistic regression ignoring clustering;

Analysis of Maximum Likelihood Estimates

Parameter	DF	Estimate	Standard Error	Wald χ^2	Pr $> \chi^2$
Intercept	1	−1.4012	0.1165	144.6401	<0.0001
X	1	0.6334	0.1372	21.3253	<0.0001

Odds Ratio Estimates

Effect	Point Estimate	95% Wald Confidence Limits	
X	1.884	1.440	2.465

Model 2: Marginal Model: Logistic regression accounting for clustering using Rao–Scott's weights.

Analysis of Maximum Likelihood Estimates

Parameter	DF	Estimate	Standard Error	Wald χ^2	Pr > χ^2
Intercept	1	−1.4247	0.1752	66.1522	<0.0001
X	1	0.6354	0.2126	8.9351	0.0028

Odds Ratio Estimates

Effect	Point Estimate	95% Wald Confidence Limits	
X	1.888	1.245	2.864

Model 3: Marginal Model: Logistic regression accounting for clustering using Donner's weights.

Analysis of Maximum Likelihood Estimates

Parameter	DF	Estimate	Standard Error	Wald χ^2	Pr > χ^2
Intercept	1	−1.4058	0.1934	52.8505	<0.0001
X	1	0.6180	0.2287	7.3015	0.0069

Odds Ratio Estimates

Effect	Point Estimate	95% Wald Confidence Limits	
X	1.855	1.185	2.905

Model 4: Cluster specific GEE model using exchangeable correlation structure.

Criteria for Assessing Goodness of Fit

Criterion	DF	Value	Value/DF
Deviance	65	168.1053	2.5862
Scaled deviance	65	168.1053	2.5862
Pearson χ^2	65	159.5761	2.4550
Scaled Pearson χ^2	65	159.5761	2.4550
Log likelihood		−237.4111	

Analysis of GEE Parameter Estimates

Empirical Standard Error Estimates

Parameter	Estimate	Standard Error	95% Confidence Limits		Z	Pr > |Z|
Intercept	−1.4012	0.1733	−1.7409	−1.0615	−8.08	<0.0001
X	0.6334	0.2171	0.2078	1.0589	2.92	0.0035

Model 5: Cluster-specific GLIMMIX model using exchangeable correlation structure.

Fit Statistics

−2 Res log pseudo-likelihood	2411.02
Generalized χ^2	355.66
Generalized χ^2/DF	0.72

Solutions for Fixed Effects

Effect	Estimate	Standard Error	DF	t-Value	Pr > |t|
Intercept	−1.5939	0.2003	65	−7.96	<0.0001
X	0.6631	0.2343	432	2.83	0.0049

The R code to set up the data for analysis and run the models 1–5 is shown below.

```
group <- c(rep("con",27),rep("low",19),rep("med",21))
litter <- 1:67
y <- c(1, 1, 4, 0, 0, 0, 0, 0, 1, 0, 2, 0, 5, 2, 1, 2, 0, 0, 1,
       0, 0, 0, 0, 3, 2, 4, 0, 0, 1, 1, 0, 2, 0, 1, 0, 1, 0, 0,
       3, 0, 0, 1, 5, 0, 0, 3, 2, 3, 2, 1, 2, 3, 0, 4, 0, 0, 4,
       0, 0, 6, 6, 5, 4, 1, 0, 3, 6)
n <- c(12, 7, 6, 6, 7, 8,10, 7, 8, 6,11, 7, 8, 9, 2, 7, 9, 7,11,
       10, 4, 8,10,12, 8, 7, 8, 5,11, 7, 9,12, 8, 6, 7, 6, 4, 6,
       9, 6, 7, 5, 9, 1, 6, 9, 4, 4, 9, 8, 9, 7, 8, 9, 6, 4, 6,
       7, 3,13, 6, 8,11, 7, 6,10, 6)
x    <- c(rep(-1,27),rep(0,19),rep(1,21))
d    <- c(rep(2.34,27),rep(1.94,19),rep(2.41,21))
raoscott=1/d
donner=1/(1+(n-1)*0.261)
data.frame(group,litter,x,y,n,raoscott,donner)
outcome <- cbind(y,n-y)
```

```
# Model 1
logistic1 <-glm(outcome~x,family=binomial("logit"))
summary(logistic1)

# Model 2
logistic2 <-glm(outcome~x,family=binomial("logit"),weights=raoscott)
summary(logistic2)

# Model 3
logistic3 <-glm(outcome~x,family=binomial("logit"),weights=donner)
summary(logistic3)

# Model 4
gee4 <-gee(outcome~x,id=litter,family=binomial("logit"),
corstr="exchangeable")
summary(gee4)

# Model 5
glmm5 <-glmmPQL(outcome~x,random=~1|litter,family=binomial
("logit"))
summary(glmm5)
```

The odds ratios, if desired, may be computed as shown in Example 3.2.

The point estimates of slope and intercept are almost the same across models 1–5; however, model 1 produces the smallest standard error for the estimated slope because it ignores the within-litter correlation. The other four models provide almost similar standard error for the slope after adjusting for the within-litter correlation. The differences between population average model and the cluster-specific or random effects models are documented in literature, and the reader can find a lucid discussion in the articles by Zeger et al. (1988) and Neuhaus et al. (1991).

3.3.5   Multiple Levels of Clustering

As we have demonstrated in the previous section, clustered data may exhibit more than two levels of hierarchy, e.g., radon—a naturally occurring radioactive gas known to cause lung cancer in high concentration. The distribution of radon varies considerably among homes, with some homes, having considerably high levels of consideration. The data are organized in several levels: regions, counties, and households within counties. It is important to identify the level of hierarchy at which the intervention should be directed.

The following example illustrates this situation within an experimental setting.

Example 3.4

The following data are taken from Schall (1991). Four hundred cells were placed on a dish and three dishes were irradiated at a time. After the cells were irradiated, the surviving cells were counted. Since cells would also die naturally, dishes with cells were put in the radiation chamber without being irradiated to establish the natural mortality. For the purpose of this example, only these zero-dose data are analyzed. Twenty-seven dishes on nine time points, or three per time point, were available. The resulting 27 binomial observations are given in Table 3.10.

TABLE 3.10

Cell Irradiation Data

Occasion	Cells Surviving Out of 400 Placed	Occasion	Cells Surviving Out of 400 Placed
1	178	6	115
1	193	6	130
1	217	6	133
2	109	7	200
2	112	7	189
2	115	7	173
3	66	8	88
3	75	8	76
3	80	8	90
4	118	9	121
4	125	9	124
4	137	9	136
5	123		
5	146		
5	170		

The GLIMMIX SAS code is

```
data dish;
input time dish y @@;
n=400; noty = 400-y;
cards;
1 1 178 1 2 193 1 3 217 2 4 109 2 5 112 2 6 115 3 7 66
3 8 75 3 9 80 4 10 118 4 11 125 4 12 137 5 13 123 5 14 146
5 15 170 6 16 115 6 17 130 6 18 133 7 19 200 7 20 189 7 21 173
8 22 88 8 23 76 8 24 90 9 29 121 9 30 124 9 31 136
;

data cell; set dish;
do i=1 to y; r=1; output; end;
do i=1 to noty; r = 0; output; end;
run;

* Model 1: One random effect;
proc glimmix data=cell;
```

```
  class time;
  model r = /solution;
  random intercept/ subject=time;
run;

* Model 2: Two random efects;
proc glimmix data=cell;
  class time dish;
  model r = /solution;
  random time dish/subject=time;
run;
```

The GLIMMIX procedure output with one random effect:

Fit Statistics

−2 Res log likelihood	13892.10
AIC (smaller is better)	13896.10

Covariance Parameter Estimates

Cov Parm	Subject	Estimate	Standard Error
Intercept	Time	0.01036	0.005269
Residual		0.2111	0.002874

Solutions for Fixed Effects

Effect	Estimate	Standard Error	DF	t-Value	Pr > |t|
Intercept	0.3277	0.03422	8	9.58	<0.0001

The GLIMMIX procedure output with two random effects:

Fit Statistics

−2 Res log likelihood	13886.93
AIC (smaller is better)	13892.93

Covariance Parameter Estimates

Cov Parm	Estimate	Standard Error
Time	0.01019	0.005270
Dish (time)	0.000507	0.000345
Residual	0.2108	0.002872

Solutions for Fixed Effects

Effect	Estimate	Standard Error	DF	*t*-Value	Pr > |*t*|
Intercept	0.3277	0.03422	8	9.58	<0.0001

The above two models do not have fixed effects except the intercept parameter. One way to select the model that provides the best fit is to compare the (−2 RES LIKELIHOOD) with the smaller value indicting a better fit. Since for the model with one variance component, −2*reslikelihood* = 13892.1, and the model with two variance components, −2*reslikelihood* = 13886.93, the second model is a better model.

Important Remark
Note that we used the *residual likelihood* (or restricted maximum likelihood, REML) to compare the models in terms of their variance components. Once a model has been selected, the model-building strategy with regard to the fixed effects cannot proceed using the model fitted with the REML. The model should be refitted using the option *method=ml* in the model statement of the GLIMMIX. That is requesting that the model be fitted using the method of maximum likelihood. Therefore, only the difference between "−2 log likelihood" of two nested models can be used to assess the goodness of fit in the "generalized linear mixed model" with components of variance. It should also be noted that this remark holds true for the linear mixed model of Chapter 1.

The following R code may be used to enter the tabular data that are then expanded to run the generalized linear mixed model using the function glmm-PQL. Lastly, the two models are fitted. Slight differences in the estimated parameters are due to different estimation methods used and different methods to compute the degrees of freedom. The interested reader may refer to the relevant documentation in R and SAS.

```
time <- c(1,1,1,2,2,2,3,3,3,4,4,4,5,5,5,6,6,6,7,7,7,8,8,8,9,9,9)
dish <- 1:27
y<-c(178,193,217,109,112,115,66,75,80,118,125,137,123,146,170,115,130,
133,200,189,173,88,76,90,121,124,136)
dishn <- data.frame(time,dish,y)
```

```
r1 <- data.frame(lapply(dishn, function(x) rep(x,dishn$y)), r=1)[,c(1,2,4)]
r0 <- data.frame(lapply(dishn, function(x) rep(x,(400-dishn$y))),
r=0)[,c(1,2,4)]
dish <- rbind(r1,r0)
glmm1 <-glmmPQL(r~1, random=~1|factor(time), family=
gaussian(link = "identity"), data=dish)
summary(glmm1)
```

glmm2 <-glmmPQL(r~1, random=~time+dish(time)| factor(time),
family=gaussian(link = "identity"), data=dish)
summary(glmm2)

3.4 Logistic Regression for Case–Control Studies

3.4.1 Cohort versus Case–Control Models

Although initial applications of the logistic regression model were specific to cohort studies, this model can be applied to the analysis of data from case–control studies. The specification of the logistic model for case–control studies in which the presence or absence of exposure is taken to be the dependent variable was given by Prentice (1976). His approach assumes that we are interested in the effect of one factor. Suppose that the exposure factor, which is the focus of interest, is dichotomous, say x_1, where $x_1 = 1$ (exposed) and $x_1 = 0$ (unexposed) and that x_2 is another potential risk factor or a confounder. Hence, the prospective logistic model corresponding to the retrospective study is such that

$$\text{logit}[\Pr(X_1 = 1|y, X_2)] = \beta_0 + \beta_1 y + \beta_2 X_2$$

The relative odds of exposure among diseased as compared to the nondiseased may be given as

$$\text{OR} = \frac{e^{\beta_0 + \beta_1(1) + \beta_2 X_2}}{e^{\beta_0 + \beta_1(0) + \beta_2 X_2}}$$

$$= e^{\beta_1}$$

The above odds ratio is mathematically equivalent to the relative odds of disease among the exposed subjects as compared to the unexposed, as we have already shown in Chapter 2.

The rationale behind this argument was provided by Mantel (1973) as follows: let f_1 denote the sampling fraction of cases; that is, if n_1 cases were drawn from a population of size N_1, then $f_1 = n_1/N_1$. Similarly, we define f_0 as the sampling fraction of control. It is assumed that neither f_1 nor f_0 depend on the covariate vector x. Now consider the following Table 3.11 in a 2×2 layout.

TABLE 3.11

Description of Sampling and Disease Occurrence in a 2×2 Layout

	Case–Control		
	$Y = 1$	$Y = 0$	Total
Sampled (s)	$f_1 p_x$	$f_0 q_x$	$f_1 p_x + f_0 q_x$
Not sampled ($\bar{s}$)	$(1 - f_1)p_x$	$(1 - f_0)q_x$	$(1 - f_1)p_x + (1 - f_0)q_x$
All	p_x	q_x	1

where $p_x = \Pr[y = 1|x]$. In a case–control study we wish to model $\mathrm{logit}[y = 1|x,$ sampled] as a linear function of the covariate vector x.
Since

$$\Pr[y = 1|x, \text{sampled}] = \frac{\Pr[y = 1, s|x]}{\Pr(s)}$$

$$= \frac{f_1 p_x}{f_1 p_x + f_0 q_x}$$

and

$$\Pr[y = 0|x, \text{sampled}] = \frac{f_0 q_x}{f_1 p_x + f_0 q_x}$$

Then

$$\mathrm{logit}(\Pr[y = 1|x, \text{sampled}])$$

$$= \log\left(\frac{f_1 p_x}{f_0 q_x}\right)$$

$$= \log\frac{f_1}{f_0} + \mathrm{logit}(\Pr[y = 1|x])$$

$$= \log\frac{f_1}{f_0} + \beta_0 + \beta_1 x_1 + \cdots + \beta_k x_k$$

$$= \beta_0^* + \sum_{j=1}^{k} \beta_j x_j$$

where

$$\beta_0^* = \log\frac{f_1}{f_0} + \beta_0 \qquad\qquad (3.15)$$

As can be seen from the last equation, the logistic model for the case–control study has the same form as that of the logistic model for cohort study. This means that the regression parameters, which measure the joint effects of groups of covariates on the risk of disease, can be estimated from the case–control study. The following remarks are emphasized:

- If $\beta_0^*, \beta_1, \ldots, \beta_k$ are estimated from a case–control study, and since β_0^* depends on the ratio f_1/f_0, the risk of disease p_x (which depends on β_0) cannot be estimated unless f_1/f_0 is known. The situations in which f_1/f_0 is known are quite uncommon.
- For a given x, Equation 3.15 represents the log odds of disease in the sample of cases and controls, which is related to the log odds of

disease in the target population by the factor $(\log f_1/f_0)$. However, if we estimate the log odds of disease in the sample of cases for a subject with covariate pattern X^*, relative to the sampled control whose covariate pattern is $\hat{X}$, then

$$\psi(X^*; \hat{X}) = \log \left(\frac{e^{\beta_0} + \sum_{j=1}^{k} \beta_j X_j^*}{e^{\beta_0} + \sum_{j=1}^{k} \beta_j \hat{X}_j} \right)$$

$$= \exp \sum_{j=1}^{k} \beta_j (X_j^* - \hat{X}_j)$$

This means that the estimate of β_0^* is irrelevant to the estimation of the odds ratio.

3.4.2 Matched Analysis

We saw how data from a case–control study can be analyzed using the logistic regression model to measure the effect of a group of covariates on the risk of disease, after adjusting for potential confounders. We have also indicated (Chapter 2) that the primary objective of matching is the elimination of the biased comparison between cases and controls that results when confounding factors are not properly accounted for. A design that enables us to achieve this control over such factors is the "matched case–control study." Unless the logistic regression model properly accounts for the matching used in the selection of cases and controls, the estimated odds ratios can be biased. Thus, matching is only the first step in controlling for confounding. To analyze matched case–control study data using logistic regression, we will discuss two situations. The first is called 1:1 matching (which means that each case is matched with one control) and the other is 1:M matching (which means that each case is matched with M controls). Before we show how the data analysis is performed, we describe the general setup of the likelihood function.

Suppose that controls are matched to cases on the basis of a set of variables $x_1, x_2, \ldots, x_k$. These variables may represent risk factors and those potential confounders that have not been used in the matching procedure. Moreover, the risk of disease for any subject may depend on the "matching variable" that defines a "matched set" to which an individual belongs. The values of these matching variables will generally differ between each of the n matched sets of individuals.

Let $p_j(x_{ij})$ denote the probability that the ith person in the jth matched set is a case (or diseased), $i = 0, 2, \ldots, M$, and $j = 1, 2, \ldots, n$. The vector of explanatory variables for the case is x_{0j}, while the vector x_{ij} denotes the explanatory variables for the Mth control in the jth matched set. The disease risk $p_j(x_{ij})$ will be modeled as

$$p_j(x_{ij}) = \frac{e^{\alpha_j} + \sum_{l=1}^{k} \beta_l x_{lij}}{1 + e^{\alpha_j} + \sum_{l=1}^{k} \beta_1 x_{lij}}$$

(3.16)

Here, x_{lij} is the value of the lth explanatory variable $l = 1, 2, \ldots, k$ for the ith individual in the jth matched set. The term α_j represents the effects of a particular configuration of matching variables for the jth matched set on the risk of disease. It can be seen from Equation 3.16 that the relationship between each explanatory variable and the risk of disease is the same for all matched sets.

From Equation 3.16, the odds of disease are given by

$$\frac{p_j(x_{ij})}{1 - p_j(x_{ij})} = \exp\left(\alpha_j + \sum_{l=1}^{k} \beta_l x_{lij}\right)$$

In particular, for two individuals from the same matched set, the odds of disease for a subject with explanatory variable x_{1j} relative to one with explanatory variable x_{2j} is

$$\left[\frac{p_j(x_{1j})}{1 - p_j(x_{1j})}\right]\left[\frac{p_j(x_{2j})}{1 - p_j(x_{2j})}\right] = \exp[\beta_1(x_{11j} - x_{12j}) + \cdots + \beta_k(x_{k1j} - x_{k2j})]$$

(3.17)

Clearly, Equation 3.17 is independent of α_j. This means that the odds of disease for two matched individuals with different explanatory variables do not depend on the actual values of the matching variables.

3.4.3 Fitting Matched Case–Control Study Data in SAS

The likelihood function based on matched case–control studies is known as "conditional likelihood." For 1:M matched case–control study, where the jth matched set contains M controls ($j = 1, 2, \ldots, n$), we denote by x_{0j}, the vector of the explanatory variables for the case and $x_{1j}, x_{2j}, \ldots, x_{Mj}$, the vectors of explanatory variables for the M controls in the jth matched set. Breslow et al. (1978) derived the likelihood function under this setup and showed that it can be written as

$$L = \prod_{j=1}^{n} \left\{1 + \sum_{i=1}^{M} \exp[\beta_1(x_{1ij} - x_{10j}) + \beta_2(x_{2ij} - x_{20j}) + \cdots + \beta_k(x_{kij} - x_{k0j})]\right\}^{-1}$$

(3.18)

The main purpose of this section is to discuss, through an example, how the parameters of the conditional likelihood (Equation 3.18) are estimated. For the matched pair design, $M = 1$, the conditional likelihood (Equation (3.18)) reduces to

$$L = \prod_{i=1}^{n} \left\{ 1 + \exp\left[\sum_{r=1}^{k} \beta_r (x_{rij} - x_{r0j}) \right] \right\}^{-1}$$

$$= \prod_{i=1}^{n} \left\{ 1 + \exp\left[-\sum_{r=1}^{k} \beta_r z_{rj} \right] \right\}^{-1} \tag{3.19}$$

where $z_{rj} = x_{r0j} - x_{r1j}$.

This likelihood (Equation 3.19) is identical to the likelihood function of a logistic regression for n binary observations y_i such that $y_i = 1$ for $i = 1, 2, ..., n$. Note that the explanatory variables here are $z_{1j}, z_{2j}, ..., z_{kj}$, and there is no intercept. Therefore, using SAS, PROC LOGISTIC fits the 1:1 matched data by following these steps:

1. The number of matched sets n is the number of observations.
2. The response variable $y_i = 1$ for all $i = 1, 2, ..., n$.
3. The explanatory variable $z_{rj} = x_{r0j} - x_{r1j}$ ($r = 1, 2, ..., k$ and $j = 1, 2, ..., n$) is the difference between the value of the rth explanatory variable for a control and the rth explanatory variable for a case within the same matched set. Note that if qualitative or factor variables are used, the explanatory variables in Equation 3.19 will correspond to dummy variables. Consequently, variables are the differences between the dummy variables of the case and control in the matched pair. Note also that the interaction terms can be included in the model by representing them as products of the corresponding main effects. The differences between these products for the case and control in a matched pair are included in the model.

Example 3.5 "Hypothetical Data"

In an investigation aimed at assessing the relationship between somatic cell counts (SCC) and the occurrence of mastitis, a 1:1 matched case–control study was postulated. A "case" cow was matched with a control cow from the same farm based on breed, number of lactations, and age as a possible confounder. The data summary is given in Table 3.12.

In this simple example, we have one risk factor, namely the SCC that was dichotomized as "high" and "low." Since it is believed that the incidence rate of the disease in younger cows is different from older cows, the matching variable age was divided into two distinct strata, the first for cows

TABLE 3.12

Hypothetical Mastitis Data

		Case		
		High	Low	
Control	High	5	110	age <4
	Low	216	40	
Control	High	5	212	age ≥4
	Low	308	21	

whose age is less than 4 years, and the second for those that are at least 4 years old.

As already mentioned, we cannot investigate the association between the disease and the age variable since age is a matching variable. However, we shall investigate the possible interaction between the SCC and age. Since the risk factor and the confounder are factor variables and each factor has two levels, we define a single dummy variable for each factor. Let X_1 be the indicator variable for SCC and X_2 for age, where

$X_1 = 1$ if the cow has high SCC
$\quad = 0$ if the cow has low SCC
$X_2 = 1$ if the cow's age is <4
$\quad = 0$ if the cow's age is ≥4

we also define a third dummy variable X_3, obtained by multiplying X_1 and X_2 for each individual animal in the study.

With this coding, the data are structured as in Table 3.13.

TABLE 3.13

Coded Variable for the Data in Table 3.12

X_1 (Case)	X_1 (Control)	X_2 (Case)	X_2 (Control)	X_3 (Case)	X_3 (Control)	Matched Pairs
1	1	0	0	0	0	5
1	0	0	0	0	0	216
0	1	0	0	0	0	110
0	0	0	0	0	0	40
1	1	1	1	1	1	5
1	0	1	1	1	0	308
0	1	1	1	0	1	212
0	0	1	1	0	0	21

The input variables $(Z_1, Z_2,$ and $Z_3)$ shown in Table 3.14 are created using variables as set up in Table 3.13, where

$$Z_1 = X_1(\text{Case}) - X_1(\text{Control})$$

$$Z_2 = X_2(\text{Case}) - X_2(\text{Control})$$

$$Z_3 = X_3(\text{Case}) - X_3(\text{Control})$$

TABLE 3.14

Variables for the Logistic Regression Model

y	Z_1	Z_2	Z_3	Count
1	0	0	0	5
1	1	0	0	215
1	−1	0	0	110
1	0	0	0	40
1	0	0	0	5
1	1	0	1	308
1	−1	0	−1	212
1	0	0	0	21

The following SAS statements describe how the logistic regression model can be fitted.

```
data match;
input y z1 z3 count @@;
cards;
1 0 0 5 1 1 0 216 1 -1  0 110 1 0 0 40
1 0 0 5 1 1 1 308 1 -1 -1 212 1 0 0 21
;

proc logistic data = match;
freq count;
model y = z1 z3/noint covb;
run;
```

Note that the response variable $y_i = 1$ for all $i = 1, 2, \ldots, 8$. In the model statement of the SAS program, we did not include the matching variable z2 since it is not possible to investigate its association with the disease status. Moreover, the option *noint* is specified, so that the logistic regression is fitted without the intercept parameter.

Selected SAS output is shown below:

Analysis of Maximum Likelihood Estimates

Parameter	DF	Estimate	Standard Error	Wald χ^2	$Pr > \chi^2$
z1	1	0.6747	0.1171	33.1793	<0.0001
z3	1	−0.3012	0.1473	4.1836	0.0408

Odds Ratio Estimates

Effect	Point Estimate	95% Wald Confidence Limits	
z1	1.963	1.561	2.470
z3	0.740	0.554	0.988

Estimated Covariance Matrix

Parameter	z1	z3
z1	0.01372	−0.01372
z3	−0.01372	0.021684

The results indicate that there is a significant association between SCC ($\hat{\beta}_1$) and the disease. There is also significant interaction between the SCC and age ($\hat{\beta}_2$) on the risk of mastitis.

The following R code reads the data and runs the desired analysis.

```
y <- rep(1,8)
z1 <- c(0, 1, -1, 0, 0, 1, -1, 0)
z3 <- c(0, 0, 0, 0, 0, 1, -1, 0)
count <- c(5, 216, 110, 40, 5, 308, 212, 21)

match <-glm(y ~ -1+z1+z3,family=binomial("logit"),weights=count)
summary(match)$coef

# Computing the odds ratio
sum.coef<-summary(match)$coef

est<-exp(sum.coef[,1])
upper.ci<-exp(sum.coef[,1] + 1.96*sum.coef[,2])
lower.ci<-exp(sum.coef[,1]-1.96*sum.coef[,2])

cbind(est,upper.ci,lower.ci)

# Estimated covariance matrix
summary(match)$cov.scaled
```

Remark

For *N:M* matching, where each case is matched with an arbitrary number of controls, the PROC PHREG in SAS can be used to fit the model. The data should be put in a special format. The following SAS code shows how to analyze the data in Example 3.6 using the proportional hazard Cox regression model. As expected, there are some differences between the two models, and this is attributed to difference in the methods of parameters estimation.

Example 3.6 Analysis of Matched Data Using Proportional Hazard Regression

```
data ph_match;
input age scc case count;
agescc=age*scc;
time=2-case;
cards;
0 1 1 50 1 0  50 1 1  216 0 0 0  216
0 0 1 110 0 1 0 110 0 0 1 40 0 0 0 40
1 1 1  51 1 0  51 1 1 308 1 0 0 308
1 0 1 212 1 1 0 212 1 0 1 21 1 0 0 21
;
proc phreg data=ph_match;
model time*case(0)=scc agescc / ties=discrete;
freq count;
strata age;
run;
```

Selected SAS output is shown below:

Summary of the Number of Events and Censored Values

Stratum	Age	Total	Event	Censored	Percent Censored
1	0	742	371	371	50.00
2	1	1092	546	546	50.00
Total		1834	917	917	50.00

Model Fit Statistics

Criterion	Without Covariates	With Covariates
−2 LOG L	2527.954	2432.091
AIC	2527.954	2436.091
SBC	2527.954	2445.733

Analysis of Maximum Likelihood Estimates

Variable	DF	Parameter Estimate	Standard Error	χ^2	$Pr > \chi^2$	Hazard Ratio
scc	1	1.18599	0.15413	59.2107	<0.0001	3.274
agescc	1	−0.47533	0.19717	5.8120	0.0159	0.622

The proportional hazard regression (PHREG) models will be discussed in detail in Chapter 7, and the reader may delay reading the last example until then. However, it can seen that the coefficients estimates are slightly different from Example 3.7. One explanation is that, while the logistic regression is fitted using the method of maximum likelihood, the PHREG is fitted using the method of partial likelihood (see Cox, 1972).

3.5   Sample-Size Calculations for Logistic Regression

As shown in Chapters 1 and 2, sample-size determination is dominated by work concerned with calculating sample sizes required for comparing means or proportions in two groups. Statistical literature gives little guidance on how to use additional information that may often be available. Gail (1973) specifies calculations for trials with dichotomous exposure and outcome that are stratified on a third variable. Whittemore (1981) gave approximate sample sizes for logistic regression with small probability when there are covariates. This approach is based on an approximation to Fisher's information matrix for the estimated parameters in a multiple logistic regression. Wilson and Gordon (1986) showed that approximate sample size can be obtained from Fisher's information matrix without the restriction that the response probability is small.

It has been shown (see McCullagh and Nelder, 1989) that if the GLM is valid, the maximum likelihood estimator of $\hat{\beta}$ is asymptotically normal and variance–covariance matrix $V(\hat{\beta}) = (I(\beta))^{-1}$, where $I(\beta)$ is Fisher's information matrix, whose (r, s) element is

$$I_{rs}(\beta) = \sum_{i=1}^{n} \left(\frac{\partial \mu_i}{\partial \eta_i}\right)^2 x_{ir} x_{is} (V(y_i))^{-1}$$

In discussing sample size required to detect, for example, significant values of β_1, only the corresponding diagonal element v_{11} of $V(\hat{\beta})$ is relevant. In the next section, we discuss the contributions made by Wilson and Gordon (1986).

Suppose that without loss of generality we are interested in testing $H_0: \beta_1 = \beta_1^{(0)}$, with level of significance α and Power $1 - \delta$ for specified alternative $H_1: \beta_1 = \beta_1^{(1)}$. Let $\hat{\beta}_1^{(k)}$ be the value of the maximum likelihood estimator of

β_1 under H_k, where $k = 0, 1$. Further, let $\Phi(z_t) = 1 - t$, where Φ is the standard normal cumulative distribution function. Moreover, let $u_k = [nv_{11}(\hat{\beta})^{(k)}]^{\frac{1}{2}}$, u_k does not involve n. By the standard power calculations, we have

$$n \geq \frac{(z_\alpha u_0 + z_\delta u_1)}{(\beta_1^{(1)} - \beta_1^{(0)})^2} \tag{3.20}$$

Example 3.7

As an example we consider the case of a prospective study discussed by Schlesselman (1982). The main interest in the study was whether there is an increased risk of giving birth to a child with a congenital heart defect among mothers who have oral contraceptive exposure 3 months prior to or after conception. Both outcome (y) and exposure (x) are binary variables. Let P_0 represent the proportion in the control population of unexposed subjects who develop the disease and P_1 the corresponding proportion in the exposed population. We assume the logistic model

$$\mu = E[y|x] = \frac{\exp(\beta_0 + \beta_1 x)}{1 + \exp(\beta_0 + \beta_1 x)}$$

Under the null hypothesis $\beta_1^{(0)} = 0$, and under the alternative hypothesis $\beta_0^{(1)} = \log(P_1 q_0 / P_0 q_1)$ and $\beta_1^{(1)} = \log(p_1 q_0 / p_0 q_1)$, where $q_j = 1 - p_j$, $j = 0, 1$, and β_1 is the log-odds ratio. Therefore, the total number of subjects in each group is $n/2$, where

$$n \geq \frac{\{z_\varepsilon (4/\overline{pq})^{1/2} + z_\delta [(2/p_0 q_0) + (2/p_1 q_1)]^{1/2}\}^2}{[\log(p_1 q_0 / p_0 q_1)]^2} \tag{3.21}$$

and $\overline{p} = (p_0 + p_1)/2$.

As an illustration, if the incidence of all congenital heart diseases among controls is $p_0 = 0.008$, the relative risk of disease is p_1/p_0. If we assume that the meaningful relative risk to detect is 3, then $p_1 = 3(0.008) = 0.024$. Taking $\alpha = 0.025$ and power 0.90, we get $n \cong 2416$ for each group.

Exercises

3.1 Let y_i be the binomially distributed random variable ($i = 1, 2, \ldots, k$). Show $E(y_i) = n_i P_i$ and $var(y_i) = n_i P_i (1 - P_i)$. Use the delta method to derive the variance of $z_i = \log\left(\frac{y_i}{n_i - y_i}\right)$.

3.2 The mycotoxin data have only group-level covariates. Use PROC Reg in SAS to fit linear regression, using the method of weighted least squares, $w_i = [var(z_i)]^{-1}$ as weights. Compare the fitting of this linear regression model to the results of fitting logistic regression model. Comment on your findings.

3.3 In a regression model, when two covariates have zero correlation they are said to be orthogonal. For the logistic regression model, the concept or orthogonality is absent. Show that, using any of the examples, the order in which terms are included in a model is important (in some cases).

3.4 Consider the data reported in Elston (1977), where 12 strains of mice were treated with a carcinogen and the numbers with and without tumors were noted. The results are shown in the following table.

Strain	1	2	3	4	5	6	7	8	9	10	11	12
y_i # with tumor	26	27	35	18	33	11	11	13	13	5	5	2
$n_i - y_i$ # without tumor	1	3	14	9	20	11	11	15	22	19	30	24

Construct on 95% confidence interval on the tumor proportion.

3.5 Tarone (1979) constructed a one-degree-of-freedom χ^2 test on the null hypothesis that data are independently binomially distributed versus a correlated binomial alternative. His test statistic is given by

$$X_T^2 = \frac{\left[\hat{p}\hat{q}\sum_{i=1}^{k}(y_i - n_i\hat{p})^2 - N\right]^2}{\left(2\sum_{i=1}^{j}n_i^2 - N\right)}$$

where $\hat{p}_i = y_i/n_i$, $\hat{p} = \sum y_i / \sum n_i$, $N = \sum n_i$, and $\hat{q} = 1 - \hat{p}$.
Show that

(i) $\hat{p} = 0.526$
(ii) $X_T^2 = 315.11$

What do you conclude?

3.6 Use PROC GLM to fit a one-way random effects model. Show that
(i) MSB (mean-square between strains) $= 2.35$
(ii) MSW (mean-square within strains) $= 0.187$
(iii) Intrastrain correlation $= 0.27$

3.7 In a study of the relationship between endometrial cancer and history of gall bladder, 70 matched case–control pairs yielded the following data:

(a) Find an estimate of odds ratio. Construct 95% confidence interval on the population odds ratio.

(b) Use McNemar's test to verify the null hypothesis H_0 = odds ratio = 0.

	Cases		
Control	Exposed	Unexposed	Total
Exposed	5	6	11
Unexposed	15	44	59
Total	20	50	70

3.8   The data of Exercise 3.7 were further classified according to age as given in the following table:

Cancer and History of Gall Bladder

		Cases		
	Controls	Exposed	Unexposed	Total
Age ≥ 65	Exposed	3	3	6
	Unexposed	7	27	34
	Total	10	30	40
Age < 65	Exposed	2	3	5
	Unexposed	8	17	25
	Total	10	20	30

(a) Calculate the odds ratio for the two groups (group $1 \equiv$ age ≥ 65, group $2 \equiv$ age < 65) and produce the p-values on the significance of each p-value.

(b) Test the equality of odds ratios in the two groups.

(c) Is age an effect modifier?

3.9   Fit the above data, first using logistic regression, and then using PHREG in SAS.

3.10   You are given the results of a logistic regression analysis with linear predictor

$$\hat{\eta} = -22.91 + 0.31X_1 + 0.52X_2 + 0.16X_3$$

The SAS output produced the following variance–covariance matrix of the estimated regression parameters:

$$\begin{bmatrix} 11 & -1 & -4 & 3 \\ -1 & 9 & -3 & -2 \\ -4 & -3 & 4 & 0 \\ 3 & -2 & 0 & 5 \end{bmatrix}$$

Construct 95% on the odds ratio for someone whose covariate profile is $\hat{X} = (3,2,0)$ is relative to someone whose covariate profile is $X^* = (0,0,1)$.

4

Analysis of Clustered Count Data

4.1   Introduction

In Chapters 2 and 3, we discussed the statistical analysis and modeling of binary and binomial data and discussed some of the techniques designed to deal with clustered data. In this chapter, we deal with the situations when the response variable is an integer nonnegative random quantity representing counts. Such variables are of common occurrence, for example, in biological, medical, agricultural, and environmental fields. The book by Cameron and Trivedi (1998) is the most recent reference that describes statistical analysis and regression models for count data in full detail.

As an example, consider the data in Table 4.1 from Janardan et al. (1979) showing the distribution of sow bugs under boards. Here, the response variable is a nonnegative integer that takes the values 0, 1, 2, and 3. The frequencies of these counts are given in the second row.

As another example, the data displayed in Table 4.2 show the relationship between virus concentration and pock counts, which is a convenient technique for the estimation of virus titers.

TABLE 4.1

Distribution of the Number of Sow Bugs

Number of spiders per board	0	1	2	3
Frequency	159	64	13	4

TABLE 4.2

Pock Count Data Corresponding to Each
Concentration Level

Concentration Factor	Pock Count
1	5, 6, 9, 10, 11, 11, 12, 13
2	18, 23, 26, 31, 33, 34, 47, 53
4	32, 32, 37, 42, 48, 53, 54, 58
8	79, 88, 103, 107

Roizman et al. (1960) estimated the relationship between virus concentration and pock counts using linear and parabolic regression, assuming that the pock counts follow a Poisson distribution.

The fundamental aim of this chapter is to model count data as functions of several covariates, particularly when the sampling units are clusters.

4.2 Poisson Regression

A random variable Y has a Poisson distribution with mean μ, if the probability that Y equals y is given by

$$\Pr(Y = y) = e^{\mu} \mu^{y}/y! \quad \text{for } y = 0, 1, \dots \text{ and } \mu > 0 \tag{4.1}$$

The Poisson distribution enjoys a variety of desirable properties that account for its popularity. The most important feature is the widespread situations where count data arise. Bishop et al. (1975) have focused their investigations almost exclusively on the analysis of data obtained from sampling models based on the Poisson, multinomial, and product multinomial sampling schemes.

To illustrate the application of Poisson model and to describe the impact of explanatory variables on the mean count, we use the data in Table 4.2 to define a Poisson regression model, assuming that (i) the number of pocks (Y) is a random variable distributed as Poisson with mean μ, and (ii) μ is some function of the virus concentration X. Plotting logarithms of counts against the virus concentration (see Figure 4.1) suggests a relationship of the form:

$$\log \mu_i = \alpha + \beta x_i \tag{4.2}$$

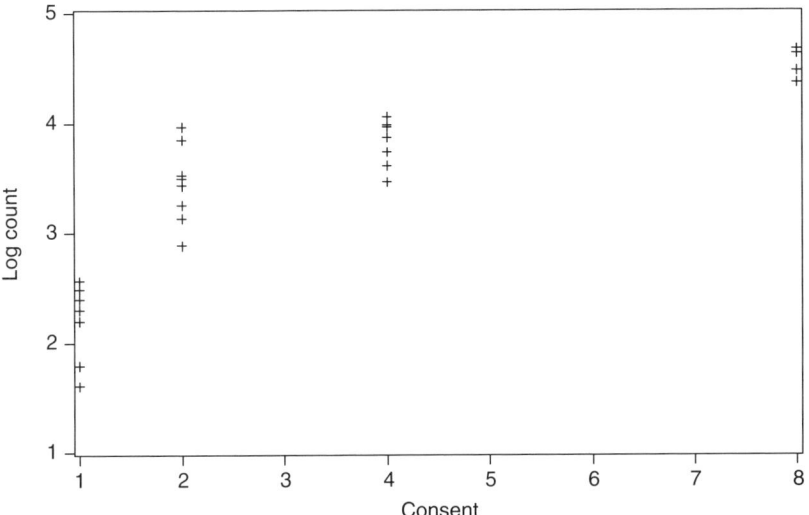

FIGURE 4.1
Scatter plot of log count against concentration.

For this log-linear model, the mean satisfies the relationship:

$$\mu_i = e^{\alpha + \beta x_i} = e^\alpha (e^\beta)^{x_i}$$

The above equation means that a unit increase in X has a multiplicative effect of e^β on μ, i.e., the mean of Y at $X + 1$ equals the mean of Y at X multiplied by e^β.

The case of multiple explanatory covariates is treated within the framework of generalized linear model (GLM) as discussed in Chapter 1. For the Poisson model, the log link is

$$\log \mu_i = \sum_{j=1}^{p} x_{ij} \beta_j$$

When employing a specific parametric model, it is natural to estimate the parameters of the model by maximizing the likelihood function. The likelihood function contains all the relevant information about the mechanism that generated the data. For the Poisson regression model, the maximum likelihood estimation is the most often used method.

The log-likelihood function of the Poisson regression model is given by

$$l(\beta) = \sum_{i=1}^{n} \{y_i \log[\eta_i(\beta)] - \eta_i(\beta)\} \qquad (4.3)$$

where

$$\mu_i = \eta_i(\beta) = \exp\left(\sum_{j=1}^{p} x_{ij} \beta_j\right) \qquad (4.4)$$

The estimating equations are obtained by differentiating Equation 4.3 with respect to the model parameters.

$$U_j(\beta) = \frac{\partial l(\beta)}{\partial \beta_j} = \sum_{i=1}^{n} \frac{\partial \eta_i(\beta)}{\partial \beta_j} \left(\frac{y_i - \eta_i(\beta)}{\eta_i(\beta)} \right) = 0$$

The above equations are solved to obtain the estimates of the regression parameters. When the log-link function 4.4 is used, $U_j(\beta)$ reduces to

$$U_j(\beta) = \sum_{i=1}^{n} \left[y_i - \exp \left(\sum_{j=1}^{p} x_{ij}\beta_j \right) \right] x_{ij} = 0$$

The GENMOD procedure in SAS can be used to estimate the parameters of a Poisson model with logarithmic link transformation.

Example 4.1

Consider the pock count data shown in Table 4.2. The following SAS code reads the data and runs the Poisson regression models.

```
data pock;
input concent count @@;
logcount=log(count);
cards;
1 5 1 6 1 9 1 10 1 11 1 11 1 11 1 12
1 13 2 18 2 23 2 26 2 31 2 33 2 34
2 47 2 53 4 32 4 32 4 37 4 42 4 48
4 53 4 54 4 58 8 79 8 88 8 103 8 107
;
* Plotting log count vs. concent;
proc gplot;
plot logcount*concent/vaxis=axis1 haxis=axis2 hminor=0 frame;
    axis1 label=(angle=-90 rotate=90 'Log count')
        order=(1 to 5 by 1) minor=none
        offset=(0.5)pct;
    axis2 label=('Concent') order=(1 to 8 by 1);
    run;

* Linear regression;
proc reg data=pock;
model logcount=concent;
run;

* Poisson model with log link;
proc genmod data=pock;
model count=concent /dist=poisson link=log scale=deviance type3;
output out=virus pred=predicted resdev=resid;
run;
```

The following is the partial output of the SAS program for fitting simple linear regression.

Parameter Estimates

Variable	DF	Parameter Estimate	Standard Error	t-Value	Pr > $|t|$
Intercept	1	2.39515	0.15532	15.42	<0.0001
concent	1	0.30192	0.03991	7.56	<0.0001

The following is the SAS output running GENMOD when the dispersion parameter is estimated as the square root of deviance divided by the number of degrees of freedom.

The GENMOD Procedure

Criteria for Assessing Goodness of Fit

Criterion	DF	Value	Value/DF
Deviance	26	134.2770	5.1645
Scaled deviance	26	26.0000	1.0000
Pearson χ^2	26	135.6029	5.2155
Scaled Pearson χ^2	26	26.2567	1.0099
Log likelihood		591.2394	

Analysis of Parameter Estimates

Parameter	DF	Estimate	Standard Error	Wald 95% Confidence Limits		χ^2	Pr > χ^2
Intercept	1	2.7418	0.1371	2.4732	3.0105	400.14	<0.0001
concent	1	0.2340	0.0252	0.1846	0.2834	86.32	<0.0001
Scale	0	2.2726	0.0000	2.2726	2.2726		

Note: The scale parameter was estimated by the square root of DEVIANCE/DF.

In the first model, we fitted linear regression using the log count as the dependent variable, and the second model fits the Poisson model with logarithmic link transformation. If the scale = pearson option is specified, another Poisson model may be fitted where dispersion parameter is estimated by Pearson's χ^2 statistic divided by its degrees of freedom and the parameter estimates are adjusted accordingly. When we compare the outputs of the three models, we find no real differences among them. Slight difference between the two Poisson models is because of the way the scale parameter is estimated. In one, the scale parameter is estimated as $\sqrt{5.1645}$, whereas in the other it is estimated as $\sqrt{5.2115}$.

There is no real quantitative measure according to which a specific model is preferred to the other. However, the most common approach to estimating the scale parameter is the square root of DEVIANCE/DF.

The following R code reads the pock count data and runs the linear regression and the Poisson models.

```
# Entering the data
concent <- c(rep(1,8),rep(2,8),rep(4,8),rep(8,4))
count <- c( 5, 6, 9,10,11,11,12,13,18,23,26,31,33,34,
           47,53,32,32,37,42,48,53,54,58,79,88,103,107)
logcount=log(count)
pock <- data.frame(concent,count,logcount)

# Plotting log count vs. concentration;
plot(logcount~concent,xlab="Concentration",ylab="Log Count",
data=pock)

# Linear regression
summary(lm(logcount ~ concent, data=pock))

# Poisson model with log link
pock.glm <- glm(count ~ concent,data=pock,family=poisson(link="log"))
summary(pock.glm)
```

4.3 Model Inference and Goodness of Fit

Similar to the logistic regression, one may compare models using $-2l$. This kind of analysis is done in SAS using the "type 3" option in the model statement (see the above output of the GENMOD procedure). The degrees of freedom for these "type 3" tests are simply the difference in the number of parameters estimated in the two competing nested models. In these models and the remainder of this chapter, hypothesis testing on regression coefficients and dispersion parameters in count data involves the application of the large sample theory of the likelihood inference. A general approach is Wald's test calculated from the z-score of the estimated parameter, that is, $z = $ estimate/SE(estimate). Large sample confidence intervals are computed as: estimate $\pm z_{\alpha/2}$SE(estimate), where $z_{\alpha/2}$ is the $(1 - \alpha/2)100\%$ cutoff point of the standard normal distribution.

A statistic capable of measuring the amount of support given by the data to a particular value of the parameter compared to its maximum likelihood estimate is the "deviance" statistic, defined as minus two times the logarithm of the normed likelihood, that is,

$$D_y(\beta) = -2[l_y(\beta) - l_y(\hat{\beta})]$$

$$= -2\sum_{i=1}^{n}\left[y_i\log\left[\frac{\eta_i(\beta)}{\eta_i(\hat{\beta})}\right] - [\eta_i(\beta) - \eta_i(\hat{\beta})]\right] \qquad (4.5)$$

Assuming β to be the true parameter, the deviance has an asymptotic χ^2 distribution with p degrees of freedom, where p is the dimension of β vector.

To obtain a measure of model "parsimony," the likelihood for the maximal model that perfectly fits the data may be compared to the likelihood of the fitted model.

The measure is written as

$$Dev_y = 2\sum_{i=1}^{n}\left[y_i\log\left(\frac{y_i}{\eta_i(\hat{\beta})}\right) - (y_i - \eta_i(\hat{\beta}))\right] \qquad (4.6)$$

The above index is known as the "deviance" as well. It can be used to compare nested models as has been described for the logistic regression model in Chapter 3.

4.4 Overdispersion in Count Data

The equality of mean and variance of the Poisson distribution places restriction on the applicability of this model to real-world data. Unfortunately, the popularity of the Poisson models and the relative ease of fitting them make it tempting to adopt these models without adequate attention for their applicability. An issue of importance is when empirical variance in the data exceeds the nominal variance under presumed model. Support for the presence of overdispersion is obtained when Pearson deviance is large. Therefore, an alternative to the Poisson distribution to model count data must be sought. It can be argued, however, if the lack of fit is negligible, and the efforts involved in fitting a more appropriate model are costly, then approximate inference under the Poisson model may still be valid.

The negative binomial distribution (NBD) has its variance larger than the mean and can be easily fitted to overdispersed count data using SAS.

DEFINITION   The random variable Y is said to follow an NBD with mean μ and dispersion parameter λ, denoted by $Y \sim \text{NBD}(\mu, \lambda)$, if

$$\Pr[Y = y] = \frac{\Gamma(y + \lambda^{-1})}{y!\Gamma(\lambda^{-1})}\left(\frac{\lambda\mu}{1 + \lambda\mu}\right)^y\left(\frac{1}{1 + \lambda\mu}\right)^{\lambda^{-1}} \qquad (4.7)$$

for $y = 0, 1, 2, \ldots$, $0 < \mu < \infty$, and $0 \leq \lambda < \infty$.

This form of the NBD reduces to the Poisson distribution when $\lambda = 0$. For the NBD $E(Y) = \mu$, and $\text{var}(y) = \mu(1 + \lambda\mu)$. It is understood by convention that $\lambda = 0$ means that as $\lambda \to 0$ the distribution in Equation 4.7 approaches Poisson with mean μ.

The problem of detecting departure from the Poisson distribution in the direction of an NBD is known as the problem of homogeneity testing.

When k groups, each of size n_i, are available, several statistical tests have been developed to test H_0: $\lambda = 0$ against H_a: $\lambda > 0$. For example, Collings (1981) showed that H_0 is rejected for large values of

$$T = \sum_{i=1}^{k}\sum_{j=1}^{n_i}\{(y_{ij} - \bar{y}_{i.})^2 - y_{ij}\} \tag{4.8}$$

Since under H_0: $\lambda = 0$, the Poisson distribution is a member of the regular exponential family, so there exists a complete sufficient statistics (see Collings and Margolin, 1985) for $(\mu_1, \mu_2, \ldots, \mu_k)$ namely $(\bar{y}_{1.}, \bar{y}_{2.}, \ldots, \bar{y}_{k.})$. Upon conditioning of the conditional statistics, one can find that large values of Equation 4.8 are equivalent to large values of

$$T_c = \sum_{i=1}^{k}\sum_{j=1}^{n_i}\left\{\frac{(y_{ij} - \bar{y}_{i.})^2}{y_{..}}\right\} \tag{4.8a}$$

where $\bar{y}_{i.} = \sum_{j=1}^{n_i} y_{ij}/n_j$ and $y_{..} = \sum_{i=1}^{k}\sum_{j=1}^{n_i} y_{ij}$.

This test statistic is valid only when all the observations are independent, and a new test statistic should be developed when observations within groups form clusters.

This test statistic can be developed using random effect models for discrete data similar to the normal random effects model.

4.5   Count Data Random Effects Models

Let y_{ij} denote independent Poisson random variables such that

$$\Pr[y_{ij}|a_i] = \frac{e^{-a_i}a_i^{y_{ij}}}{y_{ij}}, \qquad i = 1, 2, \ldots, k; \quad j = 1, 2, \ldots, n_i$$

Suppose that for some $\lambda \geq 0$

$$a_i \underset{iid}{\sim} \text{Gamma}\,(\lambda^{-1}, \mu)$$

where $\text{Gamma}(\alpha, \beta)$ represents a gamma distribution with mean $\alpha\beta$ and variance $\alpha\beta^2$.

The unconditional distribution of y_{ij} is $\text{NBD}(\mu, \lambda)$ with

$$E(y_{ij}) = \mu$$
$$\text{var}(Y_{ij}) = \mu(1 + \lambda\mu)$$
$$\text{cov}(y_{ij}, y_{il}) = \lambda\mu^2 \qquad j \neq l$$

Recall that in the one-way random effects model for normally distributed data, the hypothesis of no group effect is equivalent to

$$H_0: V(a_i) = 0.$$

In the discrete data, this is equivalent to testing $H_0: \lambda\mu^2 = 0$, which is equivalent to testing $H_0: \lambda = 0$. The test statistic in this case was developed by Collings and Margolin (1985) and is given by

$$T_r = \sum_{i=1}^{k} \left\{ \frac{(y_{i.} - n_i\tilde{\mu})^2}{y_{..}} \right\} \tag{4.9}$$

where $\tilde{\mu} = \sum_{i=1}^{k} \sum_{j=1}^{n_i} y_{ij} / \sum_{i=1}^{k} n_{i.}$.

Another way to detect overdispersion is to perform a least squares regression (without intercept)

$$\gamma_{ij} = \frac{(y_{ij} - \hat{\mu}_i)^2 - y_{ij}}{\hat{\mu}_i} = \lambda\hat{\mu}_i + u_i \tag{4.10}$$

where $\hat{\mu}_i = \frac{1}{n_i} \sum_{j=1}^{n_i} y_{ij}$ is the estimated group mean and u_i an error term (see Cameron and Trivedi, 1998). Under the hypothesis of no overdispersion, the statistic

$$t = \frac{\hat{\lambda}_{\text{ols}}}{\text{SE}(\hat{\lambda}_{\text{ols}})} \tag{4.11}$$

is asymptotically normal. In the case of Poisson regression, the fitted values $\hat{\mu}_i = \frac{1}{n_i} \sum_{j=1}^{n_i} \exp(\hat{\beta}_0 + x_{ij1}\hat{\beta}_1 + \cdots + x_{ijp}\hat{\beta}_p)$ are used in Equation 4.10.

In summary, we first fit a Poisson regression model using PROC GENMOD as shown in Section 4.2. Second, the fitted (predicted) values $\hat{\mu}_{ij}$ are saved, and with few programming statements in SAS we fit the regression equation 4.10. If t is sufficiently large (above 3, say), then we conclude that overdispersion is present, and an alternative to the Poisson regression model should be investigated.

4.5.1   Introducing the General Linear Mixed Model (GLMM)

In the previous sections, we accounted for the extra variation in count data by mixing the Poisson distribution with a gamma random variable to obtain a specific form for the NBD. Since the NBD has a closed form, the likelihood inference is possible. Shoukri et al. (2004) used the inverse Gaussian distribution as an alternative to the gamma density to obtain what was termed by them as "Poisson-inverse-Gaussian Model." They used the log-link function to model clustered count data as a function of a set of measured covariates. Such an outcome is somewhat artificially generated. In many, otherwise appealing, models a closed-form marginal density may not be generated. In this case, approximate or pseudolikelihood methods of estimation may be used. The generalized linear mixed effects models (GLMM) assume a Poisson model with normally distributed multiplicative heterogeneity term.

Assuming that $\log \mu_i = X_i^T \beta + \sigma u_i$, with $u_i \sim N(0,1)$, then conditional on u_i, y_i follows a Poisson distribution with mean $\mu_i = \exp(x_i^T \beta + \sigma u_i)$.

The marginal distribution is

$$\Pr[Y_i = y_i] = \frac{1}{\sqrt{2\pi}} \int_{-\infty}^{\infty} (y_i!)^{-1} \exp[-\exp(x_i^T \beta + \sigma u_i)] \exp[(x_i^T \beta + \sigma u_i)^{y_i}] \bar{e}^{u^2/2} du_i$$

$$(4.12)$$

There is no closed form solution for $\Pr[Y_i = y_i]$, unlike for the gamma heterogeneity term considered in Section 4.5. Two commonly used estimation procedures are (i) to approximate the objective function and (ii) to approximate the model. Algorithms in the second approach can be expressed in terms of Taylor expansion (linearization). In such an approach, we employ expansions to approximate the model by one based on pseudodata with fewer nonlinear components. The advantages of linearization-based methods include a relatively simple form of the linearized model that typically can be fit based on only the mean and variance in the linearized model. Models for which the marginal distribution is impossible to obtain can be fit with the linearization-based approach. Models with correlated errors (discussed in Chapter 5), a large number of random effects, crossed random effects, and multiple types of clusters are models where linearization is applied to.

The SAS fitting procedure that we use to fit models for clustered count data known as "GLIMMIX" fits the generalized linear mixed model based on linearization. The default estimation method in GLIMMIX for models containing random effects is a technique known as restricted pseudolikelihood estimation (see Wolfinger and O'Connell, 1993) with an expansion around the current estimate of the best linear unbiased predictors of the random effects.

4.5.2 Fitting GLMM Using SAS GLIMMIX

When non-normally distributed data with random effects are analyzed by GLIMMIX procedure in SAS, certain assumptions are made:

1. We assume that conditional on the random effect, the data have a known distribution. In models without random effects, the marginal distribution is assumed to be known so that maximum likelihood estimation is used. If quasi-likelihood methods are used, we assume that the mean and variance are known.
2. The link function is known as well.
3. Once the parameters are estimated, we assume that the large sample theory of likelihood inference applies. Tests of hypotheses for the fixed effects are based on Wald-type tests and the estimated variance–covariance matrices.
4. The link function η has the form $\eta = x\beta + z\gamma$.

The variance of the observations, conditional on the random effects, is

$$V(Y/\gamma) = A^{1/2}RA^{1/2} \tag{4.13}$$

The matrix A is a diagonal matrix and its elements are the variance functions of the model, which are determined from the specification of the distribution of the response variable Y. For example, if Y is Poisson, then the diagonal elements of A are μ (since the mean equals the variance in this case). The matrix R is a variance matrix specified by the RANDOM statement. The SAS GLIMMIX procedure distinguishes two types of random effects, the *G-side* and the *R-side*. The R-side effects are called "residual effects." In other words, if a random effect is an element of γ, it is a G-side effect, otherwise it is an R-side effect. Models without G-side effects are actually the "population-averaged" or PA models. These models have been described in detail in Chapter 3. The columns of the design matrix X are the fixed effects (covariates) specified on the right side of the MODEL statement. Columns of Z are the variance matrices G and R. These are determined from the RANDOM statement.

The R matrix is by default the scaled identity matrix, $R = \phi I$. The scale parameter ϕ is set to 1 if the distribution does not have a scale parameter, for example, in the case of the binary response, binomial, Poisson, and the geometric distribution. To specify a different R matrix, we use the RANDOM statement with the RESIDUAL keyword or the RESIDUAL option.

As a final remark, we note that the GLM (McCullagh and Nelder, 1989) is a special case of the GLMM. If the random effect $\gamma = 0$ and $R = \phi I$, GLMM reduces to the GLM or a GLM with overdispersion. For example, if A is a diagonal matrix with $E(Y) = V(y) = \mu$ on the diagonal, then the model is Poisson with $\phi = 1$, we can model Poisson data with overdispersion by adding the statement Random _ residual_;

4.5.3   Parameterization of the GLIMMIX

Similar to "PROC MIXED," the GLIMMIX constructs a linear mixed model according to the specifications in the CLASS, MODEL, and RANDOM statements. Each effect in the MODEL statement generates one or more columns in the design matrix X of the fixed effects, and each G-side effect in the RANDOM statement generates one or more columns in the Z matrix. R-side effects in the RANDOM statement do not generate model matrices; they serve only to index observations within clusters. By default, all models automatically include a column of 1s in X to estimate a fixed effect intercept parameter. Similar to "PROC MIXED" we can use the NOINT option in the model statement. The usefulness of the NOINT option has been explained in Chapter 1.

Example 4.2

Clinical mastitis (CM) is one of the endemic diseases and conditions of dairy cattle in many countries. The disease causes significant loss to the dairy industry both in terms of the reduction in output levels and wastage of resources incurred, in addition to the costs of disease prevention and treatment. Farm management practices play an important role in controlling and reducing the incidence of the disease. Hygiene is identified as an important factor. The use of organic (straw and sawdust) versus inorganic (sand) is associated with an increase in intramammary infections. Tail ducking is practiced to prevent the tail from hitting the udder and spread of the disease-causing pathogen. Milking technique is also identified as a route to spread mastitis from cow to cow. Some farmers milk the teats by hand (postmilking) after the machine milking to reduce residual milk in the quarters, and such practice might serve as an ideal growth flora for bacteria. Table 4.3 provides a summary of the data on total mastitis cases available from 57 Ontario dairy farms, each farm visited 3–6 times.

TABLE 4.3

Summary of the Mastitis Data

Visit	Number of Farms	Cultured Cows	Diseased Cows
1	57	2722	268
2	57	2916	366
3	57	2837	340
4	55	2583	262
5	48	2313	306
6	3	141	29

Let y_{ij} denote the number of mastitis cases on ith farm at jth visit. Here, the farm is a cluster ($i = 1, 2, \ldots, 57$), and the number of units within the cluster is the number of visits n_i. Note that in this example we shall assume that the within-cluster correlation is exchangeable, and we shall discuss the issue of other correlation structures in Chapter 6.

Here we model y_{ij} as a count variable using several modeling strategies: We first specify the fixed effects component of the model as

$$\log(\mu_{ij}) = \beta_0 + \beta_1 m_{ij} + \beta_0 \text{bed}_{ij} + \beta_3 pm_{ij} + \beta_4 \text{tail}_{ij}$$

where $\mu_{ij} = E(y_{ij})$, $\beta_0 = $ intercept, $m_{ij} = $ number of cows cultured on ith farm at jth visit; $\text{bed}_{ij} = 1$ if bedding is organic and is 0 otherwise; $pm_{ij} = 1$ if post-milking was not practiced, 0 otherwise; $\text{tail} = 1$ if tail docking is practiced, 0 otherwise.

The four models are

Model 1:	Poisson without overdispersion
Model 2:	Poisson with overdispersion
Model 3:	GLMMIX Poisson
Model 4:	Negative binomial

The first two models are marginal or population average, model 3 is a cluster-specific model, and the fourth is a random effects model, with a gamma distribution for the random effect.

Following Cameron and Trivedi (1998, p. 78), a test of overdispersion can empirically be carried out by using the method of least squares to fit the regression equation:

$$D_{ij} = \frac{(y_{ij} - \bar{y}_{i.})^2 - y_{ij}}{\bar{y}_{i.}} = \lambda \bar{y}_{i.} + \varepsilon_{ij}$$

where $\bar{y}_{i.} = \sum_{j=1}^{n_i} y_{ij}/n_i$ and ε_{ij} is an error term. The reported t-statistic for $\tilde{\lambda}$ is asymptotically normal under the null hypothesis $H_0: \lambda = 0$ versus $H_1: \lambda > 0$. For the mastitis data, it was found that $\tilde{\lambda} = 0.1169$ and the standard error $\text{SE}(\tilde{\lambda}) = 0.0232$, from which $t = 0.1169/0.0232 = 5.03$ (p-value < 0.001). Therefore, based on the evidence from the data, we conclude that overdispersion should not be ignored.

A short version of the SAS data step to read in the mastitis data is shown below; however, the complete dataset is available on the accompanying CD.

```
data mastitis;
input herd visit numcult y bedorg postmilk tailed;
cards;
10247 1 54 3 1 1 1
10247 2 64 6 1 1 1
10247 3 28 3 1 1 1
10247 4 3 2 1 1 1
. . . . . . .
. . . . . . .
30791 3 34 3 1 1 1
30791 5 32 2 1 1 1
;
```

Model 1: SAS code and selected output of fitting Poisson model ignoring the clustering effect and accounting for overdispersion.

```
proc genmod data=mastitis;
class herd;
model y=visit numcult bedorg postmilk tailed/ dist=poisson link=log
dscale;
run;
```

Criteria for Assessing Goodness of Fit

Criterion	DF	Value	Value/DF
Deviance	271	724.4622	2.6733
Scaled deviance	271	271.0000	1.0000
Pearson χ^2	271	781.0768	2.8822
Scaled Pearson χ^2	271	292.1779	1.0781
Log likelihood		520.1398	

Analysis of Parameter Estimates

Parameter	DF	Estimate	Standard Error	Wald 95% Confidence Limits		χ^2	Pr > χ^2
Intercept	1	0.5855	0.4748	−0.3451	1.5162	1.52	0.2175
visit	1	0.0415	0.0290	−0.0155	0.0984	2.04	0.1536
numcult	1	0.0161	0.0014	0.0133	0.0190	123.57	<0.0001
bedorg	1	1.3796	0.3749	0.6449	2.1143	13.55	0.0002
postmilk	1	−0.9117	0.1477	−1.2013	−0.6222	38.08	<0.0001
tailed	1	−0.4044	0.1098	−0.6197	−0.1892	13.56	0.0002
Scale	0	1.6350	0.0000	1.6350	1.6350		

Note: The scale parameter was estimated by the square root of DEVIANCE/DF.

Model 2: SAS code and selected output of fitting Poisson regression model accounting for the clustering effect.

```
proc genmod data=mastitis;
class herd;
model y = visit numcult bedorg postmilk tailed/ dist=poisson link=log
dscale;
repeated subject=herd/ type=cs corrw;
run;
```

Exchangeable Working Correlation

Correlation	0.4163

Analysis of GEE Parameter Estimates

Empirical Standard Error Estimates

Parameter	Estimate	Standard Error	95% Confidence Limits		Z	Pr > |Z|
Intercept	0.4237	0.5547	−0.6635	1.5109	0.76	0.4450
visit	0.0400	0.0347	−0.0281	0.1081	1.15	0.2498
numcult	0.0168	0.0019	0.0131	0.0204	8.91	<0.0001
bedorg	1.4803	0.1960	1.0962	1.8644	7.55	<0.0001
postmilk	−0.8572	0.2589	−1.3646	−0.3498	−3.31	0.0009
tailed	−0.4241	0.1504	−0.7189	−0.1292	−2.82	0.0048

Model 3: SAS code and selected output of fitting Poisson regression model using the generalized linear mixed model.

```
proc glimmix data=mastitis;
class herd;
model y = visit numcult bedorg postmilk tailed/ s dist=poisson link=log;
random intercept /subject=herd type=cs residual; run;
```

Fit Statistics

−2 Res log pseudolikelihood	585.49
Generalized χ^2	452.33
Generalized χ^2/DF	1.67

Covariance Parameter Estimates

Cov Parm	Subject	Estimate	Standard Error
CS	herd	1.2628	0.3141
Residual		1.6691	0.1595

Solutions for Fixed Effects

Effect	Estimate	Standard Error	DF	*t*-Value	Pr > |t|
Intercept	0.4157	0.7755	53	0.54	0.5942
visit	0.03998	0.02319	218	1.72	0.0861
numcult	0.01679	0.001974	218	8.50	<0.0001
bedorg	1.4856	0.6425	53	2.31	0.0247
postmilk	−0.8540	0.2553	53	−3.34	0.0015
tailed	−0.4258	0.1820	53	−2.34	0.0231

Model 4: SAS code and selected output for fitting the count data using negative binomial regression model.

```
proc glimmix data=mastitis;
class herd;
model y = visit numcult bedorg postmilk tailed/ s dist=NB link=log;
random intercept /subject=herd;
run;
```

Fit Statistics

−2 Res log Pseudolikelihood	550.09
Generalized χ^2	248.17
Generalized χ^2/DF	0.92

Solutions for Fixed Effects

Effect	Estimate	Standard Error	DF	t-Value	Pr > $|t|$
Intercept	−0.09609	0.7645	53	−0.13	0.9005
visit	0.03739	0.02391	218	1.56	0.1193
numcult	0.01980	0.002491	218	7.95	<0.0001
bedorg	1.5773	0.5459	218	2.89	0.0043
postmilk	−0.7035	0.3498	218	−2.01	0.0455
tailed	−0.3762	0.2146	218	−1.75	0.0810

Remarks on the SAS Output

1. We note that all the covariates are measured at the cluster level. Except for the visit, all covariates are significantly correlated with the response variable.
2. When the Poisson model is fitted using the generalized estimating equation (GEE), the moment estimator of the intracluster correlation (0.42) is almost identical to its restricted maximum likelihood estimate of the GLIMMIX procedure. This is obtained from the variance components estimators: $1.2628/(1.2628+1.6691)$.
3. While "tailed" was significant for the Poisson model, it was nonsignificant under the negative binomial model (NBM).
4. The dispersion parameter estimate of the NBM is $\hat{\lambda}=0.1017$ and its standard error is 0.02459. Using Wald's test on the Poisson hypothesis $H_0: \lambda=0$ against the NBM alternative, we have $z=0.1017/0.02459=4.14$ with p-value <0.001, a result that is similar to the regression test.

Models 1–3 may be fit in R as follows:

```
mastitis<-read.table("x:/xxx/mastitis.txt",header=T)
# Model 1: Poisson Model ignoring clustering effect
```

```
glm_mast<-glm(y~visit+numcult+bedorg+postmilk+tailed,
family=poisson(link="log"),data=mastitis)
summary(glm_mast)

# Model 2: Poisson Model accounting for clustering effect
gee_mast<-gee(y~visit+numcult+bedorg+postmilk+tailed,id=herd,
family=poisson(link="log"),data=mastitis,corstr="exchangeable")
summary(gee_mast)

Model 3: Fitting Poisson Model using generalized mixed modeling
cs <- corCompSymm(0.5, form = ~ 1|herd)
glmm_mast<-glmmPQL(y~visit+numcult+bedorg+postmilk+tailed,
random=~1|herd, family=poisson(link="log"),data=mastitis,cs)
summary(glmm_mast)
```

The results of fitting model 3 in R are slightly different from those in SAS because of the difference in estimation methods. The generalized linear mixed models with error term distributed as negative binomial errors are currently not available in R.

4.6 Other Models

There are many examples in the statistical literature where a mixture of count models are applied. Although the NBD is one of the most popular distributions, other distributions have been generated. For example, mixing Poisson with the inverse Gaussian distribution (Wilmot, 1987; Dean et al., 1989) and more recently the Poisson-inverse-Gaussian (PIG) distribution (Shoukri et al., 2004) were discussed.

Quite often, particularly when the sample size is small, it may be difficult to distinguish between alternative mixing distributions, and the choice may be based on the ease of computation. This issue is illustrated by comparing the Poisson-gamma (producing NBD) and Poisson-inverse-Gaussian (PIG) mixtures. Although the PIG does not have a closed form, the first two moments of the PIG mixture are the same as those of the NBD. Hence the mixing distributions can be distinguished when other information such as higher moments become available. It was conjectured by Cameron and Trivedi (1998) that in small samples such information may lead to inconclusive results. As an example, consider the "mastitis" data analyzed in Example 4.2. In that example, a comparison between the PIG and the NB regression models was made through the Q–Q plot of the residual's quantiles against the normal quantiles (see Figure 4.2 taken from Shoukri et al., 2004). Both plots are similar and one can hardly distinguish between the two models. However, because the NBD has a closed form and is programmed in commercial software, it is preferable to the PIG model.

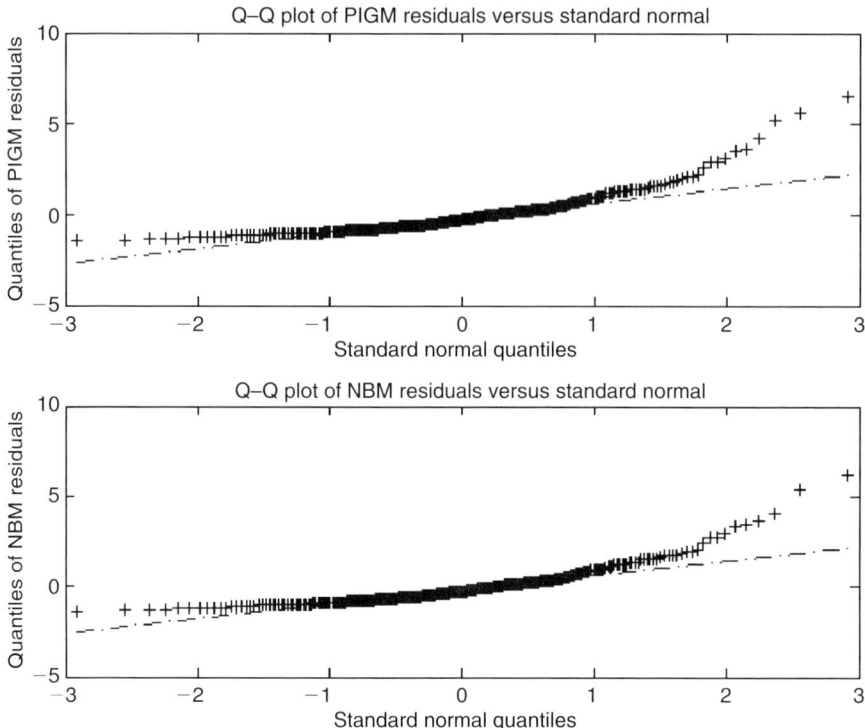

FIGURE 4.2
Q–Q plot of residuals for the Poisson-inverse-Gaussian and the negative binomial regression models.

Another issue is the comparison among nonnested models. Two models are nonnested if neither model can be represented as a special case of the other model. Note that models that have some regressors in common and some regressors not in common are overlapping models. The usual method of discriminating among models is by hypothesis test of the parameter restrictions that specialize one model to the other, for example, whether the dispersion parameter is zero in the transition from the negative binomial to the Poisson is not strictly valid. Instead, we use the Akaike (1973) information criterion to discriminate among nonnested models. Because the likelihood is expected to increase as parameters are added to the model, this criterion penalizes the likelihood with a large number of parameters (p). Akaike (1973) proposed the information criterion:

$$\text{AIC} = -2 \log l + p$$

The model with the lowest AIC is preferred. For example, the AIC for the Poisson GLMM is about 585.5, while the AIC for the NBM is about 550, indicating that the NBM provides a better fit within the class of cluster-specific models.

Another important application of count data with overdispersion is when there are excess zeros. The general term given to these models is "zero-inflated count models." The zero-inflated Poisson distribution is given by

$$Pr[y_i = 0] = \omega + (1 - \omega)e^{-\mu_i}$$
$$Pr[y_i = r] = (1 - \omega)e^{-\mu_i}\mu_i/r! \qquad r = 1, 2, \ldots$$

Here ω, the proportion of zeros, is added. Because $E(\mu_i) = \mu_i(1 - \omega)$ is smaller than $V(\mu_i) = (1 - \omega)(\mu_i + \omega\mu_i^2)$, excess zeros imply overdispersion.

Lambert (1992) introduced the zero-inflated Poisson model in which $\mu_i = \mu(x_i, \beta)$ and the probability ω is parameterized as a logistic function of the observable vector of covariates z_i, thereby insuring nonnegativity of ω; that is, $y_i = 0$ with probability ω and $y_i = e^{-\mu_i}\mu_i^{y_i}/y_i!$ with probability $1 - \omega$, and $\omega = \frac{\exp(z_i'\gamma)}{1 + \exp(z_i'\gamma)}$.

This model has been fitted to count data with zero-inflated class by several packages. The most useful fit was done by STATA when the counts are assumed to follow Poisson zero-inflated or negative binomial zero-inflated distributions.

Example 4.3

Here we analyze the motor vehicle insurance claims data from Sweden for the year 1977. The data have seven variables:

- Kilometers traveled per year: 1, <1000; 2, 1000–1500; 3, 15000–20000; 4, 20000–25000; and 5, >25000.
- Geographical zone: There are seven geographical zones.
- Bonus: No claims bonus. Equal to the number of years, plus one, since the last claim.
- Make: 1–8 represent eight different common car models. All other models are combined in class 9.
- Insured: Number of insured in policy years.
- Claims: Number of claims.
- Payment: Total value of payments in SKR.

The "claims" is a count variable and its histogram is given in Figure 4.3.

As can be seen from the histogram of the distribution of the number of claims (y), it is zero inflated and is quite skewed to the right.

Again, we shall analyze the data using a series of models. From the simple descriptive statistics, we find that the standard deviation is about four times larger than the mean. We can guess that the possible sources of this overdispersion are (1) clustering, (2) inflation in the zero class, (3) possibility of unmeasured covariates, or (4) at least one of the above reasons. We fit the data with only two covariates: "kilo" modeled as a quantitative variable and "zone" modeled as a categorical variable.

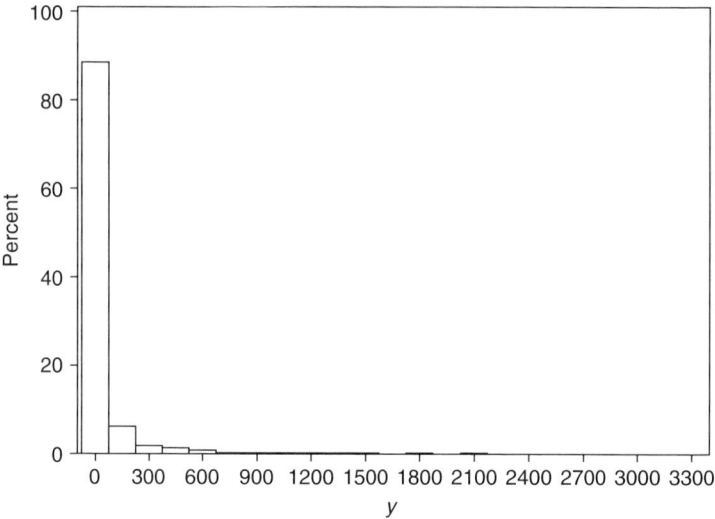

FIGURE 4.3
Histogram of the number of claims from the insurance data. (From Andrews, D.F. and Herzberg, A.M. (1985). Data: A Collection of Problems from Many Fields for the Students and Research Workers. Springer, New York.)

(I) Basic descriptive statistics and fitting Poisson regression model using GEE:

```
* Basic descriptive statistics;
proc means data=insur mean median std maxdec=2; var claims; run;

* Poisson model fitting using GEE;
proc genmod data=insur;
class make zone;
model y = kilo zone / dist=poisson link=log dscale;
repeated subject=make /type=cs;
run;
```

Analysis Variable: Claims

Mean	Median	Std Dev
51.86	5.00	201.71

Criteria for Assessing Goodness of Fit

Criterion	DF	Value	Value/DF
Deviance	2174	352784.0607	162.2742
Scaled deviance	2174	2174.0000	1.0000
Pearson χ^2	2174	984061.7447	452.6503
Scaled Pearson χ^2	2174	6064.1919	2.7894
Log likelihood		2311.2924	

Exchangeable Working Correlation

Correlation	0.3537

Analysis of GEE Parameter Estimates

Parameter		Estimate	Standard Error	95% Confidence Limits		Z	Pr > |Z|
Intercept		3.0142	0.6415	1.7570	4.2715	4.70	<0.0001
kilo		−0.3163	0.0186	−0.3529	−0.2798	−16.97	<0.0001
zone	1	2.4286	0.0741	2.2833	2.5739	32.76	<0.0001
zone	2	2.3569	0.0579	2.2435	2.4703	40.73	<0.0001
zone	3	2.3009	0.0565	2.1903	2.4116	40.76	<0.0001
zone	4	2.7054	0.0439	2.6193	2.7915	61.58	<0.0001
zone	5	1.3474	0.0366	1.2756	1.4192	36.80	<0.0001
zone	6	1.7597	0.0231	1.7145	1.8049	76.31	<0.0001
zone	7	0.0000	0.0000	0.0000	0.0000	—	—

Empirical Standard Error Estimates

(II) Fitting NBM using GEE:

```
proc genmod data=insur;
class make zone;
model y = kilo zone / dist=nb link=log dscale;
repeated subject=make /type=cs;
run;
```

Criteria for Assessing Goodness of Fit

Criterion	DF	Value	Value/DF
Deviance	2174	2572.0563	1.1831
Scaled deviance	2174	2174.0000	1.0000
Pearson χ^2	2174	6576.9273	3.0253
Scaled Pearson χ^2	2174	5559.0697	2.5571
Log likelihood		462042.7705	

Exchangeable Working Correlation

Correlation	0.4243

Analysis of GEE Parameter Estimates

Empirical Standard Error Estimates

Parameter		Estimate	Standard Error	95% Confidence Limits		Z	Pr > |Z|
Intercept		2.0253	0.7147	0.6246	3.4261	2.83	0.0046
kilo		−0.4721	0.0153	−0.5021	−0.4421	−30.82	<0.0001
zone	1	3.6308	0.0233	3.5850	3.6765	155.56	<0.0001
zone	2	3.5694	0.0219	3.5264	3.6124	162.63	<0.0001
zone	3	3.4999	0.0271	3.4469	3.5530	129.25	<0.0001
zone	4	4.0206	0.0420	3.9382	4.1030	95.66	<0.0001
zone	5	2.2214	0.0320	2.1588	2.2840	69.52	<0.0001
zone	6	2.8592	0.0587	2.7442	2.9742	48.73	<0.0001
zone	7	0.0000	0.0000	0.0000	0.0000	—	—

(III) SAS code to fit the random effects Poisson model using SAS GLIMMIX. Here "make" is used as the clustering factor.

```
* GLIMMIX fitting;
proc glimmix data=insur;
class make zone;
model y = kilo zone / s dist=poisson link=log;
random intercept/ subject=make;
run;
```

Fit Statistics

−2 Res log pseudolikelihood	121748.1
Generalized χ^2	122566.0
Generalized χ^2/DF	56.38

Covariance Parameter Estimates

Cov Parm	Subject	Estimate	Standard Error
Intercept	make	1.7092	0.8547

Solutions for Fixed Effects

Effect	Zone	Estimate	Standard Error	DF	t-Value	Pr > |t|
Intercept		0.5742	0.4377	8	1.31	0.2260
kilo		−0.3813	0.002300	2166	−165.77	<0.0001
zone	1	3.6154	0.04069	2166	88.84	<0.0001
zone	2	3.5312	0.04074	2166	86.67	<0.0001
zone	3	3.4650	0.04078	2166	84.97	<0.0001
zone	4	3.9354	0.04055	2166	97.05	<0.0001
zone	5	2.2582	0.04220	2166	53.52	<0.0001
zone	6	2.8008	0.04136	2166	67.72	<0.0001
zone	7	0	—	—	—	—

Type III Tests of Fixed Effects

Effect	Num DF	Den DF	*F*-value	Pr > F
kilo	1	2166	27480.2	<0.0001
zone	6	2166	4701.37	<0.0001

(IV) SAS code to fit the random effects NBM using SAS GLIMMIX. Here "make" is used as the clustering factor.

```
proc glimmix data=insur;
class make zone;
model y = kilo zone / s dist=nb link=log;
random make;
run;
```

Fit Statistics

−2 Res log pseudolikelihood	7897.09
Generalized χ^2	2223.39
Generalized χ^2/DF	1.02

Covariance Parameter Estimates

Cov Parm	Estimate	Standard Error
make	1.6038	0.8058
Scale	1.7335	0.06058

Solutions for Fixed Effects

Effect	Zone	Estimate	Standard Error	DF	*t*-Value	Pr > |t|
Intercept		0.6223	0.4402	8	1.41	0.1952
kilo		−0.4174	0.02151	2166	−19.40	<0.0001
zone	1	3.5942	0.1353	2166	26.56	<0.0001
zone	2	3.5682	0.1353	2166	26.36	<0.0001
zone	3	3.5551	0.1354	2166	26.26	<0.0001
zone	4	4.0803	0.1350	2166	30.23	<0.0001
zone	5	2.2952	0.1376	2166	16.68	<0.0001
zone	6	2.9745	0.1361	2166	21.86	<0.0001
zone	7	0	—	—	—	—

Type III Tests of Fixed Effects

Effect	Num DF	Den DF	*F*-value	Pr > F
kilo	1	2166	376.49	<0.0001
zone	6	2166	191.76	<0.0001

The following R code reads the data and runs models 1 and 3 above. NBMs are currently not available in R.

```
#Reading the data
insur <-read.table("x:/xxx/insur.txt",header=T)
# Generating factors and sorting the data by 'make'
insur1 <- transform(insur,zone=factor(zone),make=factor(make))
insur2 <- insur1[order(insur1[,1]) ,]
# Setting the last factor level for 'zone' as reference
insur2$zone <- relevel(insur2$zone, ref=7)


# Model 1: Poisson Model with log link
gee_insur1 <- gee(claims ~ kilo+zone, id=make,
family=poisson(link="log"), data=insur2, corstr="exchangeable")
summary(gee_insur1)$coefficients


# Model 3: Poisson Model using generalized mixed modeling
cs <- corCompSymm(0.5, form = ~ 1|make)
glmm_insur3 <- glmmPQL(claims~kilo+zone,random=~1|make,
family=poisson(link="log"),data=insur2,cs)
summary(glmm_insur3)
```

Comments on the Results

1. It is clear from all the models that the number of claims significantly depends on the number of kilometers driven. The more the car has been driven, the less the number of claims, and there are wide variations among zones. Note that a large value for the intracluster correlation (0.353 for the Poisson and 0.424 for the NBM) indicates that a significant percentage in the variability in the number of claims may be attributed to the "make" of the car.

2. If we take the deviance as a measure of goodness of fit in the GENMOD, the negative binomial provides a better fit. In fact deviance Poisson $= 352784$ and deviance negative binomial $= 2572$. The same remark holds when the models are fitted by the GLIMMIX. For the Poisson with random effect, the generalized χ^2/DF is 56.38, while the same index in the case of the negative binomial is 1.02.

3. The above fitted models do not take into account the two-part nature of the distribution of the number of claims caused by the zero inflation. Rather they deal with the issue of extra variability in the count variable.

   (a) Following Lambert (1992) approach and fitting the two-part NBM using STATA, we get

Parameter	kilo	zone 1	zone 2	zone 3	zone 4	zone 5	zone 6
Estimate	−0.46	3.25	3.19	3.12	3.64	1.85	2.48
SE	0.03	0.18	0.18	0.18	0.18	0.18	0.18

All parameter estimates are significantly different from zero. Moreover, all parameter estimates of γ in $\omega = \frac{\exp(z_i'\gamma)}{1+\exp(z_i'\gamma)}$ are not significant. It is interesting to note as well that the zero-inflated negative binomial provides information that are similar to the information obtained from the GLIMMIX negative binomial.

Exercises

4.1   The generalized Poisson distribution discussed in the article by Janardan et al. (1979) has two parameters and has its variance larger than the mean. It was first introduced to the literature by Consul and Jain (1973) and was named the generalized Poisson distribution (GPD). The probability distribution is given by

$$P_r(Y = y) = (y!)^{-1}\lambda(\lambda + y\theta)^{y-1}\exp[-(\lambda + y\theta)]$$

The mean and variance are given by $E(Y) = \lambda/(1-\theta)$ and $\text{var}(Y) = \lambda/(1-\theta)^3$, respectively. Clearly, the distribution reduces to Poisson when $\theta = 0$. Fit the Poisson and the GPD to the data in Table 4.1 using the method of moments. Using the χ^2 goodness of fit, which model fits the data better?

4.2   Suppose that $Y_i(i = 1, 2, \ldots, n)$ is a random variable whose probability distribution is Poisson with mean λ. Assume a log link $\log \lambda = \beta_0 + \beta_1 X_i$, where X is a random covariate that has a standard normal distribution. Derive the likelihood equations for estimating the parameters β_0 and β_1.

4.3   Show that the elements of Fisher's information matrix are given by

$$-E\left(\frac{\partial^2 \ell}{\partial \beta_0^2}\right) = ne^{\beta_0}E(e^{\beta_1 X}) \equiv i_{00}$$

$$-E\left(\frac{\partial^2 \ell}{\partial \beta_0 \partial \beta_1}\right) = ne^{\beta_0}E(xe^{\beta_1 X}) = i_{01}$$

and

$$-E\left(\frac{\partial^2 \ell}{\partial \beta_1^2}\right) = ne^{\beta_0}E(x^2 e^{\beta_1 X}) = i_{11}$$

4.4   Given that the moments generating function of the standard normal distribution is $E(e^{tX}) = e^{1/2t^2}$, and that differentiation is permitted inside the integration sign, show that

$$i_{00} = ne^{\beta_0 + 1/2\beta_1^2}$$

$$i_{01} = n\beta_1 e^{\beta_0 + 1/2\beta_1^2}$$

and

$$i_{11} = n(1 + \beta_1^2)e^{\beta_0 + 1/2\beta_1^2}$$

4.5   Show that by inverting Fisher's information matrix, the large sample variance of $\hat{\beta}_1$, the maximum likelihood estimation of β_1 is given by

$$n \cdot \text{var}(\hat{\beta}_1) = \bar{e}^{\beta_0 - 1/2\beta_1^2}$$

4.6   Suppose that you requested to test the hypothesis $H_0: \beta_1 = 0$ versus $H_1: \beta_1 = 0.1$. What are the values of $\text{var}(\hat{\beta}_1)$ under both hypotheses when $n = 1500$?

4.7   If you want to test the hypothesis $H_0: \beta_1 = 0$ versus a two-sided alternative $H_1: \beta_1 = 0.1$, with power $1 - \gamma$, and type I error rate α, show that the required sample size is given by

$$n \geq \frac{(Z_\gamma a_1 + Z_{\alpha/2} a_2)^2}{\beta_1^2}$$

where $a_1^{-1} = e^{1/2\beta_0 + 1/4\beta_1^2}$ and $a_2^{-1} = e^{1/2\beta_0}$.

4.8   What would be the required sample size for $\alpha = 0.05$, $\gamma = 0.20$, $\beta_0 = \log(0.07)$, and $\beta_1 = 0.1$?

4.9   Suppose that Y_{ij} has a Poisson distribution with mean:

$$\log \lambda_{ij} = \beta_0 + \beta_1 x_{ij} \qquad i = 1, 2, \ldots, n; \quad j = 1, 2, \ldots, m$$

with m being the cluster size and n the number of clusters. Assume that the intracluster correlation is ρ and we have a sample inflation factor (design effect) $D = 1 + (m - 1)\rho$. To test the hypothesis stated in Exercise 4.8, develop a sample size approach to estimate the number of clusters n taking into account the intracluster correlation.

5

Analysis of Time Series

CONTENTS

5.1   Introduction

A time series is an ordered sequence of observations. Although the ordering is usually through time, particularly in terms of some equally spaced intervals, the ordering may also be taken through other dimensions such as space.

Time series occur in a wide variety of fields. In economics, interest may be focused on the weekly fluctuations in the stock prices and their relationships to unemployment figures. Agricultural time series analyses and forecasting could be applied to annual crop yields or the prices of produce with regard to their seasonal variations. Environmental changes over time, such as levels of air and water pollution measured at different places, can be correlated with certain health indicators. The number of influenza outbreaks in successive weeks during the winter season could be approached as a time series problem by an epidemiologist. In medicine, systolic and diastolic blood pressures followed over time for a group of patients could be useful for assessing the effectiveness of a drug used in treating hypertension. Geophysical time series (Shumway, 1982) are quite important for predicting earthquakes. From these examples, one can see the diversity of fields in which time series can be applied. There are, however, some common objectives that must be achieved in collected time series data:

- *To describe the behavior of the series in a concise way.* This is done by first plotting the data and obtaining simple descriptive measures of the main properties of the series. This may not be useful for all time series because there are series that require more sophisticated techniques, and thus more complex models need to be constructed.
- *To explain the behavior of the series in terms of several variables.* For example, when observations are taken for more than one variable, it may be feasible to use the variation in one time series to explain the variation in another series.
- *We may want to predict (forecast) the future values of the series.* This is an important task for the analysis of economic and agricultural time series. It is desirable particularly if there is sufficient evidence in the system to ensure that future behavior will be similar to the past. Therefore, our ability to understand the behavior of the series may provide us with more insight into causal factors and help us make projections into the future.
- *Controlling the series by generating warning signals of future fluctuations.* For example, if we are measuring the quality of production process, our aim may be to keep the process under control. Statistical quality control provides us with the tools to achieve such an objective by constructing "control charts." More advanced strategies for control are outlined in Box and Jenkins (1970).

In the following sections we provide examples on modeling and graphing time series. We introduce simple models and the autoregressive integrated moving average (ARIMA) models. We restrict our discussion to stationary time series. Other advanced models and methods are available in many books (e.g., Anderson, 1971; Bloomfield, 1976; Cryer, 1986; and Diggle, 1990).

Example 5.1

An epidemiological time series showing the average somatic cell count (SCC) by month over a number of years is shown in Table 5.1.

TABLE 5.1

Average SCC per Farm in Cells (in 1000s) per mL of Milk

	1984	1985	1986	1987	1988	1989	1990
Jan	317	345	370	350	400	370	340
Feb	292	310	360	420	385	335	345
Mar	283	307	300	360	350	305	325
Apr	286	310	310	340	325	325	330
May	314	340	389	335	345	310	360
June	301	325	320	350	350	315	330
July	317	340	340	360	375	350	345
Aug	344	370	400	395	410	370	350
Sept	367	400	395	380	360	350	350
Oct	351	380	350	375	375	345	345
Nov	321	345	400	402	370	355	325
Dec	398	330	350	460	395	340	280

A plot of these data in Figure 5.1 shows large fluctuations in both the mean and the variance over time.

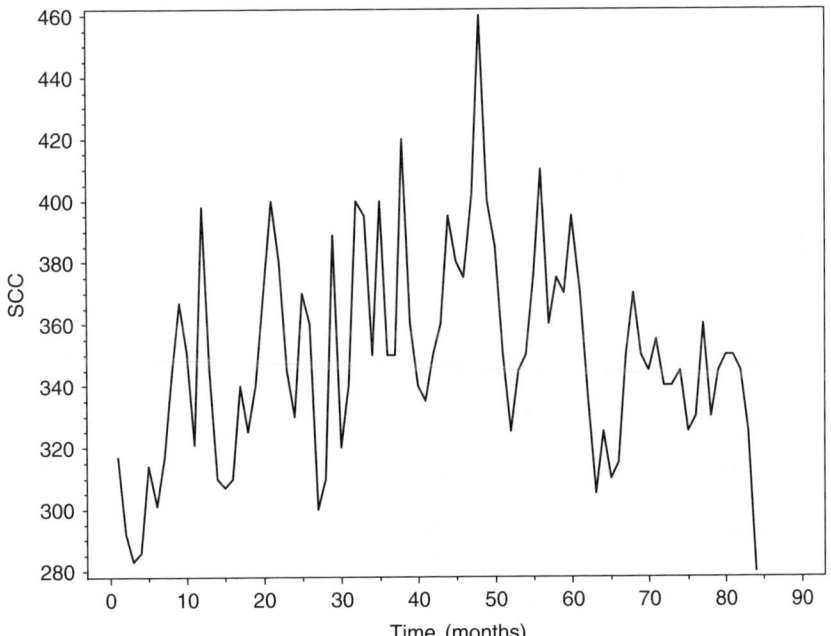

FIGURE 5.1

A time plot of average somatic cell counts per month for 84 months.

The SAS code to read the data and produce Figure 5.1 is given below.

```
data scc;
input year scc @@;
 difscc=dif(scc); time= _n_;
datalines;
84 317 84 292 84 283 84 286 84 314 84 301 84 317 84 344
84 367 84 351 84 321 84 398 85 345 85 310 85 307 85 310
85 340 85 325 85 340 85 370 85 400 85 380 85 345 85 330
86 370 86 360 86 300 86 310 86 389 86 320 86 340 86 400
86 395 86 350 86 400 86 350 87 350 87 420 87 360 87 340
87 335 87 350 87 360 87 395 87 380 87 375 87 402 87 460
88 400 88 385 88 350 88 325 88 345 88 350 88 375 88 410
88 360 88 375 88 370 88 395 89 370 89 335 89 305 89 325
89 310 89 315 89 350 89 370 89 350 89 345 89 355 89 340
90 340 90 345 90 325 90 330 90 360 90 330 90 345 90 350
90 350 90 345 90 325 90 280
;

goptions reset=global gunit=pct cback=white htitle=6 htext=3
ftext=swissb colors=(black);

* Figure 5.1: A time plot of average somatic cell counts per month;
axis1 order=(0 to 90 by 10) label=(angle=0 'Time (Month)') offset=(3)
minor=(number=1);
axis2 order=(280 to 460 by 20) label=(angle=0 'SCC') minor=
(number=3);

proc gplot data=scc;
   plot scc*time / haxis=axis1 vaxis=axis2;
   symbol1 i=join;
run; quit;
```

5.2   Simple Descriptive Methods

In this section, we describe some of the simple techniques that will detect the main characteristics of a time series. From a statistical point of view, the description of a time series is accomplished by a time plot, that is, plotting the observations against time and formulating a mathematical model to characterize the behavior of the series. This models the mechanism that governs the variability of the observations over time. Plotting the data could reveal certain features such as trend, seasonality, discontinuities, and outliers. The term "trend" usually means the upward or downward movement over a period of time, thus reflecting the long-run growth or decline in the time series.

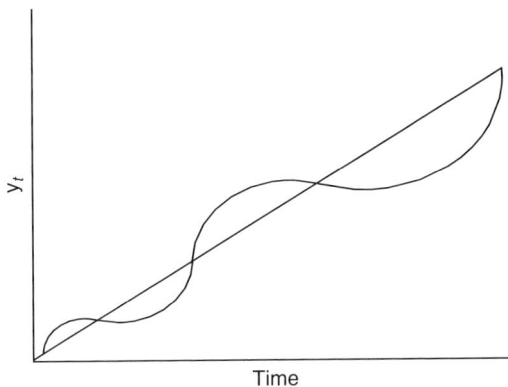

FIGURE 5.2
Additive seasonal variation model.

In addition to the effect of trend, most economic time series include seasonal variation. To include both the seasonal variation and the trend effect, there are two types of models that are frequently used. The first is the additive seasonal variation model (ASVM) and the second is the multiplicative seasonal variation model (MSVM). If a time series displays additive seasonal variation, the magnitude of the seasonal swing is independent of the mean. In contrast, in a multiplicative seasonal variation series we see that the seasonal swing is proportional to the mean. The two models are represented by the following equations:

$$y_t = T_t + S_t + \varepsilon_t \qquad \text{(ASVM)}$$
$$y_t = (T_t)(S_t) + \varepsilon_t \qquad \text{(MSVM)}$$

where y_t is the observed value at time t, T_t the mean trend factor at time t, S_t the seasonal effect at time t, and ε_t the irregular variation of the time series at time t.

The two models are illustrated in Figures 5.2 and 5.3.

Note that the MSVM has an additive irregular variation term. If such a term is multiplicative, that is, if $y_t = (T_t)(S_t)(\varepsilon_t)$, then this model can be transformed to ASVM by taking the logarithm of both sides.

5.2.1 Multiplicative Seasonal Variation Model

In this section, we will be concerned with simple methods of decomposing MSVM into its trend, seasonal, and random components. The model is somewhat different from the previous model,

$$y_t = (T_t)(S_t) + \varepsilon_t \qquad (5.1)$$

and is usually written as

$$y_t = (T_t)(S_t)(C_t)(I_t) \qquad (5.2)$$

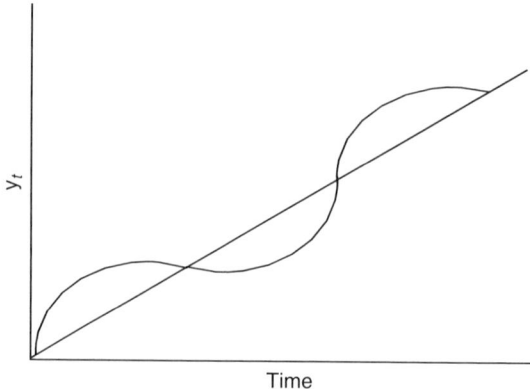

FIGURE 5.3
Multiplicative seasonal variation model.

where y_t, T_t, and S_t are as previously defined. Here, C_t represents the cyclical effect on the series at time t and I_t is the irregular variation.

We will explain how to decompose the multiplicative model in the following example.

Example 5.2

The following data represent the number of cases with bovine respiratory disease (BRD) in particular feedlots reported in eastern Alberta counties over a period of 4 years in each of the four quarters (Table 5.2).

TABLE 5.2

Cases of Bovine Respiratory Disease Reported in Eastern Alberta Counties

Quarter	Year 1	Year 2	Year 3	Year 4
1	21	25	25	30
2	14	16	18	20
3	5	7	9	10
4	8	9	13	15

The first step in the analysis of this time series is the estimation of seasonal factors for each quarter. To do this one has to calculate the moving average (MA) to remove the seasonal variation from the series. MA is calculated by adding the observations for a number of periods in the series and dividing the sum by the number of periods. In this above example, we have a four-period series since we have quarterly data. If the time series consists of data collected every 4 months, we have a three-period time series, and hence a three-period MA should be used. In the above example, the average for the four observations in the first year is

$$\frac{21 + 14 + 5 + 8}{4} = 12$$

The second average is obtained by eliminating the first observation in year 1 from the average and including the first observation in year 2 in the new average. Hence,

$$\frac{14 + 5 + 8 + 25}{4} = 13$$

The third average is obtained by dropping the second observation in year 1 and adding the second observation in year 2. This gives

$$\frac{5 + 8 + 25 + 16}{4} = 13.5$$

Continuing in this manner, these moving averages are as found in Table 5.3. Note that since the first average is the average of the observations in the four quarters, it corresponds to a midpoint between the second and third quarter.

TABLE 5.3

Moving Average of the Time Series of Table 5.2

Year (1)	Quarter (2)	y_t (3)	Moving Total (4)	MA (5)	Centered MA (6)	$S_t I_t$ (7)
1	1	21				
	2	14				
			48	12		
	3	5			12.5	0.4
			52	13		
	4	8			13.25	0.604
			54	13.5		
2	1	25			13.75	1.818
			56	14		
	2	16			14.125	1.133
			57	14.25		
	3	7			14.25	0.491
			57	14.25		
	4	9			14.5	0.621
			59	14.75		
3	1	25			15.0	1.667
			61	15.25		
	2	18			15.75	1.143
			65	16.25		
	3	9			16.875	0.533
			70	17.5		
	4	13			17.75	0.732
			72	18		
4	1	30			18.125	1.655
			73	18.25		
	2	20			18.5	1.081
			75	18.75		
	3	10				
	4	15				

To obtain the average corresponding to one of the time periods in the original time series, we calculate a centered MA. This is obtained by computing a two-period MA of the MAs previously calculated (Table 5.3).

Note that since the MA is computed using exactly one observation from each season, the seasonal variation has been removed from the data. It is also hoped that this averaging process has removed the irregular variation I_t. This means that the centered MAs in column 6 in Table 5.3 represent the trend (T_t) and cycle (C_t). Now, since

$$y_t = (T_t)(S_t)(C_t)(I_t)$$

then the entries in column 7 of Table 5.3 are computed as

$$(S_t)(I_t) = \frac{y_t}{(T_t)(C_t)} = \frac{\text{column 3}}{\text{column 6}}$$

The seasonal coefficients ($S_t I_t$) are summarized in Table 5.4.

TABLE 5.4

Seasonal Coefficients for Each Quarter by Year

Quarter 1	Quarter 2	Quarter 3	Quarter 4
1.818	1.133	0.400	0.604
1.667	1.143	0.491	0.621
1.655	1.081	0.533	0.732

The seasonal effects for each quarter can be computed by summing and dividing the number of coefficients. Thus, for quarter 1

$$\hat{S}_1 = \frac{1.818 + 1.667 + 1.655}{3} = 1.713$$

Similarly,

$$\hat{S}_2 = 1.119 \quad \hat{S}_3 = 0.475 \quad \hat{S}_4 = 0.652$$

are the estimated seasonal effects for quarters 2, 3, and 4.

Once the estimates of the seasonal factors have been calculated, we may obtain an estimate of the trend T_t of the time series. This is done by first estimating the deseasonalized observations.

The deseasonalized observations are obtained by dividing y_t by S_t. That is, deseasonalized series $= d_t = \frac{y_t}{S_t}$

These values should be close to the trend value T_t. To model the trend effect, as a first step one should plot d_t against the observation number t. If the plot is linear it is reasonable to assume that

$$T_t = \beta_0 + \beta_1 t$$

In contrast, if the plot shows a quadratic relationship then we may assume that

$$T_t = \beta_0 + \beta_1 t + \beta_2 t^2$$

and so on. Table 5.5 gives the deseasonalized observations and Figure 5.4 is a scatter plot of these observations against time.

TABLE 5.5

Deseasonalized Observations

Year	Quarter	t	y_t	S_t	$d_t = \frac{y_t}{S_t}$
1	1	1	21	1.713	12.26
	2	2	14	1.119	12.51
	3	3	5	0.475	10.53
	4	4	8	0.652	12.27
2	1	5	25	1.713	14.59
	2	6	16	1.119	23.24
	3	7	7	0.475	14.74
	4	8	9	0.652	13.80
3	1	9	25	1.713	14.59
	2	10	18	1.119	16.09
	3	11	9	0.475	12.63
	4	12	13	0.652	19.94
4	1	13	30	1.713	17.51
	2	14	20	1.119	17.87
	3	15	10	0.475	21.05
	4	16	15	0.652	23.01

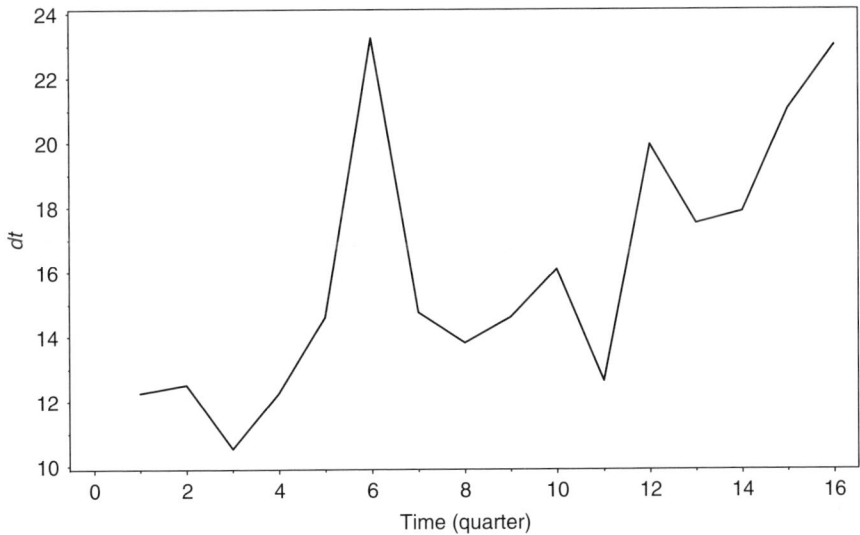

FIGURE 5.4
Deseasonalized observations over time; BRD data.

The estimated trend is found to be

$$\hat{d}_t = \hat{T}_t = 10.05 + 0.685t \qquad t = 1, 2, \ldots, 16$$

To compute the cyclical effect, recall that

$$y_t = (T_t)(S_t)(C_t)(I_t)$$

hence,

$$(C_t)(I_t) = \frac{y_t}{(\hat{T}_t)(\hat{S}_t)}$$

We summarize these computations in Table 5.6.

TABLE 5.6

Computations of Cyclical Effect and Irregular Variation

Year (1)	Quarter (2)	t (3)	y_t (4)	$T_t = 10.05 + 0.685t$ (5)	S_t (6)	$(T_t)(S_t)$ (7)	$(C_t)(I_t)$ (7)
1	1	1	21	10.74	1.713	18.39	1.14
	2	2	14	11.42	1.119	12.78	1.10
	3	3	5	12.11	0.475	5.75	0.87
	4	4	8	12.79	0.652	8.34	0.96
2	1	5	25	13.48	1.713	23.08	1.08
	2	6	16	14.16	1.119	15.85	1.64
	3	7	7	14.85	0.475	7.05	0.99
	4	8	9	15.53	0.652	10.13	0.89
3	1	9	25	16.22	1.713	27.78	0.90
	2	10	18	16.9	1.119	18.91	0.95
	3	11	9	17.59	0.475	8.35	0.72
	4	12	13	18.27	0.652	11.91	1.09
4	1	13	30	18.96	1.713	32.47	0.92
	2	14	20	19.64	1.119	21.98	0.91
	3	15	10	20.33	0.475	9.65	1.04
	4	16	15	21.01	0.652	13.70	1.10

$$C_t I_t = \frac{\text{column } 4}{\text{column } 7}$$

Once $(C_t)(I_t)$ has been obtained, a three-quarter MA may remove the effect of irregular variation. The results are summarized in Table 5.7.

The previous example shows how a time series can be decomposed into its components. Most econometricians use the trend and seasonal effect in their forecast of time series, ignoring the cyclical and irregular variations. Clearly, irregular ups and downs cannot be predicted; however, cyclical variation can be forecasted and is treated in the same manner as the seasonal effects shown in Table 5.4. In our example, the average effect of the cycle at each period is as found in Table 5.8.

TABLE 5.7

Estimated Cyclical Effect

Year	Quarter	t	$(C_t)(I_t)$	Three-Period MA C_t
1	1	1	1.14	
	2	2	1.10	1.037
	3	3	0.87	0.977
	4	4	0.96	0.970
2	1	5	1.08	1.230
	2	6	1.64	1.24
	3	7	0.99	1.173
	4	8	0.89	0.927
3	1	9	0.90	0.913
	2	10	0.95	0.857
	3	11	0.72	0.920
	4	12	1.09	0.910
4	1	13	0.92	0.973
	2	14	0.91	0.957
	3	15	1.04	1.017
	4	16	1.10	

TABLE 5.8

Cycle's Effect for Different Periods

Quarter 1	Quarter 2	Quarter 3	Quarter 4
1.23	1.04	0.98	0.97
0.92	1.24	1.17	0.93
0.97	0.86	0.92	0.91
	0.96	1.02	

It should be noted that the estimated cycles are useful if a well-defined repeating cycle of reasonable fixed duration can be recognized. In many "real-life" data this may not be possible. To obtain reliable estimates of the cyclical effect, data with several cycles should be available. Since cyclical fluctuations have a duration of 2–7 years or more, more than 25 years of data may be needed to estimate the cyclical effect and make accurate forecasts. For these reasons, the cyclical variation in time series cannot be accurately predicted. In such situations, forecasts are based on the trend and seasonal factors only. Having obtained T_t and S_t, the forecast of a future observation is given by

$$\hat{y}_t = (\hat{T}_t)(\hat{S}_t)$$

5.2.2 Additive Seasonal Variation Model

For this type of model we shall assume, for simplicity, that the series is composed of trend, seasonal effect, and error component, so that

$$y_t = T_t + S_t + I_t$$

As earlier, the trend effect can be modeled either linearly: $T_t = \beta_0 + \beta_1 t$, quadratically: $T_t = \beta_0 + \beta_1 t + \beta_2 t^2$, or exponentially: $T_t = \beta_0 \beta_1^t$ (which can be linearized through the logarithmic transformation).

The seasonal pattern may be modeled by using dummy variables. Let L denote the number of periods or seasons (quarter, month, etc.) in the year. S_t can be modeled as follows:

$$\hat{S}_t = \gamma_1 X_{1t} + \gamma_2 X_{2t} + \cdots + \gamma_{L-1} X_{L-1 t}$$

where
$$X_{1t} = \begin{cases} 1 & \text{if period } t \text{ is season 1} \\ 0 & \text{otherwise} \end{cases}$$

$$X_{2t} = \begin{cases} 1 & \text{if period } t \text{ is season 2} \\ 0 & \text{otherwise} \end{cases}$$

$$X_{L-1t} = \begin{cases} 1 & \text{if period } t \text{ is season } L - 1 \\ 0 & \text{otherwise} \end{cases}$$

For example, if $L = 4$ (quarterly data), we have

$$\begin{aligned} y_t &= T_t + S_t + I_t \\ &= T_t + \gamma_1 X_{1t} + \gamma_2 X_{2t} + \gamma_3 X_{3t} + I_t \end{aligned} \tag{5.3}$$

Similarly, if $L = 12$ (monthly data) we have

$$\begin{aligned} y_t &= T_t + S_t + I_t \\ &= T_t + \sum_{i=1}^{11} \gamma_i X_{it} + I_t \end{aligned} \tag{5.4}$$

Clearly, T_t can be represented by either a linear, quadratic, or exponential relationship.

Example 5.2 (Continued)
We now decompose an additive time series (BRD occurrence in eastern Alberta) to estimate the trend and seasonal effects under the model

$$y_t = (\beta_0 + \beta_1 t) + \gamma_1 X_{1t} + \gamma_2 X_{2t} + \gamma_3 X_{3t} \tag{5.5}$$

The following SAS program reads the data and runs the regression model. The fitted series is given by

$$\hat{y}_t = 5.6875 + 0.5563 t + 15.6688 X_{1,t} + 6.8625 X_{2,t} - 2.9438 X_{3,t}$$

from which $\hat{T}_t = 5.6875 + 0.5563t$ and $\hat{S}_t = 15.6688X_{1,t} + 6.8625X_{2,t} - 2.9438X_{3,t}$.

```
data brd;
input y x1 x2 x3 @@;
timw=_n_;
cards;
21 1 0 0 14 0 1 0 5 0 0 1 8 0 0 0
25 1 0 0 16 0 1 0 7 0 0 1 9 0 0 0
25 1 0 0 18 0 1 0 9 0 0 1 13 0 0 0
30 1 0 0 20 0 1 0 10 0 0 1 15 0 0 0
;
proc reg;
model y=time x1 x2 x3/dw;
output out=new(keep=time y x1 x2 x3 yhat yresid) p=yhat
r=yresid; run;

data new; set new; that=5.6875+0.5563*time; shat=15.6688*x1+
6.8625*x 2-2.9438*x3;

proc print data=new; run;
```

The estimated components of the series are summarized in Table 5.9.

Figure 5.5 gives the actual series and the fitted series y_t for the additive models.

TABLE 5.9

Estimated Trend and Seasonal Effect of the Series: BRD Data

Year	Quarter	t	y_t	$\hat{T}_t$	S_t	$\hat{y}_t = T_t + S_t$	$e_t = y_t - \hat{y}_t$
1	1	1	21	6.25	15.67	21.92	−0.92
	2	2	14	6.80	6.86	13.66	0.34
	3	3	5	7.36	−2.94	4.41	0.58
	4	4	8	7.91	0.00	7.91	0.09
2	1	5	25	8.47	15.67	24.14	0.86
	2	6	16	9.03	6.86	15.89	0.11
	3	7	7	9.58	−2.94	6.64	0.36
	4	8	9	10.14	0.00	10.14	−1.14
3	1	9	25	10.69	15.67	26.36	−1.36
	2	10	18	11.25	6.86	18.11	−0.11
	3	11	9	11.81	−2.94	8.86	0.14
	4	12	13	12.36	0.00	12.36	0.64
4	1	13	30	12.92	15.67	28.59	1.41
	2	14	20	13.48	6.86	20.34	−0.34
	3	15	10	14.03	−2.94	11.09	−1.09
	4	16	15	14.59	0.00	14.59	0.41

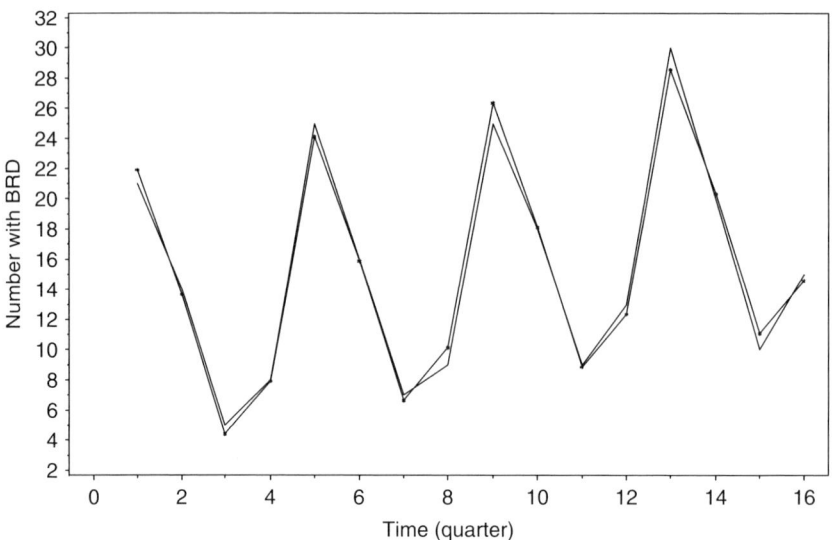

FIGURE 5.5
Observed and predicted values of y from the additive model plotted over time.

5.2.3   Detection of Seasonality: Nonparametric Test

Seasonality may be tested using a test based on ranks. The test is a simple adaptation of the nonparametric analysis of variance procedure. After removing a linear trend, if desired, we rank the values within each year from 1 (smallest) to 12 (largest) for monthly data. In general, let the years represent c columns and the months r (=12) rows. Then each column represents a permutation of the integers $1, 2, \ldots, 12$. Summing across each row gives the monthly score M_j, where $j = 1, 2, \ldots, 12$. Under the null hypothesis H_0: no seasonal pattern, the test statistic

$$T = 12 \sum_{j=1}^{r} \left\{ \frac{\left[M_j - \frac{c(r+1)}{2} \right]^2}{cr(r+1)} \right\}$$

$$= 12 \left[\sum_{j=1}^{r} \frac{M_j^2}{cr(r+1)} + \frac{c(r+1)}{4} \sum_{j=1}^{r} \frac{M_j}{r} \right] \qquad (5.6)$$

is approximately distributed as χ^2 with $(r-1)$ degrees of freedom (Kendall and Ord, 1990).

Example 5.3

The data from this example were kindly provided by J. Mallia of the Ontario Veterinary College. Cyanonsis is one of the leading causes of condemnation of poultry in Canada. To investigate seasonal patterns in the proportion of

TABLE 5.10

Number of Turkeys Condemned (per 100,000) because of Cyanosis

Month	1987	1988	1989	1990	1991	1992	1993
Jan	643.0	1168.7	1173.7	1140.4	691.2	1154.4	556.7
Feb	508.6	1422.4	1492.3	1446.4	370.9	683.0	489.3
Mar	646.2	1748.4	1600.5	1002.7	454.3	535.6	466.2
Apr	849.1	1226.9	1141.0	999.5	393.9	351.6	448.9
May	710.2	1061.0	861.0	485.1	374.0	430.2	302.1
June	653.0	905.6	706.3	416.9	253.2	371.5	260.3
July	542.2	875.7	537.7	562.6	428.2	317.1	215.6
Aug	502.6	943.0	583.3	483.7	429.5	425.2	272.9
Sept	789.5	1228.2	810.8	490.4	393.7	332.5	286.0
Oct	409.5	1286.0	750.0	670.5	387.9	327.0	270.8
Nov	836.4	1434.8	1137.6	605.6	587.0	427.6	373.3
Dec	792.4	860.3	1178.7	618.5	618.5	381.8	259.6

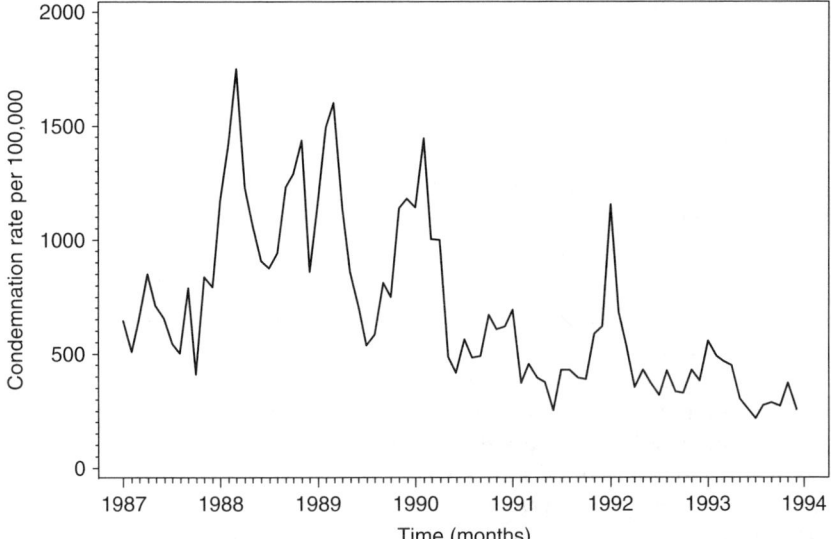

FIGURE 5.6

Time series plot of proportion of turkeys condemned.

turkeys condemned, we use the statistic (5.6). The data are summarized in Table 5.10 and plotted in Figure 5.6.

In Table 5.11 we provide the ranks, M_j and M_j^2.

$$\sum_{j=1}^{12} M_j = 546 \quad \sum_{j=1}^{12} M_j^2 = 27,750 \quad T = 31.94$$

TABLE 5.11

Ranked Values

Month	1987	1988	1989	1990	1991	1992	1993	M_j	M_j^2
1	1	6	9	11	12	12	12	63	3969
2	4	10	11	12	2	11	11	61	3721
3	6	12	12	10	9	10	10	69	4761
4	12	7	8	9	6	4	9	55	3025
5	8	5	6	3	3	9	7	41	1681
6	7	3	3	1	1	5	3	23	529
7	5	2	1	5	7	1	1	22	484
8	3	4	2	2	8	7	5	31	961
9	9	8	5	4	5	3	6	40	1600
10	2	9	4	8	4	2	4	33	1089
11	11	11	7	6	10	8	8	61	3721
12	10	1	10	7	11	6	2	47	2209

Since $\chi_{0.05,11}^2 = 19.67$, the null hypothesis of no seasonal pattern is not supported by the data.

The following SAS code is used to read the data in Table 5.10 and produce Figure 5.6.

```
data condemn;
input month:monyy5. rate @@;
rate=rate*100000;
t=_n_; year=year(month);
cards;
jan87 .006430 feb87 .005086 mar87 .006462 apr87 .008491 may87 .007102
jun87 .006530 jul87 .005422 aug87 .005026 sep87 .007895 oct87 .004095
nov87 .008364 dec87 .007924 jan88 .011687 feb88 .014224 mar88 .017484
apr88 .012269 may88 .010610 jun88 .009056 jul88 .008757 aug88 .009430
sep88 .012282 oct88 .012860 nov88 .014348 dec88 .008603 jan89 .011737
feb89 .014923 mar89 .016005 apr89 .011410 may89 .008610 jun89 .007063
jul89 .005377 aug89 .005833 sep89 .008108 oct89 .007500 nov89 .011376
dec89 .011787 jan90 .011404 feb90 .014464 mar90 .010027 apr90 .009995
may90 .004851 jun90 .004169 jul90 .005626 aug90 .004837 sep90 .004904
oct90 .006705 nov90 .006056 dec90 .006185 jan91 .006912 feb91 .003709
mar91 .004543 apr91 .003939 may91 .003740 jun91 .002532 jul91 .004282
aug91 .004295 sep91 .003937 oct91 .003879 nov91 .005870 dec91 .006185
jan92 .011544 feb92 .006830 mar92 .005356 apr92 .003516 may92 .004302
jun92 .003715 jul92 .003171 aug92 .004252 sep92 .003325 oct92 .003270
nov92 .004276 dec92 .003818 jan93 .005567 feb93 .004893 mar93 .004662
apr93 .004489 may93 .003021 jun93 .002603 jul93 .002156 aug93 .002729
sep93 .002860 oct93 .002708 nov93 .003733 dec93 .002596
;
goptions reset=global gunit=pct cback=white htitle=6 htext=3 ftext=
swissb
```

colors=(black);

*Figure 5.6: Time series plot of proportion of turkeys condemned;
axis1 order=('01jan87'd to '01jan94'd by year) label=(angle=0 'Time (Months)')
offset=(3) minor=(number = 11);
axis2 order=(0 to 2000 by 500) label=(angle=90 'Condemnation rate per 100,000');
proc gplot data=condemn;
plot rate*month / haxis=axis1 vaxis=axis2;
symbol1 i=join;
format month year4.;
run; quit;

5.2.4   Autoregressive Errors: Detection and Estimation

One of the main characteristics of a true series is that adjacent observations are likely to be correlated. One way to detect such a correlation is to plot the residuals $e_t = y_t - \hat{y}_t$ against time. This is illustrated using the additive model, where the residuals (from Table 5.9) are plotted in time order as Figure 5.7a.

From the plot one can see that the residuals have the signs $-, +, +, +, +, +, +, -, -, -, +, +, +, -, -, +$. This shows a tendency for residuals to be

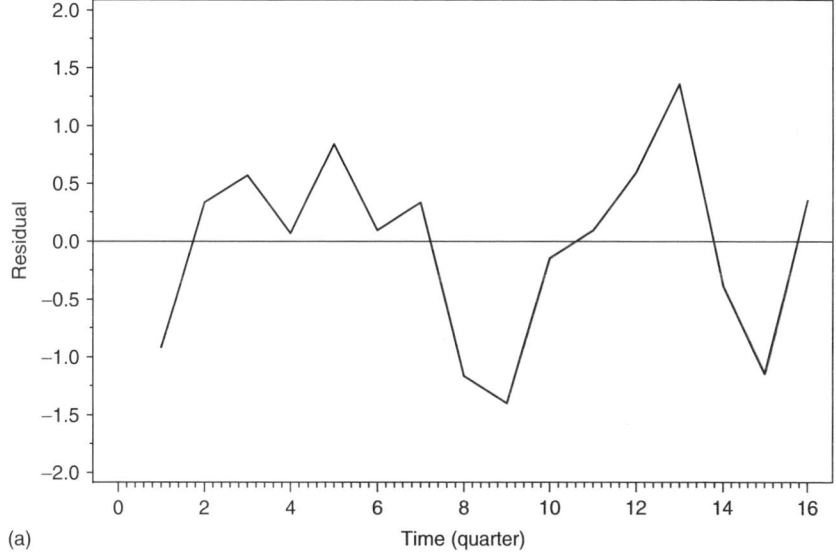

(a)

FIGURE 5.7a
Plot of residuals over time.

followed by residuals of the same sign, an indication of possible autocorrelation. Usually, the Durbin–Watson statistic (1951) given by

$$d = \frac{\sum_{t=2}^{n}(e_t - e_{t-1})^2}{\sum_{t=1}^{n} e_t^2} \tag{5.7}$$

is used to test the significance of this correlation. The sample autocorrelation is given by Equation 5.12. The Durbin–Watson option in the model statement of PROC REG would compute the Durbin–Watson d statistic to test whether the autocorrelation is zero. The relevant output is shown below.

Durbin–Watson d	1.489
Number of observations	16
First-order autocorrelation	0.201

When autocorrelation is present, ignoring its effect would produce unrealistically small standard errors for the regression estimates in the fitted model 5.5. Therefore, one has to account for the effect of this correlation to produce accurate estimates of the standard error. Our approach to modeling this autocorrelation at present will still be at a descriptive level. More rigorous treatment of the autocorrelation structure will be presented in the next section.

The simplest autocorrelation structure that we shall examine here is called the first-order "autoregression process." This model assumes that successive errors are linearly related through the relationship.

$$\varepsilon_t = \rho\varepsilon_{t-1} + u_t \tag{5.8}$$

It is assumed that $\{u_t;\ t = 1, 2, \ldots, n\}$ are independent and identically distributed $N(0,\sigma^2)$. Under the above specifications we have the model

$$y_t = \beta_0 + \beta_1 X_{1t} + \beta_2 X_{2t} + \cdots + \beta_k X_{kt} + \varepsilon_t \tag{5.9}$$

where $\varepsilon_t = \rho\varepsilon_{t-1} + u_t$ and $\rho = \mathrm{corr}(\varepsilon_t, \varepsilon_{t-1})$.

Note that

$$\rho y_{t-1} = \rho\beta_0 + \rho\beta_1 X_{1t-1} + \rho\beta_2 X_{2t-1} + \cdots + \rho\beta_k X_{kt-1} + \varepsilon_{t-1} \tag{5.10}$$

Subtracting Equation 5.10 from Equation 5.9 we have

$$\begin{aligned} y_t - \rho y_{t-1} = {} & \beta_0(1-\rho) + \beta_1(X_{1t} - \rho X_{1t-1}) + \beta_2(X_{2t} - \rho X_{2t-1}) + \cdots \\ & + \beta_k(X_{kt} - \rho X_{kt-1}) + u_t \end{aligned} \tag{5.11}$$

The last equation has u_t as an error term that satisfies the standard assumptions of inference in a linear regression model. The problem now is that the left-hand side of Equation 5.11 has a transformed response variable that depends on the unknown parameter ρ. A commonly used procedure to estimate the model parameters is to use a procedure known as Cochran and Orcutt procedure, which we outline in the following four steps.

1. Estimate the parameters of the model 5.9 using least squares or PROC REG from SAS, and compute the residuals $e_1, e_2, \ldots, e_n$.

2. From $e_1, e_2, \ldots, e_n$, evaluate the moment estimator of ρ as

$$\hat{\rho} = \frac{\sum_{t=2}^{n} e_t e_{t-1}}{\sum_{t=1}^{n} e_{t-2}^2} \tag{5.12}$$

3. Substitute $\hat{\rho}$ in place of ρ in model 5.11, which has an error term that satisfies the standard assumptions and compute revised least squares estimates.

4. From the least squares estimates obtained in step (3), compute the revised residuals and return to step (2); find an updated estimate of ρ using Equation 5.12. We iterate between step (2) and step (4) until the least squares estimate has an insignificant change between successive iterations.

5.2.5 Modeling Seasonality and Trend Using Polynomial and Trigonometric Functions

It is desirable, in many applications of time series models, to estimate both the trend and seasonal components in the series. This can be done quite effectively by expressing the series y_t as a function of polynomials in t and a combination of sine and cosine functions.

Therefore, a suggested additive model is given by

$$y_t = Q(t) + F(t) + e_t$$

where $Q(t) = \sum_{j=0}^{p} \beta_j t^j$ models the trend component and

$$F(t) = \sum_{j=1}^{q} \left[a_j \sin(2\pi jt/L) + b_j \cos(2\pi jt/L) \right]$$

models the seasonal components and L is the number of seasons in a year. Thus, $L = 4$ for quarterly data and $L = 12$ for monthly data. We may fit one of the following models, which may be suitable for modeling additive seasonal variation:

(1) $p = q = 1$

$$y_t = \beta_0 + \beta_1 t + a_1 \sin(2\pi t/L) + b_1 \cos(2\pi t/L)$$

(2) $p = 1, q = 2$

$$y_t = \beta_0 + \beta_1 t + a_1 \sin(2\pi t/L) + b_1 \cos(2\pi t/L) + a_2 \sin(4\pi t/L) + b_2 \cos(4\pi t/L)$$

Multiplicative time series may be modeled by extending either model (1) or model (2):

For model (1), a time series with multiplicative seasonal variation becomes

$$y'_t = y_t + c_1 t \sin(2\pi t/L) + c_2 t \cos(2\pi t/L)$$

whereas model (2) becomes

$$y''_t = y'_t + d_1 t \sin(4\pi t/L) + d_2 t \cos(4\pi t/L)$$

Example 5.3 (Continued)

The condemnation rate series showed significant seasonal effect. Here, we show how to model both seasonality and trend in the series. Several models were fitted using SAS PROC REG. The best model is found to be

$$\log(\text{rate}) = y_t = \beta_0 + \beta_1 t + \beta_2 t^2 + \beta_3 t^3 + a_1 \sin(2\pi t/12) + b_1 \cos(2\pi t/12)$$

The estimated coefficients are $\hat{\beta}_0 = 6.193(0.118)$, $\hat{\beta}_1 = 0.072(0.012)$, $\hat{\beta}_2 = -0.002(0.0003)$, $\hat{\beta}_3 = 14 \times 10^{-6} (2.5 \times 10^{-6})$, $\hat{a}_1 = 0.199(0.040)$, $\hat{b}_1 = 0.198(0.039)$, $R^2 = 0.769$, and the root mean square error is 0.255.

Note the PROC REG does not account for the correlation in the series. To account for such a correlation, we used PROC GENMOD. The GEE approach gave similar coefficient estimates with empirical standard errors that are robust against misspecification of the correlation structure (we assumed AR(1)).

The following SAS program will use the condemn, generate the additional variables, run the regression and GEE models, and produce Figure 5.7b.

```
data condemn; set condemn;
y=log(rate); t2=t**2; t3=t**3;
sin=sin((2*t*22)/(7*12)); cos=cos((2*t*22)/(7*12));

proc reg data=condemn noprint;
model y=t t2 t3 sin cos;
output out=new(keep=t month y yhat) p=yhat; run;

proc genmod data=condemn;
class year;
model y=t t2 t3 sin cos / dist=n link=id dscale;
```

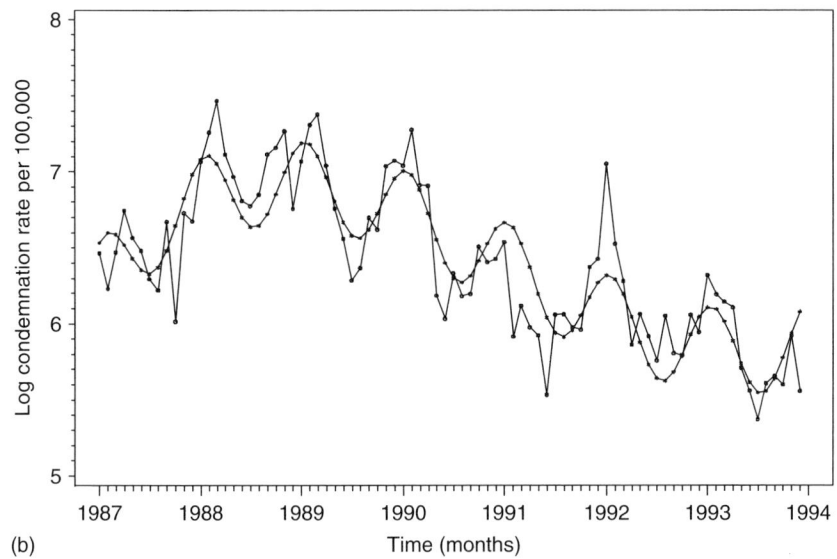

FIGURE 5.7b
Plot of the rate series with predicted series from the regression with polynomial and
trigonometric components.

```
repeated subject=year / type=ar(1);
run; quit;

axis2 order=(5 to 8 by 1) label=(angle=90 'Log condemnation rate per
100,000');
*Figure 5.7b: Plot of the rate series with predicted series from regression with
polynomial and trigonometric components;
proc gplot data=new;
symbol1 value=star i=join;
symbol2 value=circle i=join;
plot(yhat y) * month / overlay haxis=axis1 vaxis=axis2;
format month year4.;
run; quit;
```

Figure 5.7b shows the plot of the series (smooth curve) and the fitted series
using the above model.

5.3   Fundamental Concepts in the Analysis of Time Series

To establish a proper understanding of time series models, we introduce
some of the necessary fundamental concepts. Such concepts include a simple introduction to stochastic processes and autocorrelation and partial
autocorrelation functions (PACF).

5.3.1   Stochastic Processes

As earlier, y_t denotes an observation made at time t. It is assumed that for each time point t, y_t is a random variable and hence its behavior can be described by some probability distribution. We need to emphasize an important feature of time series models, which is that observations made at adjacent time points are statistically correlated. Our main objective is to investigate the nature of this correlation. Therefore, for two time points t and s, the joint behavior of (y_t, y_s) is determined from their bivariate distribution. This is generalized to the collection of observations $(y_1, y_2, \ldots, y_n)$, where their behavior is described by their multivariate joint distribution.

A stochastic process is a sequence of random variables $\{\ldots, y_{-2}, y_{-1}, y_0, y_1, y_2, \ldots\}$. We shall denote this sequence by $\{y_t; t = 0, \pm 1, \pm 2, \ldots\}$. For a given real-valued process, we define the mean function of the process:

$$\mu_t = E(y_t)$$

the variance function of the process:

$$\sigma_t^2 = E(y_t - \mu_t)^2$$

the covariance function between y_t and y_s:

$$\gamma(t, s) = E[(y_t - \mu_t)(y_s - \mu_s)]$$

and the correlation function between y_t and y_s:

$$\rho(t, s) = \frac{\gamma(t, s)}{\sqrt{\sigma_t^2 \sigma_s^2}} = \frac{\gamma(t, s)}{\sqrt{\gamma(t, t)\gamma(s, s)}}$$

From this definition it is easily verified that

$$\rho(t, t) = 1$$
$$\rho(t, s) = \rho(s, t)$$
$$|\rho(t, s)| \leq 1$$

Values of $\rho(t, s)$ near ± 1 indicate strong dependence, whereas values near zero indicate weak linear dependence.

5.3.2   Stationary Series

The notion of stationarity is quite important to make statistical inferences about the structure of the time series. The fundamental idea of stationarity is that the probability distribution of the process does not change with time. Here, we introduce two types of stationarity: the first is "strict" or "strong" stationarity and the other is "weak" stationarity. The stochastic process y_t is said to be strongly stationary if the joint distribution of $y_{t_1}, \ldots, y_{t_n}$ is the same as the joint distribution of $y_{t_1-k}, \ldots, y_{t_n-k}$ for all the choices of the points $t_1, \ldots, t_n$ and all the time lags k. To illustrate this concept, we examine the two cases $n=1$ and $n=2$. For $n=1$, the stochastic process y_t is strongly stationary if the distribution of y_t is the same as that of y_{t-k}, for any k. This implies

$$E(y_t) = E(y_{t-k})$$

and

$$V(y_t) = V(y_{t-k})$$

are constant or independent of t. For $n=2$, the process is strongly stationary if the bivariate distribution of (y_t, y_s) is the same as the bivariate distribution of (y_{t-k}, y_{s-k}), from which we have

$$\gamma(t,s) = \mathrm{Cov}(y_t, y_s) = \mathrm{Cov}(y_{t-k}, y_{s-k})$$

Setting $k=s$, we obtain

$$\gamma(t,s) = \mathrm{Cov}(y_{t-s}, y_0)$$
$$= \gamma(0, |t-s|)$$

hence

$$\gamma(t, t-k) = \gamma_k$$

and

$$\rho(t, t-k) = \rho_k$$

A process is said to be weakly stationary if

(1) $\mu_t = \mu$ for all t
(2) $\gamma(t, t-k) = \gamma(0, k)$ for all t and k

All the series that will be considered in this chapter are stationary unless otherwise specified.

5.3.3 The Autocovariance and Autocorrelation Functions

For a stationary time series $\{y_t\}$, we have already mentioned that $E(y_t) = \mu$, and $V(y_t) = E(y_t - \mu)^2$ (which are constant) and $\mathrm{Cov}(y_t, y_s)$ is a function of the time difference $|t-s|$. Hence we can write

$$\mathrm{Cov}(y_t, y_{t+k}) = E[(y_t - \mu)(y_{t+k} - \mu)] = \gamma_k$$

and

$$\rho_k = \text{Corr}(y_t, y_{t+k}) = \frac{\text{Cov}(y_t, y_{t+k})}{\sqrt{V(y_t)V(y_{t+k})}} = \frac{\gamma_k}{\gamma_0}$$

The functions γ_k and ρ_k are called the autocovariance and autocorrelation functions (ACF), respectively. Since the values of μ, γ_k, and ρ_k are unknown, the moment estimators of these parameters are as follows:

1. $\bar{y} = \frac{1}{n}\sum_{i=1}^{n} y_i$ is the sample mean estimator of μ. It is unbiased and has variance given by

$$V(\bar{y}) = \frac{1}{n^2}\sum_{t=1}^{n}\sum_{s=1}^{n}\text{Cov}(y_t, y_s)$$

From the strong stationarity assumption,

$$\text{Cov}(y_t, y_s) = \gamma(t - s)$$

Hence, letting $k = t - s$

$$V(\bar{y}) = \frac{1}{n^2}\sum_{t=1}^{n}\sum_{s=1}^{n}\gamma(t - s)$$

$$= \frac{\gamma_0}{n}\sum_{k=-(n-1)}^{n-1}\left(1 - \frac{|k|}{n}\right)\rho_k$$

$$= \frac{\gamma_0}{n}\left[1 + 2\sum_{k=1}^{n-1}\left(1 - \frac{k}{n}\right)\rho_k\right]$$

When $\rho_k = 0$ for $k = 2, 3, \ldots, n - 1$, then for large n

$$V(\bar{y}) \cong \frac{\gamma_0}{n}\left[1 + 2\left(\frac{n - 1}{n}\right)\rho_1\right] \cong \frac{\gamma_0}{n}(1 + 2\rho_1)$$

2. $\hat{\gamma}_k = \frac{1}{n}\sum_{t=1}^{n-k} (y_t - \bar{y})(y_{t+k} - \bar{y})$ is the moment estimate of the autocovariance function.

A natural moment estimator for the ACF is defined as

$$\hat{\rho}_k = \frac{\hat{\gamma}_k}{\hat{\gamma}_0} = \frac{\sum_{t=1}^{n-k} (y_t - \bar{y})(y_{t+k} - \bar{y})}{\sum_{t=1}^{n} (y_t - \bar{y})^2} \qquad k = 0, 1, 2, \ldots \qquad (5.13)$$

A plot of $\hat{\rho}_k$ versus k is sometimes called a sample correlogram. Note that $\hat{\rho}_k = \hat{\rho}_{-k}$, which means that the sample ACF is symmetric around $k = 0$.

For a stationary Gaussian process, Bartlett (1946) showed that for $k > 0$ and $k + j > 0$,

$$\text{Cov}(\hat{\rho}_k, \hat{\rho}_{k+j}) \cong \frac{1}{n} \sum_{t=-\infty}^{\infty} \left(\rho_t \rho_{t+j} + \rho_{t+j+k} \rho_{t-k} - 2\rho_k \rho_t \rho_{t-k-j} \right.$$

$$\left. -2\rho_{k+j} \rho_t \rho_{t-k} + 2\rho_k \rho_{k+j} \rho_t^2 \right) \qquad (5.14)$$

For large n, $\hat{\rho}_k$ is approximately normally distributed with mean ρ_k and variance

$$V(\hat{\rho}_k) \cong \frac{1}{n} \sum_{t=-\infty}^{\infty} \left(\rho_t^2 + \rho_{t+k} \rho_{t-k} - 4\rho_k \rho_t \rho_{t-k} + 2\rho_k^2 \rho_t^2 \right)$$

For processes with $\rho_k = 0$ for $k > l$, Bartlett's approximation becomes

$$V(\hat{\rho}_k) \cong \frac{1}{n} \left(1 + 2\rho_1^2 + 2\rho_2^2 + \cdots + 2\rho_l^2 \right) \qquad (5.15)$$

In practice, ρ_i $(i = 1, 2, \ldots, l)$ are unknown and are replaced by their sample estimates $\hat{\rho}_i$; the large sample variance of $\hat{\rho}_k$ is approximated by replacing ρ_i by $\hat{\rho}_i$ in Equation 5.15.

5.4 Models for Stationary Time Series

In this section, we consider models based on an observation made by Yule (1927) that time series in which successive values are autocorrelated can be modeled as a linear combination (or linear filter) of a sequence of uncorrelated random variables. Suppose that $\{a_t; t = 0, \pm 1, \pm 2, \ldots\}$ are a sequence of identically distributed uncorrelated random variables with $E(a_t) = 0$ and $V(a_t) = \sigma^2$, and $\text{Cov}(a_t, a_{t-k}) = 0$ for all $k \neq 0$. Such a sequence is commonly known as a "white noise." With this definition of white noise, we introduce the linear filter representation of the process y_t.

A general linear process y_t is one that can be presented as

$$y_t = a_t + \psi_1 a_{t-1} + \psi_2 a_{t-2} + \cdots$$

$$= \sum_{j=0}^{\infty} \psi_j a_{t-j} \qquad \psi_0 = 1$$

For the infinite series of the right-hand side of the above equation to be meaningful, it is assumed that

$$\sum_{j=1}^{\infty} \psi_j^2 < \infty$$

5.4.1 Autoregressive Processes

As their name implies, autoregressive processes are regressions on themselves. To be more specific, the pth order autoregressive process y_t satisfies

$$y_t = \phi_1 y_{t-1} + \phi_2 y_{t-2} + \cdots + \phi_p y_{t-p} + a_t \qquad (5.16)$$

In this model, the present value y_t is a linear combination of its p most recent values plus an "innovation" term a_t, which includes everything in the series at time t that is not explained by the past values. It is also assumed that a_t is independent of $y_{t-1}, y_{t-2}, \ldots$

Before we examine the general autoregressive process, we first consider the first-order autoregressive model that is denoted by AR(1).

5.4.1.1 AR(1) Model

Let y_t be a stationary series such that

$$y_t = \phi y_{t-1} + a_t \qquad (5.17)$$

Most textbooks write the above model as

$$y_t - \mu = \phi(y_{t-1} - \mu) + a_t$$

where μ is the mean of the series. However, we shall use Equation 5.17 assuming that the mean has been subtracted from the series. The requirement $|\phi| < 1$ is a necessary and sufficient condition for stationarity.

From Equation 5.17, $V(y_t) = \phi^2 V(y_{t-1}) + V(a_t)$ or $\gamma_0 = \phi^2 \gamma_0 + \sigma_a^2$ from which

$$\gamma_0 = \frac{\sigma_a^2}{1 - \phi^2} \qquad (5.18)$$

Multiplying both sides of Equation 5.17 by y_{t-k} and taking the expectation, the result is

$$E(y_t y_{t-k}) = \phi E(y_{t-1} y_{t-k}) + E(y_{t-k} a_t)$$

By the stationarity of the series and the independence of y_{t-1} and a_t

$$\gamma_k = \phi \gamma_{k-1}, \qquad k = 1, 2, \ldots$$

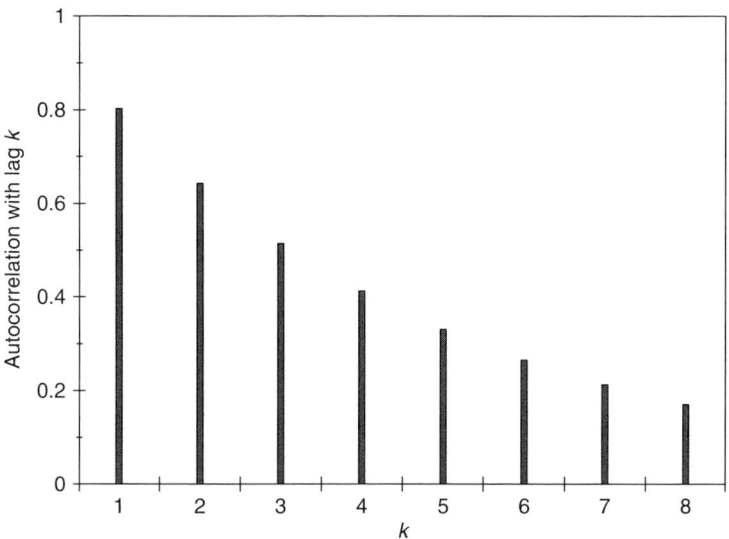

FIGURE 5.8
Autocorrelation plot for a ϕ of 0.8 and $k = 1, 2, \ldots, 8$.

For $k = 1$

$$\gamma_1 = \phi\gamma_0 = \phi\frac{\sigma_a^2}{1-\phi^2}$$

For $k = 2$

$$\gamma_2 = \phi\gamma_1 = \phi\left(\phi\frac{\sigma_a^2}{1-\phi^2}\right) = \phi^2\frac{\sigma_a^2}{1-\phi^2} = \phi^2\gamma_0$$

By mathematical induction one can show that

$$\gamma_k = \phi^k\gamma_0$$

or

$$\rho_k = \frac{\gamma_k}{\gamma_0} = \phi^k \tag{5.19}$$

Note that since $|\phi| < 1$, the autocorrelation function is exponentially decreasing in k. For $0 < \phi < 1$, all ρ_k are positive. For $-1 < \phi < 0$, $\rho_1 < 0$ and the sign of successive autocorrelations alternate (positive if k is even and negative if k is odd). Figures 5.8 and 5.9 are graphs of ρ for $\phi = 0.8$ and -0.5.

5.4.1.2 AR(2) Model (Yule's Process)

The second-order autoregressive process AR(2) is a stationary series y_t that is a linear combination of the two preceding observations and can be written as

$$y_t = \phi_1 y_{t-1} + \phi_2 y_{t-2} + a_t \tag{5.20}$$

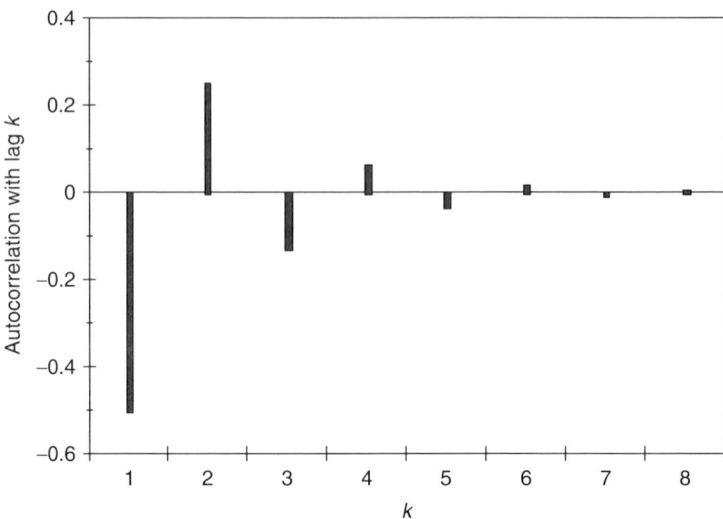

FIGURE 5.9
Autocorrelation plot for a ϕ of -0.5 and $k = 1, 2, \ldots, 8$.

To ensure stationarity, the coefficients ϕ_1 and ϕ_2 must satisfy

$$\phi_1 + \phi_2 < 1$$
$$\phi_2 - \phi_1 < 1$$
$$-1 < \phi_2 < 1$$

The above conditions are called the stationarity conditions for the AR(2) model.

To derive the autocorrelation function for the AR(2), we multiply both sides of Equation 5.20 by y_{t-k} ($k = 1, 2, \ldots$) and take the expectations. Under the assumptions of independence of y_t and a_t and the stationarity of the series, we have

$$E(y_t y_{t-k}) = \phi_1 E(y_{t-1} y_{t-k}) + \phi_2 E(y_{t-2} y_{t-k}) + E(a_t y_{t-k})$$

from which

$$\gamma_k = \phi_1 \gamma_{k-1} + \phi_2 \gamma_{k-2} \qquad\qquad (5.21)$$

and dividing by γ_0 we get

$$\rho_k = \phi_1 \rho_{k-1} + \phi_2 \rho_{k-2} \qquad\qquad (5.22)$$

Equation 5.22 is called the Yule–Walker equation. For $k = 1$,

$$\rho_1 = \phi_1 \rho_0 + \phi_2 \rho_{-1}$$

Since $\rho_0 = 1$ and $\rho_{-1} = \rho_1$ we have

$$\rho_1 = \frac{\phi_1}{1 - \phi_2}$$

For $k = 2$

$$\rho_2 = \phi_1 \rho_1 + \phi_2$$

or

$$\rho_2 = \phi_2 + \frac{\phi_1^2}{1 - \phi_2}$$

Note also that the variance of the AR(2) process can be written in terms of the model parameters. In fact, from Equation 5.20 we have

$$V(y_t) = \phi_1^2 V(y_{t-1}) + \phi_2^2 V(y_{t-2}) + 2\phi_1\phi_2 \text{Cov}(y_{t-1}, y_{t-2}) + \sigma_a^2$$

or

$$\gamma_0 = \phi_1^2 \gamma_0 + \phi_2^2 \gamma_0 + 2\phi_1\phi_2\gamma_1 + \sigma_a^2 \tag{5.23}$$

Setting $k = 1$ in Equation 5.21 we have

$$\gamma_1 = \phi_1 \gamma_0 + \phi_2 \gamma_{-1}$$
$$= \phi_1 \gamma_0 + \phi_2 \gamma_1$$

which gives

$$\gamma_1 = \phi_1 \frac{\gamma_0}{1 - \phi_2} \tag{5.24}$$

Substituting in Equation 5.23,

$$\gamma_0 = (\phi_1^2 + \phi_2^2)\gamma_0 + 2\phi_1^2\phi_2 \frac{\gamma_0}{1 - \phi_2} + \sigma_a^2$$

and hence

$$\gamma_0 = \frac{\sigma_a^2(1 - \phi_2)}{(1 - \phi_2)(1 - \phi_1^2 - \phi_2^2) - 2\phi_1^2\phi_2} \tag{5.25}$$

It should be noted that for $-1 < \phi_2 < 0$, the AR(2) process tends to exhibit sinusoidal behavior, regardless of the value of ϕ_1. When $0 < \phi_2 < 1$, the behavior of the process will depend on the sign of ϕ_1. For $\phi_1 < 0$, the AR(2) process tends to oscillate and the series shows ups and downs.

5.4.2 Moving Average Processes

Another type of stochastic model that belongs to the class of linear filter models is called an MA process. This is given as

$$y_t = a_t - \theta_1 a_{t-1} - \theta_2 a_{t-2} - \cdots - \theta_q a_{t-q}$$

This series is called a "moving average" of order q and is denoted by MA(q).

5.4.2.1 First-Order Moving Average Process MA(1)

Here we have

$$y_t = a_t - \theta a_{t-1} \tag{5.26}$$

$$E(y_t) = 0$$

$$\gamma_0 = V(y_t) = \sigma_a^2 + \theta^2 \sigma_a^2 = \sigma_a^2(1 + \theta^2)$$

Moreover,

$$\text{Cov}(y_t, y_{t-1}) = E(y_t y_{t-1})$$

$$= E\big[(a_t - \theta a_{t-1})(a_{t-1} - \theta a_{t-2})\big]$$

$$= E(a_t a_{t-1}) - \theta\Big[E(a_{t-1}^2) + E(a_t a_{t-2})\Big] + \theta^2 E(a_{t-1} a_{t-2})$$

Since $a_1, a_2, \ldots$ are independent with $E(a_t) = 0$ for all t, then

$$\gamma_1 = \text{Cov}(y_t, y_{t-1}) = -\theta \sigma_a^2$$

$$\text{Cov}(y_t, y_{t-k}) = 0, \quad k = 2, 3, \ldots$$

Furthermore, the autocorrelation function is

$$\rho_1 = \frac{\gamma_1}{\gamma_0} = -\frac{\theta}{1 + \theta^2} \tag{5.27}$$

$$\rho_k = 0 \quad k = 2, 3, \ldots$$

Note that if θ is replaced by $1/\theta$ in Equation 5.27, we get exactly the same autocorrelation function. This lack of uniqueness of MA(1) models must be rectified before we estimate the model parameters.

Rewriting Equation 5.26 as

$$a_t = y_t + \theta a_{t-1}$$

$$= y_t + \theta(y_{t-1} + \theta a_{t-2})$$

$$= y_t + \theta y_{t-1} + \theta^2 a_{t-2}$$

and continuing this substitution,

$$a_t = y_t + \theta y_{t-1} + \theta^2 y_{t-2} + \cdots$$

or

$$y_t = -(\theta y_{t-1} + \theta^2 y_{t-2} + \cdots) + a_t \tag{5.28}$$

If $|\theta| < 1$, we see that the MA(1) model can be inverted into an infinite-order AR process. It can be shown (see Box and Jenkins, 1970) that there is only one invertible MA(1) model with the given autocorrelation function ρ_1.

5.4.2.2 Second-Order Moving Average Process MA(2)

An MA(2) process is defined by

$$y_t = a_t - \theta_1 a_{t-1} - \theta_2 a_{t-2} \tag{5.29}$$

The autocovariance functions are given by

$$
\begin{aligned}
\gamma_1 &= \text{Cov}(y_t, y_{t-1}) \\
&= E\big[(a_t - \theta_1 a_{t-1} - \theta_2 a_{t-2})(a_{t-1} - \theta_1 a_{t-2} - \theta_2 a_{t-3})\big] \\
&= -\theta_1 \sigma_a^2 + \theta_1 \theta_2 \sigma_a^2 \\
&= (-\theta_1 + \theta_1 \theta_2)\sigma_a^2
\end{aligned}
$$

$$
\begin{aligned}
\gamma_2 &= \text{Cov}(y_t, y_{t-2}) \\
&= E\big[(a_t - \theta_1 a_{t-1} - \theta_2 a_{t-2})(a_{t-2} - \theta_1 a_{t-3} - \theta_2 a_{t-4})\big] \\
&= -\theta_2 \sigma_a^2
\end{aligned}
$$

and

$$
\begin{aligned}
\gamma_0 &= V(y_t) \\
&= \sigma_a^2 + \theta_1^2 \sigma_a^2 + \theta_2^2 \sigma_a^2 \\
&= (1 + \theta_1^2 + \theta_2^2)\sigma_a^2
\end{aligned}
$$

Therefore, for an MA(2) process

$$\rho_1 = \frac{\gamma_1}{\gamma_0} = \frac{-\theta_1 + \theta_1 \theta_2}{1 + \theta_1^2 + \theta_2^2} \tag{5.30}$$

$$\rho_2 = \frac{\gamma_2}{\gamma_0} = -\frac{\theta_2}{1 + \theta_1^2 + \theta_2^2} \tag{5.31}$$

$$\rho_k = 0 \qquad k = 3, 4, \ldots$$

5.4.3   The Mixed Autoregressive Moving Average Processes

In modeling time series, we are interested in constructing a parsimonious model. One type of such a model is obtained from mixing an AR(p) with an MA(q). The general form of this is given by

$$y_t = (\phi_1 y_{t-1} + \phi_2 y_{t-2} + \cdots + \phi_p y_{t-p}) + (a_t - \theta_1 a_{t-1} - \theta_2 a_{t-2} - \cdots - \theta_q a_{t-q}) \quad (5.32)$$

The process y_t, defined in Equation 5.32, is called the mixed autoregressive MA process of orders p and q, or ARMA (p,q).

An important special case of the ARMA(p,q) is ARMA(1,1) which can be obtained from Equation 5.32 for $p = q = 1$. Therefore, an ARMA(1,1) is

$$y_t = \phi y_{t-1} + a_t - \theta a_{t-1} \quad (5.33)$$

For stationarity we assume that $|\phi| < 1$ and for invertibility, we require that $|\theta| < 1$. When $\phi = 0$, Equation 5.33 is reduced to an MA(1) process, and when $\theta = 0$, it is reduced to an AR(1) process. Thus, the AR(1) and MA(1) may be regarded as special processes of the ARMA(1,1).

To obtain the autocovariance for the ARMA(1,1), we multiply both sides of Equation 5.33 by y_{t-k} and take the expectations

$$E(y_t y_{t-k}) = \phi E(y_{t-1} y_{t-k}) + E(a_t y_{t-k}) - \theta E(a_{t-1} y_{t-k})$$

from which

$$\gamma_k = \phi \gamma_{k-1} + E(a_t y_{t-k}) - \theta E(a_{t-1} y_{t-k}) \quad (5.34)$$

For $k = 0$

$$\gamma_0 = \phi \gamma_1 + E(a_t y_t) - \theta E(a_{t-1} y_t) \quad (5.35)$$

and

$$E(a_t y_t) = \sigma_a^2$$

Noting that

$$E(a_{t-1} y_t) = \phi E(a_{t-1} y_{t-1}) + E(a_t a_{t-1}) - \theta E(a_{t-1}^2)$$
$$= \phi \sigma_a^2 - \theta \sigma_a^2 = (\phi - \theta) \sigma_a^2$$

and substituting in Equation 5.35 we see that

$$\gamma_0 = \phi \gamma_1 + \sigma_a^2 - \theta(\phi - \theta) \sigma_a^2 \quad (5.36)$$

and from Equation 5.34 when $k = 1$,

$$\gamma_1 = \phi \gamma_0 + E(a_t y_{t-1}) - \theta E(a_{t-1} y_{t-1})$$
$$= \phi \gamma_0 + E(a_t y_{t-1}) - \theta \sigma_a^2 \quad (5.37)$$

But

$$E(a_t y_t) = \phi E(a_t y_{t-1}) + E(a_t^2) - \theta E(a_t a_{t-1})$$

or

$$a_a^2 = \phi E(a_t y_{t-1}) + a_a^2$$

so

$$E(a_t y_{t-1}) = 0 \tag{5.38}$$

Substituting Equation 5.38 in Equation 5.37,

$$\gamma_1 = \phi \gamma_0 - \theta \sigma_a^2 \tag{5.39}$$

and using this in Equation 5.36 we have

$$\gamma_0 = \phi^2 \gamma_0 - \phi \theta \sigma_a^2 + \sigma_a^2 - \phi \theta \sigma_a^2 + \theta^2 \sigma_a^2$$

from which

$$\gamma_0 = \frac{1 + \theta^2 - 2\phi\theta}{1 - \phi^2} \sigma_a^2$$

Thus,

$$\gamma_1 = \phi \left(\frac{1 + \theta^2 - 2\phi\theta}{1 - \phi^2} \right) \sigma_a^2 - \theta \sigma_a^2$$

$$= \frac{(\phi - \theta)(1 - \phi\theta)}{1 - \phi^2} \sigma_a^2$$

From Equation 5.34, we have

$$\gamma_k = \phi \gamma_{k-1}$$

Hence, the ARMA(1,1) has the following ACF

$$\rho_k = \begin{cases} 1 & k = 0 \\ \dfrac{(\phi - \theta)(1 - \phi\theta)}{1 + \theta^2 - 2\phi\theta} & k = 1 \\ \phi \rho_{k-1} & k \geq 2 \end{cases} \tag{5.40}$$

5.5 ARIMA Models

A series y_t is said to follow an ARIMA model of order d if the dth difference denoted by $\nabla^d y_t$ is a stationary ARMA model. The notation used for this model is ARIMA (p,d,q), where p is the order of the autoregressive component, q the order of the MA component, and d the number of differences performed to produce a stationary series. Fortunately, for practical reasons we can take $d = 1$ or 2.

An ARIMA $(p,1,q)$ process can be written as

$$w_t = \phi_1 w_{t-1} + \phi_2 w_{t-2} + \cdots + \phi_p w_{t-p} + a_t - \theta_1 a_{t-1} - \theta_2 a_{t-2} - \cdots - \theta_q a_{t-q} \quad (5.41)$$

where

$$w_t = y_t - y_{t-1}$$

As an example, the ARIMA $(0,1,1)$ or the IMA$(1,1)$ is given by

$$\begin{aligned} w_t &= a_t - \theta_1 a_{t-1} \qquad \text{or} \\ y_t &= y_{t-1} + a_t - \theta_1 a_{t-1} \end{aligned} \qquad (5.42)$$

which means that the first difference $(d = 1)$ would produce a stationary MA(1) series as long as $|\theta_1| < 1$.

Example 5.1 (Continued)

Using the SCC data, we will fit two models: the AR(1) and the MA(1). This will be accomplished by running the PROC ARIMA in SAS/ETS. The data were differenced once so as to stabilize the mean.

The following SAS/PROC ARIMA code produces the plots of the ACF and the partial correlation function and forecasts for the AR(1) and MA(1) models.

```
* fitting an AR(1) model;
proc arima data=scc;
identify var=scc(1) nlags=20;
estimate p=1/plot;
forecast lead=12 id=time interval=month;
run; quit;
```

```
* fitting an MA(1) model;
proc arima data=scc;
identify var=scc(1) nlags=20;
estimate q=1/plot;
forecast lead=12 id=time interval=month;
run; quit;
```

Note that $p(1)$ is replaced by $q(1)$ to fit an MA(1) seasonal model.

The partial SAS output is shown below.

		Autocorrelations	
Lag	Covariance	Correlation −1 9 8 7 6 5 4 3 2 1 0 1 2 3 4 5 6 7 8 9 1	Std Error
0	1007.500	1.00000 | |********************|	0
1	−207.536	−0.20599 | ****| . |	0.109764
2	−293.539	−0.29135 | ******| . |	0.114327
3	177.445	0.17612 | . |****. |	0.122948
4	16.087389	0.01597 | . | . |	0.125951
5	−196.800	−0.19533 | .****| . |	0.125975
6	43.477143	0.04315 | . |* . |	0.129573
7	−110.087	−0.10927 | . **| . |	0.129746
8	−90.458840	−0.08979 | . **| . |	0.130850
9	129.236	0.12827 | . |***. |	0.131590
10	15.333874	0.01522 | . | . |	0.133088
11	−103.832	−0.10306 | . **| . |	0.133109
12	244.896	0.24307 | . |***** |	0.134067
13	186.837	0.18545 | . |****. |	0.139276
14	−175.962	−0.17465 | . ***| . |	0.142219
15	−86.242765	−0.08560 | . **| . . |	0.144781
16	44.315590	0.04399 | . |* . |	0.145389
17	12.768269	0.01267 | . | . |	0.145549
18	−114.418	−0.11357 | . **| . |	0.145563
19	−65.211117	−0.06473 | . *| . |	0.146626
20	−3.510942	−0.00348 | . | . |	0.146970

Note: . marks two standard errors.

The maximum likelihood and the least squares estimates of the parameters of the AR(1) and MA(1) models are shown below.

AR(1)

	Parameter	Estimate	Std Error
Least square	μ	−0.309	2.854
	AR1,1	−0.211	0.110
MLE	μ	−0.301	2.855
	AR1,1	−0.210	0.110

MA(1)

	Parameter	Estimate	Std Error
Least square	μ	−0.01804	1.71859
	MA1,1	0.49064	0.09976
MLE	μ	−0.02744	1.73327
	MA1,1	0.48592	0.10055

Remarks

The ACF lists the estimated autocorrelation coefficients at each lag. The value of the ACF at lag 0 is always 1. The dotted lines provide an approximate

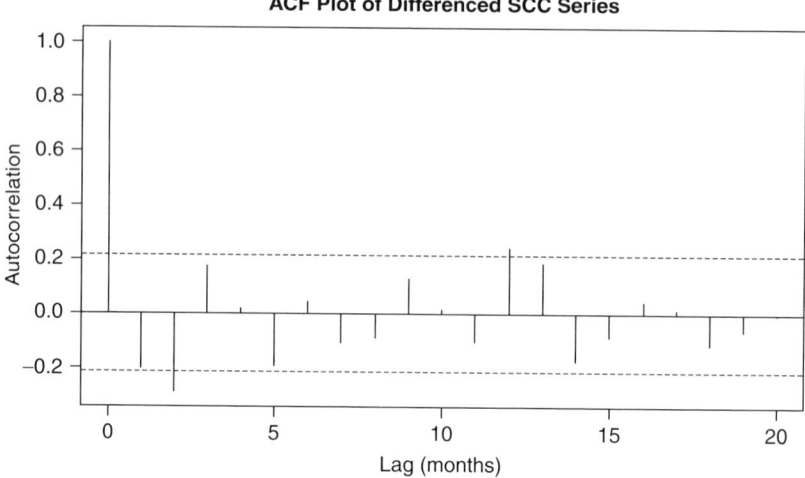

FIGURE 5.10
The ACF plot of the differenced series.

95% confidence limit for the autocorrelation estimate at each lag. If none of
the autocorrelation estimates fall outside the strip defined by the two dotted
lines (and no outliers in the data), one may assume the absence of serial correlation. In effect, the ACF is a measure of how important the sequence of
distant observations $y_{t-1}, y_{t-2}, \ldots$ are to the current time series value y_t.

The PACF is the ACF at lag p accounting for the effects of all intervening
observations. Thus, the PACF at lag 1 is identical to the ACF at lag 1, but they
are different at higher lags.

The following R code may be used to produce the autocorrelations and the
ACF plot and to fit the AR(1) model by the conditional least squares method
(Figure 5.10).

```
scc <- c(317,292,283,286,314,301,317,344,367,351,321,398,
    345,310,307,310,340,325,340,370,400,380,345,330,
    370,360,300,310,389,320,340,400,395,350,400,350,
    350,420,360,340,335,350,360,395,380,375,402,460,
    400,385,350,325,345,350,375,410,360,375,370,395,
    370,335,305,325,310,315,350,370,350,345,355,340,
    340,345,325,330,360,330,345,350,350,345,325,280)

scc.acf <- acf(diff(scc), lag.max = 20, type ="correlation",plot=F)
scc.acf
plot(scc.acf,ylab="Autocorrelation",xlab="Lag (in Months)", main=
"ACF Plot of Differenced SCC Series")
scc.ar1 <- arima(scc, order = c(1,1,0), method ="CSS")
scc.ar1
```

5.6 Forecasting

One of the most important objectives of time series analysis is to forecast the future values of the series. The term forecasting is used more frequently in recent time series literature than the term prediction. However, most forecasting results are derived from a general theory of linear prediction developed by Kolmogorov (1939, 1941), Kalman (1960), Whittle (1983), and many others.

Once a good time series model has become available, it can be used to make inferences about future observations. What we mean by a good model is that identification, estimation, and diagnostics have been completed. Even with good time series models, the reliability of the forecast is based on the assumption that the future behaves like the past. However, the nature of the stochastic process may change in time and the current time series model may no longer be appropriate. If this happens, the resulting forecast may be misleading. This is particularly true for forecasts with a long lead time.

Let y_n denote the last value of the time series, and let us suppose that we are interested in forecasting the value that will be observed l time periods ($l > 0$) in the future and also that we are interested in forecasting the future value y_{n+l}. We denote the forecast of y_{n+l} by $y_n(l)$, where the subscript denotes the forecast origin and the number in parentheses denotes the lead time. Box and Jenkins (1970) showed that the "best" forecast of y_{n+l} is given by the expected value of y_{n+l} at time n, where best is defined as that forecast that minimizes the mean square error,

$$E[y_{n+l} - \hat{y}_n(l)]^2$$

It should be noted that the above expectation is in fact a conditional expectation since, in general, it will depend on $y_1, y_2, \ldots, y_n$. This expectation is minimized when

$$\hat{y}_n(l) \cong E(y_{n+l})$$

We now show how to obtain the forecast for the time series models AR(1), AR(2), and MA(1).

5.6.1 AR(1) Model

$$y_t - \mu = \phi(y_{t-1} - \mu) + a_t \tag{5.43}$$

Consider the problem of forecasting 1 time unit into the future. Replacing t by $t+1$ in Equation 5.43 we have

$$y_{t+1} - \mu = \phi(y_t - \mu) + a_{t+1} \tag{5.44}$$

Conditional on $y_1, y_2, \ldots, y_{t-1}, y_t$, the expectation of both sides of Equation 5.44 is

$$E(y_{t+1}) - \mu = \phi\{E(y_t|y_t, y_{t-1}, \ldots, y_1) - \mu\} + E(a_{t+1}|y_t, y_{t-1}, \ldots, y_1)$$

Since

$$E(y_t|y_t, y_{t-1}, \ldots, y_1) = y_t$$
$$E(a_{t+1}|y_t, y_{t-1}, \ldots, y_1) = E(a_{t+1}) = 0$$

and

$$E(y_{t+1}) = \hat{y}_t(1)$$

then

$$\hat{y}_t(1) - \mu = \mu + \phi(y_t - \mu) \tag{5.45}$$

For a general lead time l, we replace t by $t + l$ in Equation 5.43 and taking the conditional expectation we get

$$\hat{y}_t(l) = \mu + \phi(y_t(l-1) - \mu) \qquad l \geq 1 \tag{5.46}$$

It is clear now that Equation 5.46 is recursive in l. It can also be shown that

$$\hat{y}_t(l) = \mu + \phi^l(y_t - \mu) \qquad l \geq 1 \tag{5.47}$$

Since $|\phi| < 1$, we may simply have

$$\hat{y}_t(l) \cong \mu \qquad \text{for large } l$$

Now let us consider the one step-ahead, forecast error, $e_t(1)$. From Equation 5.44 and 5.45

$$
\begin{aligned}
e_t(1) &= y_{t+1} - \hat{y}_t(1) \\
&= \mu + \phi(y_t - \mu) + a_{t+1} - \left[\mu + \phi(y_t - \mu)\right] \\
&= a_{t+1}
\end{aligned}
\tag{5.48}
$$

This means that the white noise a_{t+1} can now be explained as a sequence of one-step-ahead forecast errors. From Equation 5.48

$$V[e_t(1)] = V(a_{t+1}) = \sigma_a^2$$

It can be shown (see Abraham and Ledolter, 1983, p. 241) that for the AR(1)

$$V[e_t(l)] = \frac{1 - \phi^{2l}}{1 - \phi^2}\sigma_a^2 \tag{5.49}$$

and for large l,

$$V[e_t(l)] \cong \frac{\sigma_a^2}{1 - \phi^2} \tag{5.50}$$

5.6.2 AR(2) Model

Consider the AR(2) model

$$y_t - \mu = \phi_1(y_{t-1} - \mu) + \phi_2(y_{t-2} - \mu) + a_t$$

Setting $t = t + l$, the above equation is written as

$$y_{t+l} - \mu = \phi_1(y_{t+l-1} - \mu) + \phi_2(y_{t+l-2} - \mu) + a_{t+l}$$

For the one-step-ahead forecast (i.e., $l = 1$)

$$y_{t+1} = \mu + \phi_1(y_t - \mu) + \phi_2(y_{t-1} - \mu) + a_{t+1} \tag{5.51}$$

From the observed series, y_t and y_{t-1} are the last two observations in the series. Therefore, for given values of the model parameters, the only unknown quantity on the right-hand side of Equation 5.51 is a_{t+1}. Therefore, conditional on $y_t, y_{t-1}, \ldots, y_1$ we have

$$E(y_{t+1}) = \mu + \phi_1(y_t - \mu) + \phi_2(y_{t-1} - \mu) + E(a_{t+1})$$

By assumption, $E(a_{t+1}) = 0$, and hence the forecast of y_{t+1} is

$$\hat{y}_t(1) = E(y_{t+1})$$
$$= \mu + \phi_1(y_t - \mu) + \phi_2(y_{t-1} - \mu)$$

where μ, ϕ_1, and ϕ_2 are replaced by their estimates. In general, we have

$$\hat{y}_t(l) = E(y_{t-l})$$
$$= \mu + \phi_1(\hat{y}_t(l-1) - \mu) + \phi_2(y_t(l-2) - \mu) \qquad l > 3 \tag{5.52}$$

The forecast error is given by

$$e_t(l) = y_t(l) - \hat{y}_t(l)$$

For $l = 1$

$$V[e_t(l)] = \sigma_a^2 \left[1 + \psi_1^2 + \psi_2^2 + \cdots + \psi_{l-1}^2 \right] \tag{5.53}$$

where

$$\psi_1 = \phi_1 \quad \psi_2 = \phi_1^2 + \phi_2$$
$$\psi_j = \phi_1 \psi_{j-1} + \phi_2 \psi_{j-2} \qquad j > 2$$

For $l = 1$

$$V[e_t(1)] = \sigma_a^2 [1 + \phi_1^2 + (\phi_1^2 + \phi_2)^2] \tag{5.54}$$

(see Abraham and Ledoter, 1983, p. 243).

5.6.3 MA(1) Model

In a similar manner, we show how to forecast an MA(1) time series model

$$y_t = \mu + a_t - \theta a_{t-1}$$

First, we replace t by $t + l$ so that

$$y_{t+l} = \mu + a_{t+l} + \theta a_{t+l-1} \qquad (5.55)$$

Conditional on the observed series we have

$$\hat{y}_t(l) = \mu + a_{t+l} + \theta a_{t+l-1} \qquad (5.56)$$

because for $l > 1$ both a_{t+l} and a_{t+l-1} are independent of $y_t, y_{t-1}, \ldots, y_1$. Hence

$$\hat{y}_t(l) = \begin{cases} \mu & l > 1 \\ \mu - \theta a_t & l = 1 \end{cases}$$

$$V[\hat{y}_t(l)] = \begin{cases} \sigma_a^2(1 + \theta) & l > 1 \\ \sigma_a^2 & l = 1 \end{cases} \qquad (5.57)$$

The above results allow constructing $(1 - \alpha)100\%$ confidence limits on the future observations y_{t+l} as

$$\hat{y}_t(l) \pm Z_{1-\alpha/2}\sqrt{V[e_t(l)]} \qquad (5.58)$$

Example 5.1 (Continued)

Again, using the SCC data of Example 5.1, we can compute forecasts for the variable SCC by employing the time series programs in SAS. The following estimates and 95% upper and lower confidence limits are obtained for the AR(1) model.

Forecasts for Variable SCC

Obs	Forecast	Std Error	95% Confidence Limits	
85	289.1262	31.4242	227.5360	350.7164
86	286.8251	40.0251	208.3773	365.2729
87	286.9365	47.8325	193.1866	380.6865
88	286.5386	54.3920	179.9324	393.1449
89	286.2483	60.2682	168.1247	404.3718
90	285.9352	65.6151	157.3319	414.5385
91	285.6269	70.5591	147.3337	423.9202
92	285.3176	75.1784	137.9708	432.6645
93	285.0086	79.5298	129.1330	440.8842
94	284.6995	83.6553	120.7382	448.6608
95	284.3904	87.5866	112.7238	456.0569
96	284.0812	91.3489	105.0407	463.1218

The R code and the resulting output of the forecast of the SSC series are displayed below.

```
> scc.pr <- predict(scc.ar1,n.ahead=12)
> U=scc.pr$pred+2*scc.pr$se
> L=scc.pr$pred-2*scc.pr$se
> cbind(L,scc.pr$pred,U)
Time Series:
Start = 85
End = 96
Frequency = 1
        L scc.pr$pred    U
85 227.2818  289.5057 351.7296
86 208.2472  287.4977 366.7483
87 193.2132  287.9219 382.6306
88 180.1368  287.8323 395.5279
89 168.5212  287.8512 407.1813
90 157.9308  287.8472 417.7637
91 148.1431  287.8481 427.5531
92 138.9971  287.8479 436.6987
93 130.3816  287.8479 445.3143
94 122.2135  287.8479 453.4824
95 114.4298  287.8479 461.2661
96 106.9807  287.8479 468.7152
```

5.7 Modeling Seasonality with ARIMA: The Condemnation Rates Series Revisited

The ARIMA models presented in this chapter assume that seasonal effects are removed or that the series is nonseasonal. However, in many practical situations it is important to model and quantify the seasonal effects. For example, it might be of interest to poultry producers to know which months of the year the condemnation rates are higher. This is important to avoid potential losses if the supply falls short of the demand due to excess condemnation.

Box and Jenkins (1970) extend their ARIMA models to describe and forecast time series with seasonal variation. Modeling of time series with seasonal variation using ARIMA is quite complicated, and detailed treatment of this topic is beyond the scope of this chapter. However, we shall outline the steps of modeling seasonality in the condemnation rates data of Example 5.3.

Example 5.3 (Continued)

First, we examine the monthly means of the series (Table 5.12):

TABLE 5.12

Monthly Means of Condemnation Rates per 100,000 Birds

Jan	Feb	Mar	Apr	May	Jun	Jul	Aug	Sep	Oct	Nov	Dec
932.58	916.13	921.99	772.99	603.37	509.54	497.01	520.03	618.73	585.96	771.76	672.83

The data suggest that the condemnation rates tend to be relatively high in the winter and low in the summer. Figure 5.11 shows the sample ACF of the series for lags 0 through 20.

The sample autocorrelations beyond lag 13 are insignificant. Moreover, we can see that (i) the autocorrelations are not tailing off, which indicates that the series is nonstationary and (ii) there is a sinusoidal pattern confirming a seasonal pattern in the series. Note that an AR(1) series $y_t = \mu + \phi y_{t-1} + \rho_t$ is nonstationary if $\phi = 1$. To confirm the nonstationarity of our series, we fitted an AR(1) model. The maximum likelihood estimator of ϕ was $\hat{\phi} = 0.961$ with SE $= 0.03$, and hence a value of 1.0 for ϕ seems acceptable. To remove nonstationarity, we formed the series $w_t = y_t - y_{t-1}$. Figure 5.12 is the time series plot of w_t.

In modeling seasonality, we decided to choose between two models. The first is an MA with one nonseasonal component and several seasonal components and the second being an AR with similar structure.

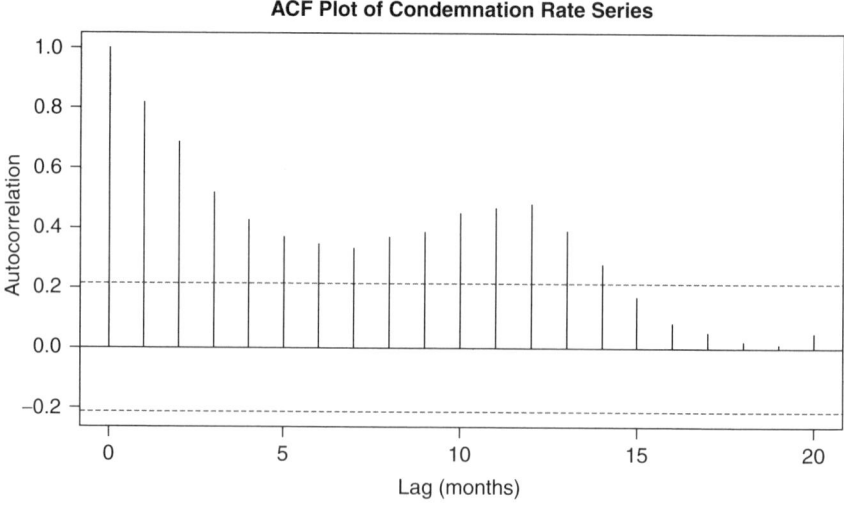

FIGURE 5.11

The autocorrelation function of rate.

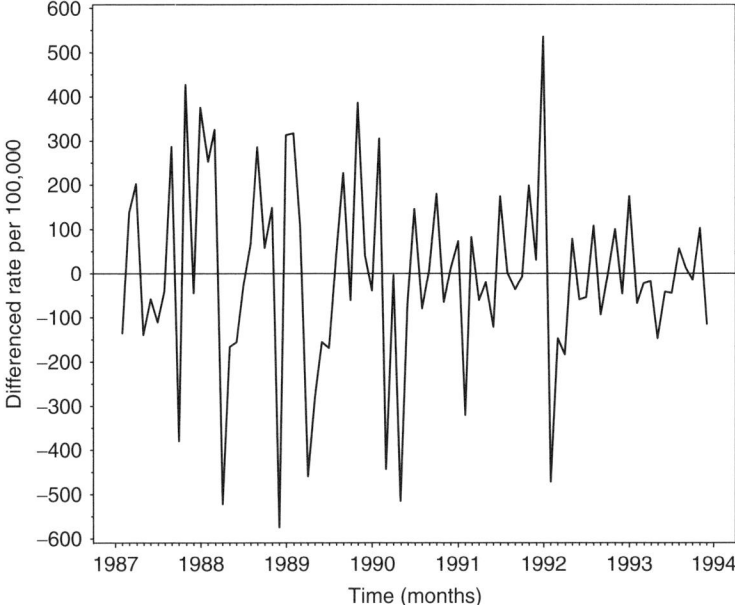

FIGURE 5.12
The time series plot after differencing.

Since the series is monthly, it has 12 periods. Accordingly, we constructed the series with 12 periods of differencing. The ACF plot of this series is given below.

			Autocorrelations	
Lag	Covariance	Correlation	−1 9 8 7 6 5 4 3 2 1 0 1 2 3 4 5 6 7 8 9 1	Std Error
0	67754.388	1.00000	| |********************|	0
1	−18042.711	−0.26630	| *****| . |	0.118678
2	362.343	0.00535	| . | . |	0.126815
3	−9104.458	−0.13437	| .***| . |	0.126818
4	−6323.896	−0.09334	| .**| . |	0.128808
5	−101.925	−0.00150	| . | . |	0.129757
6	−413.938	−0.00611	| . | . |	0.129757
7	333.580	0.00492	| . | . |	0.129761
8	17370.707	0.25638	| . |***** |	0.129764
9	−8973.790	−0.13245	| .***| . |	0.136712
10	1977.626	0.02919	| . |* . |	0.138508
11	−2154.738	−0.03180	| . *| . |	0.138594
12	−19482.516	−0.28755	| ******| . |	0.138697

Note: . marks two standard errors.

This plot shows significant autocorrelations at lags 1, 8, and 12. The candidate model for this situation is an additive AR model:

$$y_t = \mu + \phi_1 y_{t-1} + \phi_2 y_{t-3} + \phi_3 y_{t-8} + \phi_4 y_{t-12} + a_t$$

or an additive MA model:

$$y_t = \mu + a_t - \theta_1 a_{t-1} - \theta_2 a_{t-3} - \theta_3 a_{t-8} - \theta_4 a_{t-12}$$

Our choice of an additive structure is for simplicity. The fitted seasonal AR model is

$$y_t = -10.03 - 0.26 y_{t-1} - 0.16 y_{t-3} + 0.22 y_{t-8} - 0.29 y_{t-12}$$
$$\quad\ \, (18.76)\ \ (0.12)\qquad (0.12)\qquad\ \ (0.12)\qquad\ \ (0.13)$$

and the fitted seasonal MA model is

$$y_t = -9.43 + 0.33 \varepsilon_{t-1} + 0.23 \varepsilon_{t-3} - 0.16 \varepsilon_{t-8} + 0.63 \varepsilon_{t-12}$$
$$\quad (7.95)\ \ (0.11)\qquad\ (0.11)\qquad\ \ (0.11)\qquad\ \ (0.10)$$

The bracketed numbers are the standard errors of the estimates. Parameters of both models were estimated via conditional least squares.

As a diagnostic tool that may be used to check the model adequacy, we use the Q statistic of Box and Pierce (1970), later modified by Ljung and Box (1978). They suggested a test to contrast the null hypothesis

$$H_0\colon \rho_1 = \rho_2 = \cdots = \rho_k = 0$$

against the general alternative

$$H_1\colon \text{not all } \rho_i = 0$$

Based on the autocorrelation between residuals, they suggested the statistic

$$Q = Q(k) = n(n+2) \sum_{j=1}^{k} \frac{r_j^2}{n-j}$$

where n is the length of the series after any differencing and r_j the residual autocorrelation at lag j. Box and Pierce (1970) showed that under H_0, Q is asymptotically distributed as chi-squared with $(k - p - q)$ degrees of freedom.

Typically, the statistic is evaluated for several choices of k. Under H_0, for large n

$$E[Q(k_2) - Q(k_1)] = k_2 - k_1$$

so that different sections of the correlogram can be checked for departures from H_0.

The following tables (Tables 5.13 and 5.14) gives the Box–Pierce–Ljung (BPL) statistics for the condemnation rates using the AR and MA models.

TABLE 5.13

BPL Statistic Using AR Seasonal Model

Lag(k)	$Q(k)$	DF	Pr ob	Autocorrelations r_j					
6	2.57	2	0.2762	−0.062	−0.142	−0.046	−0.088	−0.015	0.011
12	3.09	8	0.9287	0.019	0.033	−0.036	−0.008	0.001	−0.057
18	5.14	14	0.9838	0.093	−0.076	−0.001	−0.078	0.041	0.012
24	18.31	20	0.5673	−0.067	0.022	0.170	0.050	0.181	−0.231

$p = 4, q = 0, \mathrm{DF} = k - 4.$

TABLE 5.14

BPL Statistic Using MA Seasonal Model

Lag(k)	$Q(k)$	DF	Pr ob	Autocorrelations r_j					
6	0.88	2	0.6435	0.018	−0.099	0.006	−0.028	0.022	−0.015
12	3.32	8	0.9129	0.031	0.048	−0.095	−0.022	−0.036	0.120
18	5.63	14	0.9750	0.053	−0.121	−0.012	−0.067	0.056	−0.004
24	12.50	20	0.8978	−0.035	0.035	0.163	0.090	0.151	−0.072

$p = 0, q = 4, \mathrm{DF} = k - 4.$

Note that all the Q statistics of the two models are nonsignificant. This means that the models captured the autocorrelation in the data and that the residual autocorrelations are nonsignificant. Therefore, both models provide good fit to the condemnation rate's times series process. However, we might argue that the MA seasonal model gives a better fit owing to the fact that it has smaller Akaike information criterion (AIC = 978.07 for the MA and AIC = 982.25 for the AR).

The following SAS program produces the parameter estimates, the Q statistics, and the AICs.

```
* fitting the MA seasonal model;
proc arima;
identify var = rate (1,12) nlag = 12;
estimate q=(1,3,8)(12);
run; quit;
```

Note that $q(1,3,8)$ is replaced by $p(1,3,8)$ to fit an AR seasonal model.

Exercises

5.1   The table below shows the average air temperature at a capital city in a Middle East country from 1960 to 1969.

Year	Jan	Feb	Mar	Apr	May	Jun	Jul	Aug	Sep	Oct	Nov	Dec
1960	27.1	27	28	29.2	32	35	42	49.1	38	36	32	26.9
1961	27.1	27.1	28.1	29.1	34.1	36.1	42	49.2	38.1	35.6	31	27.2
1962	28.1	27.2	27.9	29.1	35.1	37.2	41	48.1	39.1	35.5	29.2	27.6
1963	27.2	27.1	26.9	28.2	35.2	37	43	47.2	41.2	36.5	29.7	28.6
1964	26.8	27.9	30.1	30.1	36.1	37	44	47	41.1	34.2	28.9	28.6
1965	27.0	26.8	30.1	30.1	37.1	37	45	47	41.6	34.1	29.6	27.5
1966	27.0	27.3	30.2	28.1	37.2	38	45	48	41.7	34.2	28.6	25.6
1967	28.1	28.3	29.9	29.2	38	39	46.1	49	42.6	35.1	27.6	27.6
1968	26.8	28.2	29.9	31.2	39	39	47	48	41.2	36.1	30.1	28.6
1969	26.9	29.9	31.9	33.2	39	39	46.1	46	41.7	36	30.1	29.6

(a) Plot the data.

(b) Using a nonparametric test for seasonality, what do you conclude?

(c) Calculate the overall January average, the overall February average, and so on. Subtract each individual value from the corresponding monthly average. Test for seasonality of the resulting data.

(d) Assuming a multiplicative model, evaluate the seasonal coefficients.

(e) After fitting a linear trend model, what is the predicted temperature in the month of February 1961?

5.2   Suppose that you are given the series
63, 54, 75, 50, 52, 54, 6.6, 5.5, 6.0, 50, 70, 50, 60, 65, 40, 66, 60, 62, 42, 62, 70, 44, 62, 49, 71, 50, 63, 55, 75, 54

(a) Plot the series.

(b) What is the approximate value of the first log autocorrelation coefficient ρ_1?

(c) Plot y_t against y_{t+1}. What is the approximate value of ρ_1 from the scatter plot?

(d) Calculate and plot the sample ACF $\hat{\rho}_k$ for $k = 0, 1, 2, 3, 4, 5$.

5.3   Consider a stationary time series with theoretical autocorrelation function

$$\rho_k = \alpha \pi^{k-1} \qquad k = 1, 2, \ldots$$

What is $\text{var}(\hat{\rho}_k)$ using Bartlett's approximation using Equations 5.14 and 5.15.

5.4   Find the ACF and plot ρ_k for $k = 0, 1, 2, 3$, and 4 for each of the following models:

$$(1) \quad y_t - 0.5y_{t-1} = a_t$$

$$(2) \quad y_t - 1.5y_{t-1} + 0.5y_{t-2} = a_t$$

5.5   For the AR(2) model

$$y_t - 0.6y_{t-1} - 0.3y_{t-2} = a_t$$

Calculate $\text{var}(y_t)$ assuming that $\sigma_a^2 = 1$.

5.6   Find the AR representation of the MA(1) process $y_t = a_t - 0.4a_{t-1}$.

6

Repeated Measures and Longitudinal Data Analysis

CONTENTS

6.1 Introduction

Experimental designs with repeated measures over time are very common in biological and medical research. This type of design is characterized by repeated observations on a large number of individuals for a relatively small number of time points, where each individual is observed at such points. The repeated measures design has several advantages over completely randomized designs, the most important of which is the ability to control biological heterogeneity between individuals by measuring individuals repeatedly over time. This reduction in heterogeneity makes the repeated measures design more efficient than completely randomized designs.

Longitudinal and repeated measures data are very frequent in almost all scientific fields, including agriculture, biology, medicine, epidemiology, geography, demography, and many other disciplines. It is not the aim of this chapter to provide a comprehensive coverage of the subject. We refer the reader to many excellent texts such as Crowder and Hand (1990), Lindsay (1993), and Diggle et al. (1994), and many articles that have appeared in scientific journals (*Biometrics* and *Statistics in Medicine*). In this chapter, we describe the statistical methodologies that are used to answer the scientific questions posed. Detailed examples on repeated measures and longitudinal data using the population-averaged "generalized estimating equations (GEE)" models and the subject-specific "generalized mixed" models are provided to illustrate the utility of these models in the context of repeated measures or longitudinal studies that include covariate effects. In the following section, we provide examples of repeated measures experiments that are frequently encountered.

6.1.1 Examples

6.1.1.1 *Experimental Studies*

6.1.1.1.1 *Liver Enzyme Activity*

Frison and Pocock (1992) describe a clinical trial in which 152 patients with heart disease were randomly allocated to treatment using an active drug or a placebo during a 12-month follow-up period. The concentration of the liver enzyme creatine phosphokinase (CPK) in the patient's serum was measured as an indicator of liver damage arising as a side effect of the treatment. Each patient had three pretreatment measurements, which were taken 2 months before, 1 month before, and at the time of randomization. They also had eight posttreatment measurements taken every 1.5 months after randomization. The main objective of the study was to see how the enzyme level varied over time before and after treatment.

6.1.1.1.2 *Effect of Mycobacterium Inoculation on Weight*

An experiment was conducted in a veterinary microbiology lab with the main objective to determine the effect of Mycobacterium inoculation on the weight of immune-deficient mice. Severely immune-deficient beige mice (6–8 weeks old) were randomly allocated to the following groups:

1. Control group where animals did not receive any inoculation.
2. Animals were inoculated intraperitoneally with live *Mycobacterium paratuberculosis* (MPTB) and transplanted with peripheral blood leucocytes (PBL) from humans with Crohn's disease.

3. Animals were inoculated with live MPTB and transplanted with PBL from bovine.

In each group, the mice were weighed at baseline (week 0), week 2, and week 4. The question of interest concerns differences between the mean weights among the three groups. The data are given in Table 6.1.

TABLE 6.1

Weights in Grams of Inoculated Immunodeficient Mice

			Time in Weeks	
Group	Mice	0	2	4
1	1	28	25	45
2	1	40	31	70
3	1	31	40	44
4	1	27	21	26
5	1	27	25	40
6	2	34	25	38
7	2	36	31	49
8	2	41	21	25
9	2	28	22	10
10	2	29	24	22
11	2	31	18	36
12	2	31	16	5
13	3	28	28	61
14	3	27	23	63
15	3	31	30	42
16	3	19	16	28
17	3	20	18	39
18	3	22	24	52
19	3	22	22	25
20	3	28	26	53

6.1.2 Observational Studies

6.1.2.1 Variations in Teenage Pregnancy Rates (TAPR) in Canada

Table 6.2 shows teenage pregnancy rates (per 1000 females aged 15–17 and 18–19). These rates include live births, therapeutic abortions, hospitalized cases of spontaneous and other unspecified abortions, and registered still-births with at least 20 weeks' gestation at pregnancy termination. The Newfoundland data are not included. It is important to detect variations regionally and over time in TAPR.

Longitudinal surveys are also common in medical research. Laird and Ware (1982), for example, described a survey in which pulmonary function in about 200 schoolchildren was examined under normal conditions, then during an air pollution alert, and later on three successive weeks following the alert. The main aim of the study was to determine whether the volume of air exhaled in

TABLE 6.2

Teenage Pregnancy Rates per 1000 Females Aged 15–17 and 18–19

Year	Age Group	East					West				Territories	
		PEI	NS	NB	QU	ONT	MAN	SASK	ALTA	BC	Y	NWT
1975	15–17	41.6	43.4	40.5	12.8	39	41.7	48.5	50.5	48.6	70	77.5
	18–19	96.6	98.6	103.7	43.4	91.5	98.8	116.1	120.9	102	110	192.5
1980	15–17	28	34.9	28.9	12.9	32.8	34.2	46.3	43.2	41.0	65	104
	18–19	59.6	81.4	73.6	39.8	74.4	85.4	106.6	111.4	89.4	105	165
1985	15–17	20.3	28.6	21.6	11.9	26	35.4	37.9	34.5	29.9	50	109.3
	18–19	64.5	65.8	59.5	37.7	63	88.9	88.4	85.8	72	77.5	186
1989	15–17	21.1	30.8	22.6	16.6	27.2	40.5	37.7	64.4	31.6	38.3	97.8
	18–19	60.5	69.4	56.4	48.0	64.8	96.9	95.0	87.6	77.2	120	220

PEI, Prince Edward Island; NS, Nova Scotia; NB, New Brunswick; QU, Quebec; ONT, Ontario; MAN, Manitoba; SASK, Saskatchewan; ALTA, Alberta; BC, British Columbia; Y, Yukon; NWT, North West Territories.

Source: Health Report; Statistics Canada 1991, Vol. 3, No. 4.

the first second of a forced exhalation (FEV_1) was depressed during the alert. The analysis of repeated categorical measures has been illustrated by Ware et al. (1988). Children were assessed annually at ages 9–12 to evaluate the potential effects of air pollution on persistent wheezeing. Parents were asked about wheezing by their children during the previous year, and responses were grouped into three mutually exclusive categories or states: no wheeze, wheeze with colds, or wheeze apart from colds.

6.2　Methods for the Analysis of Repeated Measures Data

In the analysis of repeated measures or longitudinal data, the critical feature to recognize is that, since sets of measures are obtained from the same subjects, these measures are likely to be correlated and can rarely be considered as independent. How that dependence is dealt with is a principal distinguishing feature of different methods of analysis. However, before we discuss in detail this fundamental feature, more preliminary examination of the data must be considered.

Such examination includes the graphical display of the data, an important step before modeling and data analyses are performed.

Diggle et al. (1994) give the following simple guidelines for the exploration of repeated measures data using graphical displays:

1. Show as much of the relevant data as possible rather than data summaries.
2. Highlight aggregate patterns of potential scientific interest.

3. Identify both cross-sectional and longitudinal patterns in the data.
4. Make easy the identification of unusual individuals or unusual observations.

6.2.1 Basic Models

Suppose that observations are obtained on n time points for each of the k subjects that are divided into h groups, with k_j subjects in the jth group.

Let y_{hij} denote the jth measurement made on the ith subject within the hth group. The analysis of data from the repeated measures designs considered in this chapter will be dealt with linear mixed model analysis of variance. As for Chapter 1, the linear model representation of the observations y_{hij} is as follows:

$$y_{hij} = \mu_h + \alpha_{ij} + e_{hij} \tag{6.1}$$

where

(i) μ_h is the overall mean response in the hth group. The μ_h is called the fixed effect because it takes one unique value irrespective of the subject being observed and irrespective of the time point.

(ii) α_{ij} represents the departure of y_{hij} from μ_h for a particular subject; this is called a random effect.

(iii) e_{hij} is the error term representing the discrepancy between y_{hij} and $\mu_h + \alpha_{ij}$.

Further to the above setup, some assumptions on the distributions of the random components of the mixed model 6.1 are needed. These assumptions are

A. $E(\alpha_{ij}) = E(e_{hij}) = 0$.
B. $V(\alpha_{ij}) = \sigma_\alpha^2$, $V(e_{ij}) = \sigma_e^2$, $\text{Cov}(\alpha_{ij}, \alpha_{i'j'}) = 0$, and $\text{Cov}(\alpha_{ij}, \alpha_{ij'}) = \sigma_\alpha^2$.
C. $\text{Cov}(e_{hij}, e_{h'i'j'}) = 0$ $i \neq i'$ or $j \neq j', h \neq h'$.
D. The random effect α_{ij} is uncorrelated with e_{hij}.
E. α_{ij} and e_{ij} are normally distributed.

Consequently, it can be shown that the covariance between any pair of measurements is

$$\text{Cov}(y_{hij}, y_{h'i'j'}) = \begin{cases} 0 & i \neq i' \\ \sigma_\alpha^2 & i = i' \text{ and } j \neq j' \\ \sigma_\alpha^2 + \sigma_e^2 & i = i' \text{ and } j = j' \end{cases} \tag{6.2}$$

Therefore, any pair of measurements on the same individual are correlated, and the correlation is given by

$$\text{Corr}(y_{hij}, y_{h'i'j}) = \rho = \frac{\sigma_\alpha^2}{\sigma_\alpha^2 + \sigma_e^2} \tag{6.3}$$

which we have already discussed in Chapters 1 and 2 (known as the intraclass correlation). The assumptions of common variance of the observations and common correlation among all pairs of observations on the same subject can be expressed as an $n_i \times n_i$ matrix Σ, where n_i is the number of observations taken repeatedly on the ith subject and

$$\text{Cov}(y_{hij}, y_{h'i'j}) = \sum = \sigma^2 \begin{bmatrix} 1 & \rho & \cdots & \rho \\ \rho & 1 & \cdots & \rho \\ \cdot & \cdot & \cdots & \cdot \\ \cdot & \cdot & \cdots & \cdot \\ \cdot & \cdot & \cdots & \cdot \\ \rho & \rho & \cdots & 1 \end{bmatrix} \tag{6.4}$$

where $\sigma^2 = \sigma_\alpha^2 + \sigma_e^2$.

A matrix of the form (6.4) is said to possess the property of compound symmetry or uniformity or exchangeable correlation structure (Geisser, 1963).

Unfortunately, the data obtained in many repeated measures or longitudinal settings rarely satisfy the assumption of compound symmetry. In such designs, it is common to find that the adjacent observations or successive measurements on adjacent time points are more highly correlated than nonadjacent time points, with the correlation between these measurements decreasing the measurement further apart.

It would become apparent that for analyzing longitudinal data, although the main interest may lie in estimating the effects of risk factors and exposures on the expected value of the response, it often seems necessary to expend more effort to ensure that the model for the variance and covariance among the response is correct. Huber (1967) proposed a heteroscedastic consistent "sandwich" estimator for the parameter covariance matrix. Variants of this covariance estimator are available among many of the software implementations of procedures described in this chapter. At the cost of reduced efficiency—often trivial but sometimes large—the use of this method provides some relief from an excessive concern that the nonsystematic component of the adopted model needs to be correctly specified in every detail. Summarizing the objectives of analyzing longitudinal data includes

- Measurement of the average treatment effect over time.
- Assessment of treatment effects separately at each time point and testing whether treatment interacts with time.
- Identification of any covariance patterns in the repeated measurements.
- Determination of a suitable model to describe the relationship of a measurement with time.

6.2.2 The Issue of Missing Observations

Missing data are quite common for longitudinal and repeated measures data. It is important to consider the reasons behind the missing observations.

If the reason that an observation is missing is related to the response variable that is missed, the analysis will be biased. Rubin (1976, 1994) discusses the concept of data that are missing at random in a general statistical setting. Little and Rubin (1987) distinguish between observations that are missing completely at random, where the probability of missing an observation is independent of both the observed responses and the missing responses, and missing at random, where the probability of missing an observation is independent of the responses. Laird (1988) used the term "ignorable missing data" to describe observations that are missing at random.

Diggle (1989) discussed the problem of testing whether dropouts in repeated measures investigations occur at random. Dropouts are a common source of missing observations, and it is important for the analysis to determine if the dropouts occur at random. In the data analysis sections, we will assume that the mechanism for missing observations is ignorable.

6.3 Mixed Linear Regression Models

6.3.1 Formulation of the Models

A general linear mixed model for the analysis of longitudinal data has been proposed by Laird and Ware (1982):

$$Y_i = Z_i\beta + Z_i\alpha_1 + \varepsilon_i \tag{6.5}$$

where Y_i is an $n_i \times 1$ column vector of measurements for subject (cluster) i, X_i an $n_i \times p$ design matrix, β a $p \times 1$ vector of regression coefficients assumed to be fixed, Z_i an $n_i \times q$ design matrix for the random effects α_i, which are assumed to be independently distributed across subjects with distribution $\alpha_i \sim N(0, \sigma^2 G)$, where G is an arbitrary covariance matrix. The within-subjects errors ε_i are assumed to be distributed $\alpha_i \sim N(0, \sigma^2 R_i)$. It is also assumed that ε_i and α_i are independent of each other. The fact that Y_i, X_i, Z_i, and R_i are indexed by i means that these matrices are subject specific. Note that the model 6.1 is a special case of model 6.5.

Mixed models have the following advantages:

- A single model can be used to estimate the overall treatment effects and to estimate treatment effects at each time point. There is no need to calculate mean values across all time points (to obtain the overall treatment effects) or to analyze time points separately (to obtain treatment effects at each time point). Standard errors for treatment effects at individual time points are calculated using information from all time points and are therefore more robust than standard errors calculated from separate time points.

- The presence of missing data causes no problems provided they can be assumed missing at random. This assumption will be assumed to hold throughout this chapter.
- The covariance pattern of the repeated measurements can be determined and properly accounted for.

There are several ways a mixed model can be used to analyze repeated measures data. The simplest approach is to use a random effects model with subjects' effects considered as random. This will allow for a constant correlation between all observations on the same patient. When the relationship of the response variable with time is of interest, a random coefficients model is appropriate. Here, regression curves are fitted for each patient and the regression coefficients are allowed to vary randomly between the patients. These models are considered in the following sections.

6.3.2   Covariance Patterns

A large selection of covariance patterns is available for use in mixed models. Most of the patterns are dependent on measurements being taken at fixed times, and some are also easier to justify when the observations are evenly spaced. There are also other patterns where covariances are based on the exact value of time, and these are most useful in situations where the time intervals are irregular.

Some simple covariance patterns for the R_i matrices for a trial with four time points are shown below. In the general pattern (i), sometimes also referred to as "unstructured," the variances of responses σ_i^2 differs for each time period i, and the covariance θ_{jk} differs between each pair of periods j and k. For the first-order autoregressive model (ii), the variances are equal and the covariance decreases exponentially depending on their separation $|j - k|$, so $\theta_{jk} = \rho^{|j-k|}\sigma^2$. This is sometimes an appropriate model when time periods are evenly spaced. It can then be seen as a "natural" model from a time series viewpoint. However, it may be justified empirically in circumstances where the observations are not evenly spaced.

For the compound symmetry covariance model (iii), all covariances are equal. Other covariance patterns are possible, but we shall restrict our presentations to these three commonly occurring patterns. These are

(i) General (unstructured): UN

$$R_i = \begin{pmatrix} \sigma_1^2 & \theta_{12} & \theta_{13} & \theta_{14} \\ \theta_{12} & \sigma_2^2 & \theta_{23} & \theta_{24} \\ \theta_{13} & \theta_{23} & \sigma_3^2 & \theta_{34} \\ \theta_{14} & \theta_{24} & \theta_{34} & \sigma_4^2 \end{pmatrix}$$

(ii) First-order autoregressive: AR

$$R_i = \sigma^2 \begin{pmatrix} 1 & \rho & \rho^2 & \rho^3 \\ \rho & 1 & \rho & \rho^2 \\ \rho^2 & \rho & 1 & \rho \\ \rho^3 & \rho^2 & \rho & 1 \end{pmatrix}$$

(iii) Compound symmetry: CS

$$R_i = \begin{pmatrix} \sigma^2 & \theta & \theta & \theta \\ \theta & \sigma^2 & \theta & \theta \\ \theta & \theta & \sigma^2 & \theta \\ \theta & \theta & \theta & \sigma^2 \end{pmatrix}$$

There are many covariance patterns available and choosing the most appropriate one is not always easy. The ideal is to select the pattern that best fits the true covariance of data and provide appropriate standard errors for fixed effects estimates. There are two alternative approaches to making a model choice. One is to compare models based on measures of fit that are adjusted for the number of covariance parameters. Another is to use likelihood ratio tests to find whether additional parameters cause a statistically significant improvement in the model.

The likelihood statistics is expected to become larger as more parameters are included in the model. The two statistics below are based on the likelihood but make allowance for the number of covariance parameters fitted. They can be used to make direct comparisons between models that fit the same fixed effects. Akaike's information criterion (AIC) (Akaike, 1973) is given by

$$\text{AIC} = -2\log(L) + 2p$$

where p is the number of covariates, including the intercept. Schwarz's information criterion (SIC) (Schwarz, 1978) takes into account the number of fixed effects p and the number of observations n, and is given by

$$\text{SIC} = -2\log(L) + p\log(N)$$

Models with smaller values of AIC and SIC denote better fits. However, it is unclear to us which criterion is preferable. Both the criteria are calculated within PROC MIXED and PROC GLIMMIX.

6.3.3 Statistical Inference and Model Comparison

Models can be compared statistically using likelihood ratio tests provided that they fit the same fixed effects and their covariance parameters are nested. Nesting of covariance parameters occurs when the covariance parameters in the simpler model can be obtained by restricting some of the parameters in the more complex model (e.g., compound symmetry pattern is nested within a Toeplitz pattern, but it is not nested within a first-order autoregressive pattern). The likelihood ratio test statistic is given by

$$2(\log(L_1) - \log(L_2)) \sim \chi^2_{DF}$$

where DF = difference in the number of covariance parameters fitted.

If the covariance parameters in the models compared are not nested, statistical comparison using a likelihood ratio test is not valid. Akaike's or Schwarz's criteria defined above could be used.

As a simple strategy, we find that in many datasets, especially those with only a few repeated measurements, estimates of overall group differences will differ little between models using different covariance patterns. If obtaining a reliable treatment estimate and standard error is the only objective, a compound symmetry pattern is likely to be robust. A rough check can be made of this by comparing the results with those obtained using a general pattern. If the differences are small, then the compound symmetry pattern can be used with reasonable confidence. These strategies will be explored in Section 6.5.

6.3.4 Estimation of Model Parameters

The estimation of the parameters of the general normal mixed model 6.5 is obtained using the method of maximum likelihood, which is described in full detail in Jones (1993). The solutions of the likelihood equations are

$$\hat{\beta} = \sum_j (X_j' V_j^{-1} X_j)^{-1} \left(\sum_j X_j' V_j^{-1} X_j \right) \tag{6.6}$$

and

$$\text{Cov}(\hat{\beta}) = \hat{\sigma}^2 \left(\sum X_j' V_j^{-1} X_j \right)^{-1} \tag{6.7}$$

for given G and R_j, where

$$V_j = Z_j G Z_j' + R_j$$

is the covariance matrix for the jth subject. The maximum likelihood estimator (MLE) of the scale parameter σ^2 is

$$\hat{\sigma}^2 = \frac{1}{N} \sum_j (Y_j - X_j \hat{\beta})' V_j^{-1} (Y_j - X_j \hat{\beta}) \tag{6.8}$$

where $N = \sum_j n_j$ is the total number of observations on all subjects. When the number of parameters is not small relative to the total number of observations, the estimated variances of the maximum likelihood estimators become seriously biased. To reduce the bias, the restricted maximum likelihood (REML) is used. For repeated measures experiments, Diggle (1988) showed that the REML estimate of β is the same as in Equation 6.6; however, the unbiased estimate of σ^2 is

$$\hat{\sigma}^2 = \frac{1}{n-p} \sum_j (Y_j - X_j\hat{\beta})' V_j^{-1} (Y_j - X_j\hat{\beta}) \qquad (6.9)$$

6.4 Examples Using the SAS Mixed and GLIMMIX Procedures

We shall present four examples (Examples 6.1 through 6.4) on repeated measures data. The first two examples are for normally distributed observations, the third example is for count data, and the fourth example is on repeated binary outcome measurement.

6.4.1 Linear Mixed Model for Normally Distributed Repeated Measures Data

Following the approach in Chapter 1, we shall first start with models with two levels: level-1 model is a linear model that has "time" as an independent variable and level-2 model relates the variability in the parameters as random coefficients unrelated to any subject covariates. To be able to extend our argument to a 3-level hierarchical model, in which subjects within treatment groups are followed over time, we represent the parameters in level-1 (within subject) model using γ and the parameters in level-2 (between subjects) model using β. Let y_{ij} denote the measurement taken from the ith subject at the jth time point t_{ij}:

$$y_{ij} = \gamma_{0i} + \gamma_{1i} t_{ij} + e_{ij}$$

where $e_{ij} \sim N(0, \sigma^2)$.

Moreover, we assume that

$$\gamma_{0i} = \beta_0 + u_{0i}$$
$$\gamma_{1i} = \beta_1 + u_{1i}$$

where $u = \begin{pmatrix} u_{0i} \\ u_{1i} \end{pmatrix} \sim BVN \left[\begin{pmatrix} 0 \\ 0 \end{pmatrix}, \begin{pmatrix} \tau_{00} & \tau_{01} \\ \tau_{10} & \tau_{11} \end{pmatrix} \right]$ is independent of e_{ij}

Therefore,

$$y_{ij} = \beta_0 + u_{01} + (\beta_1 + u_{1i}) t_{ij} + e_{ij}$$

or

$$y_{ij} = (\beta_0 + \beta_1 t_{ij}) + (u_{0i} + u_{1i} t_{ij} + e_{ij}) \qquad (6.10)$$

There is a similarity between this model and the unconditional mean model of Chapter 1. The multilevel model 6.10 has two components: a fixed component, which contains "intercept" and "t"; and a random component, which contains three random effects.

Example 6.1

The arrhythmogenic dose of epinephrine (ADE) is determined by infusing epinephrine into a dog until arrhythmia criterion is reached. The arrhythmia criterion was the occurrence of four intermittent or continuous premature ventricular contractions. Once the criterion has been reached, the infusion required to produce the criteria is recorded. The ADE is then calculated by multiplying the duration of the infusion by the infusion rate. The following table gives the ADE for six dogs measured at the 0, $\frac{1}{2}$, 1, $1\frac{1}{2}$, 2, $2\frac{1}{2}$, 3, $3\frac{1}{2}$, 4, and $4\frac{1}{2}$ h.

					Time					
Dog	**0**	**½**	**1**	**1½**	**2**	**2½**	**3**	**3½**	**4**	**4½**
1	5.7	4.7	4.8	4.9	3.88	3.51	2.8	2.6	2.5	2.5
2	5.3	3.7	5.2	4.9	5.04	3.5	2.9	2.6	2.4	2.5
3	4.0	4.6	4.1	4.58	3.58	4.0	3.6	2.5	3.5	2.1
4	13.7	8.9	9.6	8.6	7.5	4.0	3.1	4.1	4.08	3.0
5	5.0	4.0	4.1	3.9	3.4	3.39	2.95	3.0	3.1	2.0
6	7.1	3.0	2.4	3.3	3.9	4.0	3.0	2.4	2.1	2.0

The ADE data are analyzed to monitor the levels of ADE across time.
    Figure 6.1 displays the ADE data over time.

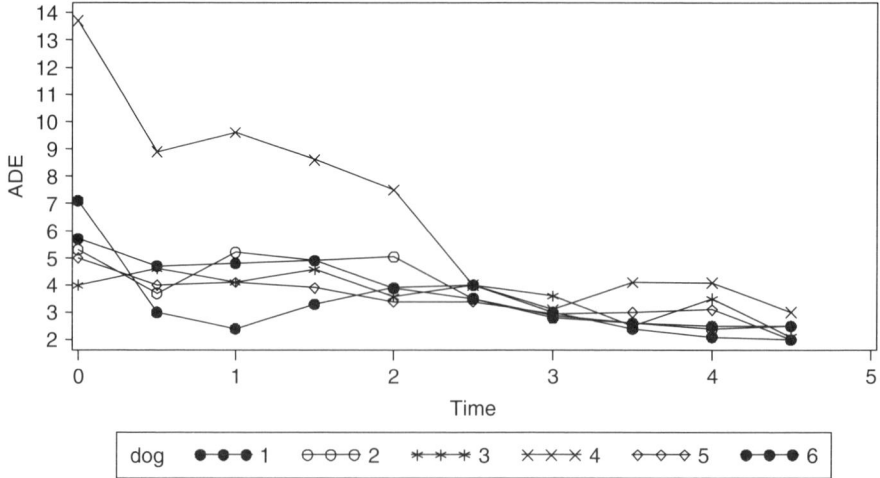

FIGURE 6.1
ADE data for six dogs over time.

Three mixed models will be fit to these data:

data ade; set ade; period=time;

* Model 1: Random coefficient model without exploring the error
covariance structure;
proc mixed covtest data=ade;
   class dog;
   model ade=time/ s ddfm=bw notest;
   random intercept time / type=un sub=dog g;
run;

* Model 2: Exploring the correlation structures within a subject;
proc mixed covtest data=ade;
   class dog period;
   model ade=time/ s ddfm=bw notest;
   repeated period / type=ar(1) sub=dog r;
run;

* Model 3: Modeling between and within subject covariance;
proc mixed covtest data=ade;
   class dog period;
   model ade=time/ s ddfm=bw notest;
   random intercept time / type=un sub=dog g;
   repeated period / type=ar(1) sub=dog r;
run;

The SAS output of the ADE example is listed below.
   Model 1: Unstructured correlation

Covariance Parameter Estimates

Cov Parm	Subject	Estimate	Standard Error	Z-Value	Pr > |Z|
UN(1,1)	dog	6.9941	4.5965	1.52	0.0641
UN(2,1)	dog	−1.6450	1.0973	−1.50	0.1339
UN(2,2)	dog	0.3775	0.2631	1.43	0.0757
Residual		0.7906	0.1614	4.90	<0.0001

Fit Statistics

−2 Res log likelihood	170.5
AIC (smaller is better)	178.5
AICC (smaller is better)	179.2
BIC (smaller is better)	177.6

Solution for Fixed Effects

Effect	Estimate	Standard Error	DF	t-Value	Pr > |t|
Intercept	6.0468	1.1005	5	5.49	0.0027
time	−0.8570	0.2633	53	−3.26	0.0020

Model 2: Autocorrelation structure

Covariance Parameter Estimates

Cov Parm	Subject	Estimate	Standard Error	Z-Value	Pr Z
AR(1)	dog	0.8445	0.07506	11.25	<0.0001
Residual		4.1532	1.8760	2.21	0.0134

Fit Statistics

−2 Res log likelihood	186.4
AIC (smaller is better)	190.4

Solution for Fixed Effects

Effect	Estimate	Standard Error	DF	t-Value	Pr > |t|
Intercept	6.5415	0.8144	5	8.03	0.0005
time	−0.9713	0.2307	53	−4.21	<0.0001

Model 3: Autocorrelation structure for within-subjects and unstructured correlation for between-subjects variation

Covariance Parameter Estimates

Cov Parm	Subject	Estimate	Standard Error	Z-Value	Pr Z
UN(1,1)	dog	7.1916	4.8981	1.47	0.0710
UN(2,1)	dog	−1.6627	1.1576	−1.44	0.1509
UN(2,2)	dog	0.3624	0.2759	1.31	0.0944
AR(1)	dog	0.3573	0.2222	1.61	0.1078
Residual		0.9634	0.3197	3.01	0.0013

Fit Statistics

−2 Res log likelihood	167.5
AIC (smaller is better)	177.5

Solution for Fixed Effects

Effect	Estimate	Standard Error	DF	*t*-Value	Pr > |*t*|
Intercept	6.1722	1.1358	5	5.43	0.0029
time	−0.8924	0.2691	53	−3.32	0.0017

Comments on the SAS output of Example 6.1:

1. For model 1, the average value of the intercept parameter is $\hat{\beta}_0 = 6.0468$ and $\hat{\beta}_1 = -0.857$ is the estimate of the average slope. We reject the hypothesis that either of the parameters is 0 in the population. For the random effects $\hat{\tau}_{00} = 6.9941$, $\hat{\tau}_{11} = 0.3775$, and $\hat{\tau}_{01} = -1.645$. The estimated residual variance is $\hat{\sigma}^2 = 0.7906$. Note that the test results show that there are no significant variations among subjects. The AIC of this model is 178.5.

2. Since the components of variance were not significant, model 2 fits the data with autocorrelation structure for the within-subject covariance. The autocorrelation parameter was significant. The solution for fixed effects of model 2 is not different from model 1 and there is a substantial increase in the within-residual variance. The AIC of this model is 190.4.

3. In model 3, we attempted to model both the between-subjects variations and the within-subject covariance structure. This required the inclusion of a class variable called "period" needed in the "repeated" statement of SAS. Again the fixed effects estimates were the same, with time being a significant factor. However, neither the covariance parameters nor the AR(1) correlation was significant. The AIC of this model is 177.5.

In conclusion, the first model seems to provide adequate representation of the data.

The lmer in R fits the generalized linear mixed models (GLIMMIX); however, it does not support modeling variation within experimental units or clusters. The reader is referred to the documentation for the SAS-mixed package R for a comparison of the capabilities of lmer with reference to SAS PROC MIXED. We illustrate the use of lmer function in R to fit model 1.

```
dog <- c(rep(1,10),rep(2,10),rep(3,10),rep(4,10),rep(5,10),rep(6,10))
time <- rep(c(0.0,0.5,1.0,1.5,2.0,2.5,3.0,3.5,4.0,4.5),6)
ade <- c(5.70,4.70,4.80,4.90,3.88,3.51,2.80,2.60,2.50,2.50,
        5.30,3.70,5.20,4.90,5.04,3.50,2.90,2.60,2.40,2.50,
        4.00,4.60,4.10,4.58,3.58,4.00,3.60,2.50,3.50,2.10,
        13.70,8.90,9.60,8.60,7.50,4.00,3.10,4.10,4.08,3.00,
```

5.00,4.00,4.10,3.90,3.40,3.39,2.95,3.00,3.10,2.00,
7.10,3.00,2.40,3.30,3.90,4.00,3.00,2.40,2.10,2.00)
ade <- data.frame(dog,time,ade)

(lme1 <- lmer(ade ~ time + (time | dog), ade))

There are several other facilities in R for fitting mixed effect models, the most popular is the nlme library described in detail by Pinheiro and Bates (2000). Alternative correlation structures for the random effects may be specified using the correlation argument to lme. The results of fitting the linear mixed models in R may be different than those produced by SAS. For illustration purpose, alternative models will be fit using lme in Example 6.2.

Example 6.2   Data with Subject-Level Covariate

Potthoff and Roy (1964) present a set of growth data for 11 girls and 16 boys. For each subject, the distance (mm) from the center of the pituitary to the pterygomaxillary fissure was recorded at the ages of 8, 10, 12, and 14. None of the data are missing. The questions posed by the authors were

- Should the growth curves be presented by second-degree equation in age or are linear equations adequate?
- Should two separate curves be used for boys and girls or do both have the same growth curve?
- Can we obtain confidence band(s) for the expected growth curves?

Before we address these questions, we should emphasize that little is known about the nature of the correlation between the $n_i = 4$ observations on any subject, except perhaps that they are serially correlated. The simplest correlation model is the one in which the correlation coefficient between any two observations t periods of time apart is equal to ρ^t, and in which the variance is constant with respect to time. Under this model, the covariance matrix is

$$w_i \sigma^2 = \begin{bmatrix} 1 & \rho & \rho^2 & \rho^3 \\ \rho & 1 & \rho & \rho^2 \\ \rho^2 & \rho & 1 & \rho \\ \rho^3 & \rho^2 & \rho & 1 \end{bmatrix} \sigma^2$$

This is the AR(1) correlation structure. We shall explore several covariance structures while modeling these data.

We now consider a model in which we address the possible variation in intercept and slope attributed to measured subject-level covariate x_i. We first consider the model

$$y_{ij} = \gamma_{0i} + \gamma_{1i} t_{ij} + e_{ij}$$
$$\gamma_{0i} = \beta_{00} + \beta_{01} x_i + u_{0i}$$
$$\gamma_{1i} = \beta_{10} + \beta_{11} x_i + u_{1i}$$

where the assumptions on the distributions of u_i and e_{ij} are the same as in Chapter 1. Following the argument of Singer (1998), it is convenient to centralize the covariate x_i around its mean (if it is measured on the continuous scale), so that the model is written as

$$y_{ij} = \beta_{00} + \beta_{01}(x_i - \bar{x}) + u_{0i} + (\beta_{10} + \beta_{11}(x_i - \bar{x}) + u_{1i})t_{ij} + e_{ij}$$

Arranging the terms we have

$$y_{ij} = [\beta_{00} + \beta_{01}(x_i - \bar{x}) + \beta_{10}t_{ij} + \beta_{11}(x_i - \bar{x})t_{ij}] + [u_{0i} + u_{1i}t_{ij} + e_{ij}] \quad (6.11)$$

Letting $\tilde{x} \equiv x_i - \bar{x}$, model 6.11 again has two components: a fixed component, which contains "intercept," "$\tilde{x}$," "t," and an interaction term $(\tilde{x})*(t)$; a random component, which contains intercept, time, and the error term. When a quadratic component of age was added to the model, its β-coefficient was not significant and thus a linear effect deemed sufficient.

Based on the fitted model, it seems that a linear function in age is adequate and that separate curves be used for boys and girls (significant coefficient of x_{i1}).

To address question (iii) posed by Potthoff and Roy, we follow the approach suggested by Jones (1993). Since for each subject in the study, there is an X_i matrix, let x denote a possible row of X_i for any subject. For example, for a subject who is a girl at age 14, then $x = (1\ 1\ 14)'$ or for a subject who is a boy at age 10, then $x = (1\ 0\ 10)'$. The estimated population mean for a given x vector is

$$\hat{y} = \hat{x}\hat{\beta} \quad (6.12)$$

and has estimated variance

$$V(\hat{y}) = x\text{Cov}(\hat{\beta})x'$$
$$= \hat{\sigma}^2 x \left(\sum_i x_i' V_i^{-1} x_i \right)^{-1} x' \quad (6.13)$$

By varying the elements of the x vector, estimated population curves can be generated for different values of the covariates. The $(1 - \alpha)100\%$ confidence limits are thus $\hat{y} \pm z_{\alpha/2}\sqrt{\text{var}(\hat{y})}$.

```
data growth;
input gender subject age distance @@;
wave=age; age=age-11;
cards;
1 1 8 21.0 1 1 10 20.0 1 1 12 21.5 1 1 14 23.0
1 2 8 21.0 1 2 10 21.5 1 2 12 24.0 1 2 14 25.5
1 3 8 20.5 1 3 10 24.0 1 3 12 24.5 1 3 14 26.0
1 4 8 23.5 1 4 10 24.5 1 4 12 25.0 1 4 14 26.5
```

```
1 5 8 21.5 1 5 10 23.0 1 5 12 22.5 1 5 14 23.5
1 6 8 20.0 1 6 10 21.0 1 6 12 21.0 1 6 14 22.5
1 7 8 21.5 1 7 10 22.5 1 7 12 23.0 1 7 14 25.0
1 8 8 23.0 1 8 10 23.0 1 8 12 23.5 1 8 14 24.0
1 9 8 20.0 1 9 10 21.0 1 9 12 22.0 1 9 14 21.5
1 10 8 16.5 1 10 10 19.0 1 10 12 19.0 1 10 14 19.5
1 11 8 24.5 1 11 10 25.0 1 11 12 28.0 1 11 14 28.0
2 12 8 26.0 2 12 10 25.0 2 12 12 29.0 2 12 14 31.0
2 13 8 21.5 2 13 10 22.5 2 13 12 23.0 2 13 14 26.5
2 14 8 23.0 2 14 10 22.5 2 14 12 24.0 2 14 14 27.5
2 15 8 25.5 2 15 10 27.5 2 15 12 26.5 2 15 14 27.0
2 16 8 20.0 2 16 10 23.5 2 16 12 22.5 2 16 14 26.0
2 17 8 24.5 2 17 10 25.5 2 17 12 27.0 2 17 14 28.5
2 18 8 22.0 2 18 10 22.0 2 18 12 24.5 2 18 14 26.5
2 19 8 24.0 2 19 10 21.5 2 19 12 24.5 2 19 14 25.5
2 20 8 23.0 2 20 10 20.5 2 20 12 31.0 2 20 14 26.0
2 21 8 27.5 2 21 10 28.0 2 21 12 31.0 2 21 14 31.5
2 22 8 23.0 2 22 10 23.0 2 22 12 23.5 2 22 14 25.0
2 23 8 21.5 2 23 10 23.5 2 23 12 24.0 2 23 14 28.0
2 24 8 17.0 2 24 10 24.5 2 24 12 26.0 2 24 14 29.5
2 25 8 22.5 2 25 10 25.5 2 25 12 25.5 2 25 14 26.0
2 26 8 23.0 2 26 10 24.5 2 26 12 26.0 2 26 14 30.0
2 27 8 22.0 2 27 10 21.5 2 27 12 23.5 2 27 14 25.0
;
```

We fitted three models to the data:

* Model 1: Mixed model with unstructured between subject covariance;
```
proc mixed;
  class gender subject;
  model distance = gender age gender*age / s ddfm=bw notest;
  random intercept age / type=un sub= subject gcorr;
run;
```

* Model 2: AR(1) structure for within subject variation;
```
proc mixed;
  class gender wave;
  model distance = gender age gender*age / s ddfm=bw notest;
  repeated wave / type=ar(1) sub= subject r;
run;
```

* Model 3: Combining repeated statement with the random statement;
```
proc mixed;
  class gender wave subject;
  model distance = gender age gender*age / s ddfm=bw notest;
```

```
        random intercept age / type=un sub= subject g;
        repeated wave / type=ar(1) sub= subject r;
    run;
```

The selected SAS output is given below
Model 1:

Covariance Parameter Estimates

Cov Parm	Subject	Estimate
UN(1,1)	subject	3.3501
UN(2,1)	subject	0.06814
UN(2,2)	subject	0.03252
Residual		1.7162

Fit Statistics

−2 Res log likelihood	432.6
AIC (smaller is better)	440.6

Solution for Fixed Effects

Effect	Gender	Estimate	Standard Error	DF	t-Value	$Pr > |t|$
Intercept		24.9688	0.4860	25	51.38	<0.0001
gender	1	−2.3210	0.7614	25	−3.05	0.0054
gender	2	0	—	—	—	—
age		0.7844	0.08600	79	9.12	<0.0001
age*gender	1	−0.3048	0.1347	79	−2.26	0.0264
age*gender	2	0	—	—	—	—

Model 2:

Covariance Parameter Estimates

Cov Parm	Subject	Estimate
AR(1)	subject	0.6245
Residual		5.2145

Fit Statistics

−2 Res log likelihood	444.6
AIC (smaller is better)	448.6

Solution for Fixed Effects

Effect	Gender	Estimate	Standard Error	DF	t-Value	Pr > |t|
Intercept		25.0610	0.4387	25	57.13	<0.0001
gender	1	−2.4184	0.6873	25	−3.52	0.0017
gender	2	0	—	—	—	—
age		0.7693	0.1170	79	6.58	<0.0001
age*gender	1	−0.2854	0.1832	79	−1.56	0.1233
age*gender	2	0	—	—	—	—

Model 3:

Covariance Parameter Estimates

Cov Parm	Subject	Estimate
UN(1,1)	subject	3.6778
UN(2,1)	subject	0.1150
UN(2,2)	subject	0.08455
AR(1)	subject	−0.4733
Residual		1.1924

Fit Statistics

−2 Res log likelihood	428.8
AIC (smaller is better)	438.8

Solution for Fixed Effects

Effect	Gender	Estimate	Standard Error	DF	t-Value	Pr > |t|
Intercept		24.9299	0.4876	25	51.12	<0.0001
gender	1	−2.2800	0.7640	25	−2.98	0.0063
gender	2	0	—	—	—	—
age		0.7979	0.08707	79	9.16	<0.0001
age*gender	1	−0.3222	0.1364	79	−2.36	0.0206
age*gender	2	0	—	—	—	—

Clearly, for the fixed effects estimates, there is little or no difference among the four models. Since none of the above models are considered nested within either of the others, model comparisons should be confined to the AIC. Based on the AIC values, model 3 outperforms models 1 and 2.

Note that we subtracted the mean age (11 years) from the age of each subject, so that the intercept would be interpreted as the average response for a randomly selected subject whose age is 11 years.

Now, we illustrate the use of the lme function in R to fit the linear mixed effect models. Following is the R code to set up the data for Example 6.2 and fitting alternative mixed effect models with AR(1) correlation structure. In lme1, intercept and age are the random effects, whereas in lme2 only intercept is specified as the random effect so that lme2 is nested within lme1. The likelihood ratio test is then performed to see if age as a random effect is required in the model, and it turns out that age is not required as a random effect. To see if a nonzero correlation structure is needed, lme3 was fit with the default independence correlation structure. Comparison of lme2 and lme3 by likelihood ratio test shows that the AR(1) correlation structure does not improve the fit of the model. The statistics of fitting the final model are then displayed. Lastly, the intervals function is used to display the confidence intervals for the parameters of the model.

```
> # Setting up the data for Example 6.2
> g <- factor(c(rep(1,44),rep(2,64)))
> subject <- gl(27, 4, length = 108, labels = 1:27)
> age <- rep(c(8,10,12,14),27)-11
>
> distance <-
c(21.0,20.0,21.5,23.0,21.0,21.5,24.0,25.5,20.5,24.0,24.5,26.0,
  23.5,24.5,25.0,26.5,21.5,23.0,22.5,23.5,20.0,21.0,21.0,22.5,
  21.5,22.5,23.0,25.0,23.0,23.0,23.5,24.0,20.0,21.0,22.0,21.5,
  16.5,19.0,19.0,19.5,24.5,25.0,28.0,28.0,26.0,25.0,29.0,31.0,
  21.5,22.5,23.0,26.5,23.0,22.5,24.0,27.5,25.5,27.5,26.5,27.0,
  20.0,23.5,22.5,26.0,24.5,25.5,27.0,28.5,22.0,22.0,24.5,26.5,
  24.0,21.5,24.5,25.5,23.0,20.5,31.0,26.0,27.5,28.0,31.0,31.5,
  23.0,23.0,23.5,25.0,21.5,23.5,24.0,28.0,17.0,24.5,26.0,29.5,
  22.5,25.5,25.5,26.0,23.0,24.5,26.0,30.0,22.0,21.5,23.5,25.0)
>
> # Changing the reference level as 2
> gender <- relevel(g,2)
> growth <- data.frame(gender,subject,age,distance)
>
> # Fitting the model with intercept and age as random effects and AR1
correlation structure
> lme1 <-
lme(distance~gender*age,random=~age|subject,
corr=corAR1(form=~age|subject),data=growth)
>
> # Fitting the model with intercept only as random effect and AR1
correlation structure
> lme2 <-lme(distance~gender*age,random=~1|subject, corr=corAR1(),
data=growth)
>
> # Likelihood Ratio test to test if age as random effect is required
> anova(lme1,lme2)
```

```
      Model df    AIC     BIC    logLik  Test  L.Ratio p-value
lme1   1    9  450.5817 474.3812  -216.2908
lme2   2    7  447.7081 466.2188  -216.8541  1 vs 2 1.126451  0.5694
>
> # Fittinng the model with zero random effects correlation
> lme3 <-lme(distance~gender*age,random=~1|subject,data=growth)
>
> # Likelihood Ratio test of zero random effects correlation
> anova(lme2,lme3)
      Model df  AIC     BIC    logLik     Test  L.Ratio p-value
lme2   1    7  447.7081 466.2188  -216.8541
lme3   2    6  445.7572 461.6236  -216.8786  1 vs 2 0.04913688  0.8246
>
> summary(lme3)
Linear mixed-effects model fit by REML
Data: growth
  AIC      BIC      logLik
445.7572 461.6236 -216.8786


Random effects:
Formula: ~1 | subject
        (Intercept) Residual
StdDev:  1.816214   1.386382


Fixed effects: distance ~ gender * age
                Value     Std.Error   DF    t-value   p-value
(Intercept)   24.968750  0.4860008   79   51.37595   0.0000
gender1       -2.321023  0.7614168   25   -3.04829   0.0054
age            0.784375  0.0775011   79   10.12082   0.0000
gender1:age   -0.304830  0.1214209   79   -2.51052   0.0141
Correlation:
        (Intr) gendr1 age
gender1   -0.638
age       0.000 0.000
gender1:age 0.000 0.000 -0.638
Standardized within-group residuals:
     Min          Q1           Med          Q3          Max
-3.59804400  -0.45461690  0.01578365  0.50244658  3.68620792


Number of Observations: 108
Number of Groups: 27
> intervals(lme3)
Approximate 95% confidence intervals
```

Fixed effects:

	lower	est.	upper
(Intercept)	24.0013897	24.9687500	25.9361103
gender1	-3.8891901	-2.3210227	-0.7528554
age	0.6301129	0.7843750	0.9386371
gender1:age	-0.5465118	-0.3048295	-0.0631473

attr(,"label")
[1] "Fixed effects:"

Random effects:
Level: subject

	lower	est.	upper
sd((Intercept))	1.320996	1.816214	2.497081

Within-group standard error:

lower	est.	upper
1.186215	1.386382	1.620326

It is interesting to note that the estimates of the fixed effects parameters and the log-likelihood statistics are the same as for model 2 in SAS indicating that fitting a more complicated model did not really improve the fit of the model.

6.4.2 Analysis of Longitudinal Binary and Count Data

Examples in this section will focus on the analysis of longitudinal count and binary data. We shall adopt two modeling strategies, the first being a population average (PA) approach and the second is known as subject-specific (SS) approach. Both methodologies have been discussed in previous chapters to deal with clustered data.

The PA models use the GEE (GENMOD) methodology of Liang and Zeger (1986, 1993), and the SS models use the GLIMMIX. We have demonstrated the use of both techniques on cross-sectional continuous, binary, and count data. Here, we illustrate both techniques on repeated measures non-normally distributed outcome variables. We first discuss situations where such data may be available.

Example: EPA-CHESS Study (Longitudinal Binary Data)

An asthma study conducted by the Environmental Protection Agency's Community Health and Environment Surveillance System (EPA-CHESS) was described in Korn and Whittemore (1979). Daily records of the absence/presence of an asthma attack were recorded on each participant, in addition to measurements of air pollutants and meteorological variables such as daily temperature and humidity. Here, the aerometric and meteorological variables are time-varying covariates, since they can change from one time point to another time point, whereas individual characteristics, such as sex and ethnicity, do not vary with time. One of the objectives of the study was to determine the effects of outside air quality on the rates of asthma attacks. Since we are interested in modeling the probability of disease as a function of covariates, a regression model is appropriate. However, the over-time correlation among the binary responses must be properly accounted for.

The issue of robustness, of the GEE approach, against misspecification of the correlation structure was the subject of investigation by many authors. In particular, if the correlation structure is misspecified as "independence," which assumes that the within-cluster responses are independent, the GEE has been shown to be nearly efficient relative to the maximum likelihood in a variety of settings. When the correlation between responses is not too high, Zeger et al. (1988) suggested that this estimator should be nearly efficient. MacDonald (1993), focusing on the case of clusters of size $n_i = 2$ (i.e., the bivariate case), concluded that the estimator obtained under specifying independence may be recommended whenever the correlation between the within-cluster pair is nuisance. This may have practical implications since the model can be implemented using standard software packages. In a more recent article, Fitzmaurice (1995) investigated this issue analytically. He has confirmed the suggestions made by Zeger et al. (1988) and MacDonald (1993). Furthermore, he showed that when the responses are strongly correlated and the covariate design includes a within-cluster covariate, assuming independence can lead to a considerable loss of efficiency if the GEE is used in estimating the regression parameters associated with that covariate. His results demonstrate that the degree of efficiency depends on both the strength of the correlation between the responses and the covariate design. He recommended that an effort should be made to model the association between responses, even when this association is regarded as a nuisance feature of the data and its correct nature is unknown.

Example 6.3   The Epilepsy Data

These data have been analyzed by Thall and Vail (1990) and Stukel (1993) using several models for longitudinal count data. It is a randomized clinical trial of an antiepileptic drug (Progabide), in which 59 patients were observed and the count of seizures was taken at baseline and at four follow-up visits. The main objective was to estimate the treatment effect and its possible modification by disease severity (seizure count at baseline) and age. The data are given in Table 6.3.

First, we note from Figures 6.2 and 6.3 that the number of seizures declines as time elapses. From Figure 6.4, it is clear that the two treatments (0, 1) are equally effective.

The data would be transformed into the longitudinal format so that there would be four observations for each subject corresponding to the

TABLE 6.3

Epilepsy Data

ID	Treat	Age	Base	Y1	Y2	Y3	Y4	ID	Treat	Age	Base	Y1	Y2	Y3	Y4
101	1	18	76	11	14	9	8	104	0	31	11	5	3	3	3
102	1	32	38	8	7	9	4	106	0	30	11	3	5	3	3
103	1	20	19	0	4	3	0	107	0	25	6	2	4	0	5
108	1	30	10	3	6	1	3	114	0	36	8	4	4	1	4
110	1	18	19	2	6	7	4	116	0	22	66	7	18	9	21
111	1	24	24	4	3	1	3	118	0	29	27	5	2	8	7
112	1	30	31	22	17	19	16	123	0	31	12	6	4	0	2
113	1	35	14	5	4	7	4	126	0	42	52	40	20	23	12
117	1	27	11	2	4	0	4	130	0	37	23	5	6	6	5
121	1	20	67	3	7	7	7	135	0	28	10	14	13	6	0
122	1	22	41	4	18	2	5	141	0	36	52	26	12	6	22
124	1	28	7	2	1	1	0	145	0	24	33	12	6	8	4
128	1	23	22	0	2	4	0	201	0	23	18	4	4	6	2
129	1	40	13	5	4	0	3	202	0	36	42	7	9	12	14
137	1	33	46	11	14	25	15	205	0	26	87	16	24	10	9
139	1	21	36	10	5	3	8	206	0	26	50	11	0	0	5
143	1	35	38	19	7	6	7	210	0	28	18	0	0	3	3
147	1	25	7	1	1	2	3	213	0	31	111	37	29	28	29
203	1	26	36	6	10	8	8	215	0	32	18	3	5	2	5
204	1	25	11	2	1	0	0	217	0	21	20	3	0	6	7
207	1	22	151	102	65	72	63	219	0	29	12	3	4	3	4
208	1	32	22	4	3	2	4	220	0	21	9	3	4	3	4
209	1	25	41	8	6	5	7	222	0	32	17	2	3	3	5
211	1	35	32	1	3	1	5	226	0	25	28	8	12	2	8
214	1	21	56	18	11	28	13	227	0	30	55	18	24	76	25
218	1	41	24	6	3	4	0	230	0	40	9	2	1	2	1
221	1	32	16	3	5	4	3	234	0	19	10	3	1	4	2
225	1	26	22	1	23	19	8	238	0	22	47	13	15	13	12
228	1	21	25	2	3	0	1								
232	1	36	13	0	0	0	0								
236	1	37	12	1	4	3	2								

four repeated measurements. If the dataset is stored in a temporary SAS dataset say "epilepsy," transformation may be achieved using the following code:

```
data epilepsy1; set epilepsy;
  period=1; count=y1; output; period=2; count=y2; output;
  period=3; count=y3; output; period=4; count=y4; output;
  drop y1-y4;
```

The models are now run as below.

```
* Population averaged model with exchangeable correlation structure;
proc genmod data=a;
  class id treat;
  model count = treat base age/ d=poisson;
  repeated subject=id/ corrw type=exch;
```

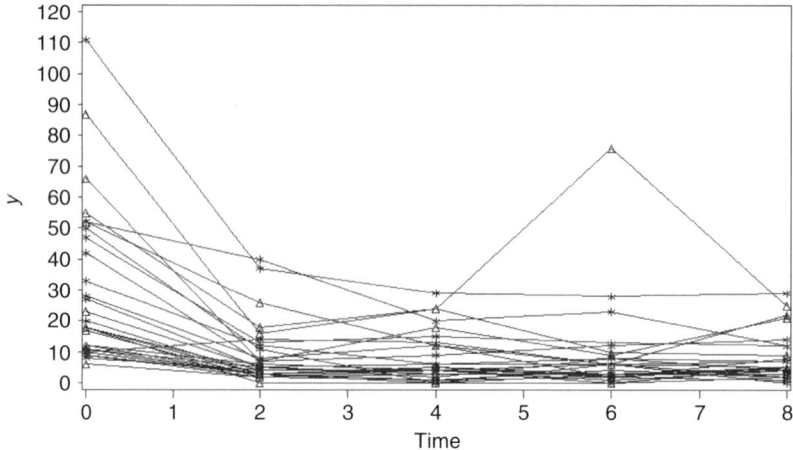

FIGURE 6.2
Plot of number of episodes by time for control group.

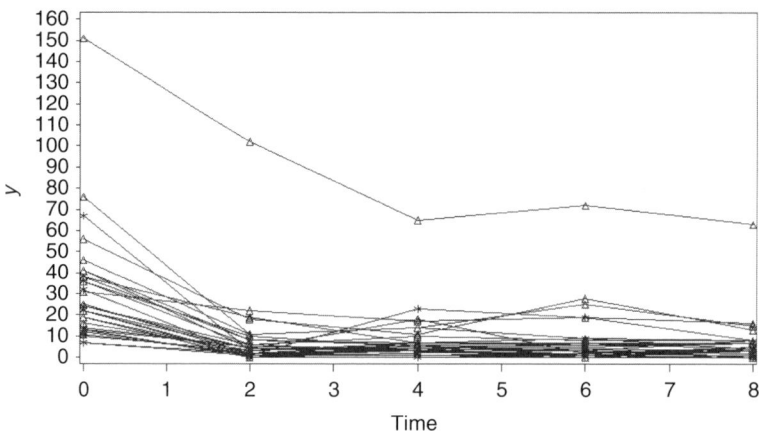

FIGURE 6.3
Plot of number of episodes by time for treatment group.

```
run;
* Subject specific model with exchangeable correlation structure;
proc glimmix data=a;
  class id treat;
  model count = treat base age / s d=poisson;
  random intercept /subject=id type=cs;
run;
```

The SAS output

The two models assume that the number of seizures follows Poisson distribution. First, we used PROC GENMOD to fit the data with exchangeable

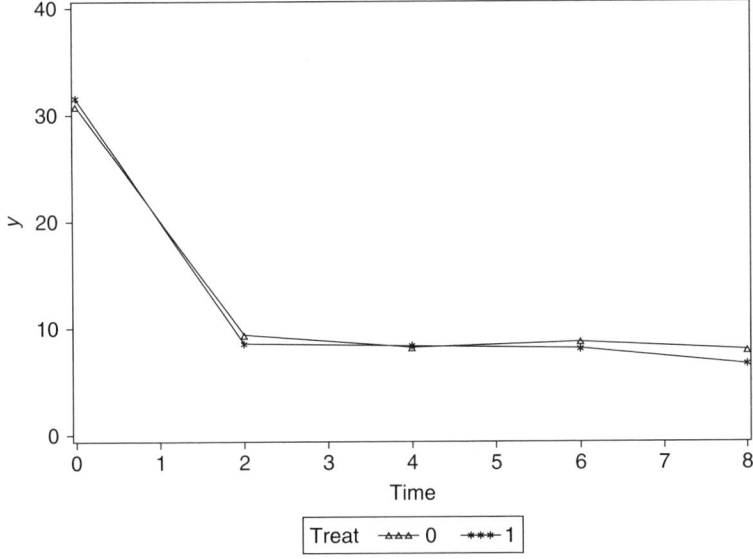

FIGURE 6.4
Plot of the average number of episodes for two groups over time.

correlation structure. We note that the value of the intrasubject correlation is quite high ($\hat{\rho} = 0.395$). Other correlation structures may be explored, but we shall leave this issue to be discussed in the exercises at the end of the chapter. Note also that we used the baseline count as a covariate. Although this is not a strictly valid approach, it is modeled as such to demonstrate the dependence of patients' profile on the baseline measurement. Again, we shall elaborate on this issue in the exercises.

The GLIMMIX results are not qualitatively different from the PROC GENMOD, although the estimated coefficients and their standard errors differ between the two models. Note that the default correlation in the GLIMMIX is the exchangeable correlation. Both models indicate that there is no significance between the treatment and the placebo. Moreover, both models indicate that the baseline counts are significant predictors. Note that the GEE identified "age" as a significant covariate, while this was not the case under the cluster-specific model.

Model 1: Population averaged model

Criteria for Assessing Goodness of Fit

Criterion	DF	Value	Value/DF
Deviance	232	958.4636	4.1313
Scaled deviance	232	958.4636	4.1313
Pearson χ^2	232	1180.7884	5.0896
Scaled Pearson χ^2	232	1180.7884	5.0896
Log likelihood		2949.5627	

Exchangeable Working Correlation

Correlation	0.3948

Analysis of GEE Parameter Estimates

Empirical Standard Error Estimates

Parameter		Estimate	Standard Error	95% Confidence Limits		Z	Pr > |Z|
Intercept		0.4098	0.3630	−0.3017	1.1214	1.13	0.2589
treat	0	0.1527	0.1711	−0.1827	0.4881	0.89	0.3722
treat	1	0.0000	0.0000	0.0000	0.0000	—	—
base		0.0227	0.0012	0.0202	0.0251	18.33	<0.0001
age		0.0227	0.0116	0.0000	0.0454	1.96	0.0496

Model 2: Subject-specific model

Fit Statistics

−2 Res log pseudolikelihood	602.13
Generalized χ^2	418.36
Generalized χ^2/DF	1.80

Covariance Parameter Estimates

Cov Parm	Subject	Estimate	Standard Error
Variance	id	0.3785	0.06921
CS	id	−0.07723	—

Solutions for Fixed Effects

Effect	Treat	Estimate	Standard Error	DF	t-Value	Pr > |t|
Intercept		0.3000	0.4000	55	0.75	0.4565
treat	0	0.2584	0.1574	177	1.64	0.1025
treat	1	0	—	—	—	—
base		0.02694	0.002862	177	9.41	<0.0001
age		0.01400	0.01283	177	1.09	0.2767

The following R code reads the epilepsy data and runs models 1 and 2.

```
e <- read.table("x:/xxx/epilepsy.txt",header=T)
c1 <- cbind(e[,c(1:5)], count=e$y1)[,c(1:4,6)]
c2 <- cbind(e[,c(1:4,6)],count=e$y2)[,c(1:4,6)]
```

```
c3 <- cbind(e[,c(1:4,7)],count=e$y3)[,c(1:4,6)]
c4 <- cbind(e[,c(1:4,8)],count=e$y4)[,c(1:4,6)]

epilepsy <- rbind(c1,c2,c3,c4)
epilepsy$treat <- factor(epilepsy$treat,levels=c(1,0))

# Model 1
gee1 <-gee(count~treat+base+age,id=factor(id),family=poisson("log"),
corstr="exchangeable",data=epilepsy,scale.fix=T)
summary(gee1)

# Model 2
glmm2 <-glmmPQL(count~treat+base+age, random=~1|id,
family=poisson("log"),correlation=corCompSymm(),data=epilepsy)
summary(glmm2)
```

Slight differences in the results of model 2 with those produced by SAS are because of different model fitting methods.

The next example is on longitudinal binary data with covariates measured at the subject level. During the past few decades, repeated binary data have been the subject of a great deal of research in the statistical literature, with special emphasis on the random effects model. In modeling such data, the central problem will be modeling the repeated responses as a function of covariates measured at several levels of hierarchies, and taking into account the interdependencies of the observations and exploring several models as we did for continuous and count longitudinal data.

Example 6.4   Hip Dysplasia in Dogs

The following data are the results of a longitudinal investigation that aimed at assessing the long-term effects of two types of treatments ($1 \equiv$ excision arthroplasty, $2 \equiv$ triple-pelvic osteotomy) for hip dysplasia in dogs. The owner's assessment was the response variable and was recorded on a binary scale at weeks 1, 3, 6, 10, and 20. Using the GEE approach, we test for treatment effect controlling for laterality and age as possible confounders.

The data in Example 6.4 have been fitted under three different specifications of the correlations among the scores in weeks 1, 3, 6, 10, and 20. The data are entered in a longitudinal format so that the new data will have six times the number of observations as in Table 6.4. The SAS programs to fit the models are given below:

```
* Model l: Fitting a PA (GEE) model with AR(1) correlation structure;
proc genmod descending;
   class dog lateral typsurg;
   model score= week lateral typsurg age / dist=binomial;
   repeated subject= dog / type=AR(1);
run;
```

TABLE 6.4

Longitudinal Data for Hip Dysplasia in Dogs

Dog No.	Laterality[a]	Age	Type of Surgery[b]	Owner's Assessment[c]				
				Week 1	Week 3	Week 6	Week 10	Week 20
1	U	6	1	1	1	1	1	1
2	U	4	1	1	1	1	1	1
3	U	7	2	1	1	1	1	1
4	B	7	2	1	1	1	1	1
5	U	4	2	1	1	1	1	1
6	U	8	2	1	1	0	1	1
7	U	7	2	1	0	1	1	1
8	U	6	2	1	1	1	0	1
9	U	8	1	1	1	1	1	1
10	U	5	2	1	1	1	1	1
11	U	6	1	1	1	1	1	1
12	U	6	2	0	0	0	1	1
13	U	7	1	1	1	1	1	1
14	U	7	1	1	1	1	1	1
15	B	7	2	1	1	1	1	1
16	B	7	2	1	1	1	0	1
17	B	5	1	1	0	1	0	1
18	B	6	1	0	0	1	1	0
19	B	8	2	1	1	0	1	0
20	B	6	1	1	1	1	0	1
21	U	8	1	1	1	1	1	1
22	B	2	2	1	1	0	0	0
23	B	1	1	0	1	1	1	1
24	U	1	1	1	1	1	1	1
25	U	1	1	1	1	1	1	1
26	B	2	2	1	0	1	0	1
27	B	2	2	0	0	0	0	0
28	B	2	2	0	0	0	0	0
29	U	1	1	1	0	1	1	1
30	B	2	2	1	1	0	1	1
31	B	2	2	0	0	0	0	0
32	B	2	2	0	0	0	1	1
33	U	1	1	1	1	1	1	1
34	U	2	2	1	1	0	1	1
35	U	1	1	1	1	1	1	1
36	U	2	2	1	0	1	1	1
37	U	1	1	0	1	1	1	1
38	U	2	2	1	1	1	1	1
39	U	6	1	1	1	1	1	1
40	U	8	1	0	0	1	0	0
41	U	8	2	1	1	0	0	0
42	U	8	1	0	1	0	0	0
43	U	2	2	1	0	0	1	0
44	U	1	1	0	0	1	1	1
45	U	1	1	1	1	1	1	1
46	U	2	2	0	0	0	1	0

Note: U ≡ unilateral, B ≡ bilateral.

[a] excision arthroplasty.

[b] Triple pelvic osteotomy (TPO).

[c] 1 ≡ good and 0 ≡ poor.

* Model 2: Fitting a PA (GEE) model with exchangeable correlation structure;
```
proc genmod descending;
  class dog lateral typsurg;
  model score= week lateral typsurg age / dist=binomial;
  repeated subject=dog / type=cs;
run;
```

* Model 3: Fitting GLMM, a cluster specific model with AR(1) correlation structure;
```
proc glimmix;
  class dog lateral typsurg;
  model score= week lateral typsurg age /s dist=binomial;
  random intercept/ subject= dog type=AR(1);
run;
```

* Model 4: Fitting GLIM, a cluster specific model compound symmetry;
```
proc glimmix;
  class dog lateral typsurg;
  model score= week lateral typsurg age /s dist=binomial;
  random intercept/ subject= dog type=cs;
run;
```

Model 1:

Criteria for Assessing Goodness of Fit

Criterion	DF	Value	Value/DF
Deviance	225	248.2603	1.1034
Scaled deviance	225	248.2603	1.1034
Pearson χ^2	225	235.1769	1.0452
Scaled Pearson χ^2	225	235.1769	1.0452
Log likelihood		−124.1301	

Analysis of GEE Parameter Estimates

				95% Confidence Limits			
Empirical Standard Error Estimates							
Parameter		Estimate	Standard Error			Z	Pr > |Z|
Intercept		0.7011	0.5773	−0.4305	1.8327	1.21	0.2246
week		0.0148	0.0179	−0.0203	0.0499	0.82	0.4101
lateral	B	−1.0174	0.4505	−1.9002	−0.1345	−2.26	0.0239
lateral	U	0.0000	0.0000	0.0000	0.0000	—	—
typsurg	1	0.7000	0.4898	−0.2600	1.6600	1.43	0.1530
typsurg	2	0.0000	0.0000	0.0000	0.0000	—	—
age		0.0585	0.1023	−0.1419	0.2590	0.57	0.5671

Model 3:

Fit Statistics

−2 Res log pseudolikelihood	1096.81
Generalized χ^2	149.80
Generalized χ^2/DF	0.67

Covariance Parameter Estimates

Cov Parm	Subject	Estimate	Standard Error
Variance	dog	1.9652	0.7513
AR(1)	dog	0	—

Solutions for Fixed Effects

Effect	Lateral	Typsurg	Estimate	Standard Error	DF	t-Value	$Pr > |t|$
Intercept			0.7694	0.6858	42	1.12	0.2682
week			0.02069	0.02612	183	0.79	0.4295
lateral	B		−1.2576	0.5898	183	−2.13	0.0343
lateral	U		0	—	—	—	—
typsurg		1	0.9772	0.5802	183	1.68	0.0938
typsurg		2	0	—	—	—	—
age			0.06153	0.1045	183	0.59	0.5566

Comments

1. All the covariates in the model are measured at the cluster (subject) level, and no time-varying covariates are included in the study. With this type of covariate design, one should expect little or no difference between the PA models. The same remark holds for the subject-specific models.
2. All the models indicate that, relative to the unilateral, lateral has a significant negative effect on the condition of the dog. However, neither age nor type of surgery has an effect on the subject's condition.
3. We noted that the results of fitting Models 2 and 4 were similar to Model 1, and therefore we did not include their output.

The R code to read the data and fit the four models is given below.

```
dogs <- read.table("x:/xxx/dogs.txt",header=T)
dogs$dog <- factor(dogs$dog)
dogs$lateral <- factor(dogs$lateral,levels=c("u","b")) # Changing
the order for reference level
```

```
dogs$typsurg <- factor(dogs$typsurg,levels=c(2,1)) # Changing
the order for reference level
# Model 1
gee1 <-
gee(score~week+lateral+typsurg+age,id=dog,family=binomial("logit"),
corstr="AR-M",Mv=1,data=dogs,scale.fix=T)
summary(gee1)
```

```
# Model 2
gee2 <-
gee(score~week+lateral+typsurg+age,id=dog,family=binomial("logit"),
corstr="exchangeable",data=dogs,scale.fix=T)
summary(gee2)
```

```
# Model 3
glmm3 <-
glmmPQL(score~week+lateral+typsurg+age,random=~1|dog,
family=binomial("logit"),correlation=corAR1(),data=dogs)
summary(glmm3)
```

```
# Model 4
glmm4 <-
glmmPQL(score~week+lateral+typsurg+age,random=~1|dog,
family=binomial("logit"),correlation=corCompSymm(),data=dogs)
summary(glmm4)
```

Slight differences in the results of models 3 and 4 with those produced by SAS are because of different model fitting methods.

Exercises

6.1 Situations in which more than two factors would be nested within each other are of frequent occurrence in repeated measures experiments. Example 6.1 illustrates this situation. Pens of animals are randomized into two diet groups. Animals in each pen are approximately of the same age and initial weight. Their weights were measured at weeks 1, 2, and 3. The data are presented in Table 6.5.

The data in Table 6.5 show that pens 1, 2, and 3 are nested within the diet group 1 while pens 4, 5, and 6 are nested in diet group 2 (i.e., different pens within each group) and animals are nested within pens. The main objectives of the trial were to see if the weights of animals differed between the diet groups, and if such differences were present over time.

6.2 Familial polyposis supplementation trial (FPST) was a 4-year random-ized double-blind placebo-controlled trial of high fiber and vitamins C and E to reduce polyps in a high-risk population (part of the data is produced here).

TABLE 6.5

Data for the Feed Trial

Animal	Diet	Pen	Weight		
			Week 1	Week 2	Week 3
1	1	1	2.5	3.0	4.0
2	1	1	2.0	2.5	2.5
3	1	1	1.5	2.0	2.0
4	1	1	1.5	2.5	3.0
5	1	2	2.0	4.0	4.0
6	1	2	2.5	3.5	2.5
7	1	2	1.5	2.0	2.5
8	1	2	1.0	1.5	1.0
9	1	3	1.5	1.5	2.0
10	1	3	2.0	2.0	2.5
11	1	3	1.5	2.0	2.0
12	2	4	3.0	3.0	4.0
13	2	4	3.0	6.0	8.0
14	2	4	3.0	4.0	7.0
15	2	4	4.0	5.0	6.0
16	2	5	3.0	3.0	5.0
17	2	5	4.0	4.5	5.5
18	2	5	3.0	3.0	4.0
19	2	6	3.0	7.0	9.0
20	2	6	4.0	6.0	7.0
21	2	6	4.0	6.0	8.0
22	2	6	4.0	6.0	7.0

Fifty-eight patients were randomized to take either placebo ($k = 22$), vitamins C and E ($k = 16$), or vitamins C and E and high fiber ($k = 20$). Subjects were examined every 3 months and rectal polyps were counted. The study was reported in detail in De Cosse et al. (1989).

   Examine the data carefully, state the hypotheses, and conduct data analysis using PA and SS models.

Data for Familial Polyposis Supplementation Trial

ID	Treatment	Sex	Baseline Polyp Count	V1	V2	V3	V4	V5
1	0	0	41	36	56	34	46	61
2	2	1	4	2	2	0	1	1
3	2	1	26	1	2	0	0	1
4	2	0	15	13	6	12	6	12
5	2	0	9	6	2	8	6	4
6	1	1	6	15	9	4	4	2
7	1	0	1	7	8	5	3	6
8	0	1	2	3	1	1	3	3
9	0	0	2	4	10	9	17	8
10	1	0	1	2	1	1	1	2
11	0	0	7	10	31	31	37	11

(Continued)

(*Continued*)

ID	Treatment	Sex	Baseline Polyp Count	V1	V2	V3	V4	V5
12	2	1	25	8	6	8	11	16
13	1	1	10	6	3	3	7	9
14	2	0	1	0	0	0	0	0
15	2	1	4	5	2	1	1	2
16	2	0	24	21	13	14	9	16
17	1	1	1	4	4	10	4	7
18	0	0	3	3	1	1	4	0
19	2	0	8	1	1	2	2	1
20	1	1	5	4	6	6	11	16
21	0	0	8	16	17	22	24	36
22	1	0	0	0	0	0	0	0
23	1	0	27	15	10	37	32	30
24	2	1	3	5	5	6	4	1
25	0	1	1	6	4	3	11	6
26	1	1	1	3	3	7	6	7
27	2	1	10	11	9	9	21	23
28	0	1	5	1	4	2	0	0
29	0	0	11	7	4	11	8	8

7

Survival Data Analysis

CONTENTS

7.1 Introduction

stewed
censored

Time to event or survival studies involve observing units until an event is experienced. In the case of medical studies, the units are humans or animals, and failure may be broadly defined as the occurrence of a prespecified event. Events of this nature include time to death, disease remission, occurrence, or recurrence.

Although survival data analysis is similar to the analysis of other types of data discussed previously (continuous, binary, time series) in that information is collected on the response variable as well as any covariates of interest, it differs in one important aspect: the anticipated event may not occur for each subject under study. Not all subjects will experience the outcome during the course of observation, resulting in the absence of a failure time for that particular individual. This situation is referred to as *censoring* in the analysis of survival data, and a study subject for which no failure time is available is referred to as *censored*.

Unlike the other types of analysis discussed previously, censored data analysis requires special methods to compensate for the information lost by not knowing the time of failure of all subjects. In addition, survival data analysis must account for highly skewed data. Often one or two individuals will experience the event of interest much sooner or later than the majority of individuals under study, giving the overall distribution of failure times a skewed appearance and preventing the use of the normal distribution in the analysis. Thus, the analysis of survival data requires techniques that are able to incorporate the possibility of skewed and censored observations.

The above paragraphs referred to censoring in a broad sense, defining censored survival data as data for which the true failure time is not known. This general definition may be broken down for three specific situations, resulting in three types of censoring:

Type I Censoring: Subjects are observed for a fixed period of time, with exact failure times recorded for those who fail during the observation period. Subjects not failing during the observation period are considered censored. Their failure times become the time at which they were last observed or the time at which the study finished.

Type II Censoring: Subjects are observed until a fixed number of failures occur. As with Type I censoring, those failing during the observation period are considered uncensored and have known failure times. Those not failing are considered censored and have failure times that become the time at which they were last observed or the time at which the longest uncensored failure occurred.

Random Censoring: Often encountered in clinical trials, random censoring occurs owing to the accrual of patients gradually over time, resulting in unequal times under study. The study takes place over a fixed period of time, resulting in exact failure times for those failing during the period of observation and censored failure times for those lost to follow up or not failing before study termination. All failure times reflect the period under study for that individual.

The three censoring situations are further elaborated in Table 7.1.

TABLE 7.1

Summary Information for Three Types of Censoring

Characteristics	Type I	Type II	Random
Duration	Study continues for a fixed period of time	Study continues until a fixed number/ proportion of failures	Study continues for a fixed period of time Unequal periods of observation possible
Uncensored failure time	Equal to the exact failure time which is known	Equal to the exact failure time which is known	Equal to the exact failure time which is known
Censored failure time	Equal to the length of the study -	Equal to the largest uncensored failure time	Calculated using time of study completion and time of subject enrollment
Lost to follow-up failure time	Calculated using time at which subject is lost and time at which study starts	Calculated using time at which subject is lost and time at which study starts	Calculated using time at which subject is lost and time of subject enrollment

If the survival time is denoted by the random variable T, then the following definitions are useful in the context of survival analysis:

1. Cumulative distribution function (CDF)—denoted by $F(t)$, this quantity defines the probability of failure before time t:

$$F(t) = \text{Pr(individual fails before time } t)$$
$$= \text{Pr}(T < t)$$

2. Probability density function (PDF)—denoted by $f(t)$, this quantity is the derivative of the CDF and defines the probability that an individual fails in a small interval per unit time:

$$f(t) = \lim_{\Delta t \to 0} \frac{\text{Pr(an individual dies in } (t, t + \Delta t))}{\Delta t}$$
$$= \frac{d}{dt} F(t)$$

As with all density functions, $f(t)$ is assumed to have the following properties:

(a) The area under the density curve equals one.

(b) The density is a nonnegative function such that

$$f(t) \begin{cases} >0 & \text{for all } t > 0 \\ =0 & \text{for all } t \leq 0 \end{cases}$$

3. Survival function—denoted by $S(t)$, this function gives the probability of survival longer than time t:

$$S(t) = \text{Pr(an individual survives longer than } t)$$
$$= \text{Pr}(T > t)$$

The survival function is assumed to have the following properties:

(a) The probability of survival at time zero is one, $S(t) = 1$ for $t = 0$.

(b) The probability of infinite survival is zero, $S(t) = 0$ for $t = \infty$.

(c) The survival function is nonincreasing.

4. Hazard function—denoted by $h(t)$, this function gives the probability that an individual fails in a small interval of time conditional on their survival at the beginning of the interval:

$$h(t) = \lim_{\Delta t \to 0} \frac{\text{Pr(an individual dies in } (t, t + \Delta t) \,|\, T > t)}{\Delta t}$$

In terms of the previously defined quantities, the hazard function may be written as

$$h(t) = \frac{f(t)}{S(t)}$$

In practice, the hazard function is also referred to as the instantaneous failure rate or the force of mortality. It represents the failure risk per unit of time during a lifetime. The cumulative hazard function is written as $H(t)$ and is the integral of the hazard function:

$$H(t) = \int_0^t h(x) \, dx$$

Although the quantities $F(t), f(t), S(t)$, and $h(t)$ may be defined for any continuous random variable, $S(t)$ and $h(t)$ are usually seen in the context of survival data since they are particularly suited to its analysis. Note as well that given any one of the four quantities, the other three are easily obtained. Thus specifying the survival function, for instance, also determines what the cumulative distribution function, probability density function, and hazard function are. The following relationships hold:

$$f(t) = -\frac{dS(t)}{dt}$$
$$S(t) = \exp[-H(t)]$$
$$f(t) = h(t)\exp[-H(t)]$$
$$h(t) = -\frac{d}{dt}\ln(S(t))$$

In the following section, we introduce four examples of survival data.

7.2 Examples

7.2.1 Cystic Ovary Data

This study examined the effectiveness of hormonal therapy for treatment of cows with cystic ovarian disease. Two groups of cows were randomized to hormonal treatment and one group to placebo. The time of cyst disappearance was then recorded with the possibility of censored data due to not all cysts disappearing. The data are shown in Table 7.2.

TABLE 7.2

Cystic Ovary Data

Treatment 1	Treatment 2	Placebo
4, 6, 8, 8, 9, 10, 12	7, 12, 15, 16, 18, 22[a]	19, 24, 18[a], 20[a], 22[a], 27[a], 30[a]

[a]Means censored observation.

7.2.2 Breast Cancer Data

An increase in the incidence of breast cancer in recent years has resulted in a substantial portion of health care dollars being directed toward research in this area. The research studies have focused on early detection through mass screening and recurrence prevention through effective treatments. The focus of one such investigation was to determine which prognostic measures were predictive of breast cancer recurrence in female patients. The dataset contains the following variables:

id	patient identification number
censor	breast cancer recurrence [0=no, 1=yes]
time	time until breast cancer recurrence in months

pag   proliferative AgNOR index [0=low, 1=high]
mag   mean AgNOR count [0=low, 1=high]
age   age at the start of the study in years
tsize   size of original tumor [small=0 or large=1]

7.2.3 Ventilating Tube Data

One-third of pediatric visits arise owing to inflammation of the middle ear, also known as otitis media, resulting in a substantial health care burden. In addition, concerns have surfaced relating to long-term language, behavior, and speech development. Unsuccessful treatment with various drug therapies often leads to surgical intervention, in which tubes are placed in the ear. It has been shown that ventilating tubes are successful in preventing otitis media as long as the tubes are in place and unblocked. Le and Lindgren (1996) studied the time of tube failure (displacement or blockage) for 78 children. Each child was randomly assigned to be treated with placebo or prednisone and sulfamethoprim. The children were observed from February 1987 to January 1990, resulting in the possibility of censored failure times for children not experiencing tube failure before the completion of the study. In addition, it is anticipated that the failure times of the two ears from one child will correlate. The analysis of these data will be discussed under the topic of correlated survival data analysis. The dataset contains the following variables:

child   4 digit ID
treat   Treatment group [2 = medical, 1 = control]
ear   Left or right ear [1 = right, 2 = left]
time   Time, in months
status Event [1 = failed, 0 = censored]

7.2.4 Age at Culling of Dairy Cows

Individual cow data were obtained from 72 Ontario farms from April 1993 to October 1994. The information included date of birth, calving and culling dates, and lactation number. During a 2½ year study, the producer recorded all occurrences of clinical diseases of cows. Culling age was calculated as the date of birth to the date the cow was culled. The definition of culling (the event of interest) was restricted to the removal of cows by slaughter. During the study, cows that were in the herd and removed for other reasons (e.g., sold) were considered lost-to-follow-up and their unobserved culling age was treated as censored observation. The three covariates believed to be prognostic indicators for culling were parity, total milk production in the previous parity, and presence or absence of clinical mastitis in the period prior to the lactation in which the cow was culled.

The datasets B, C, and D are given on the accompanying CD.

These four examples will be used throughout the chapter to demonstrate methods of survival data analysis using SAS and R.

7.3 Estimating the Survival Probabilities

Two distinct methodologies exist for the analysis of survival data: non-parametric approaches in which no distributional assumptions are made for the previously defined probability density function $f(t)$ and parametric approaches in which distributional restrictions are imposed. Each methodology will be discussed separately.

7.3.1 Nonparametric Methods

7.3.1.1 Methods for Noncensored Data

Estimates of the survival function, probability density function, and hazard function exist for the specific case of noncensored data. They are given as follows:

(i) Estimate of the survival function for noncensored data

$$\hat{S}(t) = \frac{\text{number of patients surviving longer than } t}{\text{total number of patients}}$$

(ii) Estimate of the probability density function for noncensored data

$$\hat{f}(t) = \frac{\text{number of patients dying in the interval beginning at time } t}{(\text{total number of patients})(\text{interval width})}$$

(iii) Estimate of the hazard function for noncensored data

$$\hat{h}(t) = \frac{\text{number of patients dying in the interval beginning at time } t}{(\text{number of patients surviving at } t)(\text{interval width})}$$

$$= \frac{\text{number of patients dying per unit time in the interval}}{\text{number of patients surviving at } t}$$

It is also possible to define the average hazard rate that uses the average number of survivors at the interval midpoint to calculate the denominator of the estimate:

$$\hat{h}^{\bullet}(t) = \frac{\text{number of patients dying per unit time in the interval}}{\left(\begin{array}{c}\text{number of patients}\\\text{surviving at } t\end{array}\right) - 0.5\left(\begin{array}{c}\text{number of deaths in}\\\text{the interval}\end{array}\right)}$$

The estimate given in $\hat{h}^{\bullet}(t)$ results in a smaller denominator and thus a larger hazard rate. The $\hat{h}^{\bullet}(t)$ is used primarily by actuaries.

Obviously different methods are required in the presence of censored data. These methods are now discussed.

7.3.1.2 Methods for Censored Data

The Kaplan–Meier (1958) estimate of the survival function in the presence of censored data, also known as the product-limit estimate, is given by

$$\hat{S}(k) = p_1 \times p_2 \times p_3 \times \cdots \times p_k$$

where $k \geq 2$ years and p_i denotes the proportion of patients surviving the ith year conditional on their survival until the $(i-1)$th year. In practice, $\hat{S}(k)$ is calculated using the following formula:

$$\hat{S}(t) = \prod_{t_{(r)} \leq t} \frac{n-r}{n-r+1} \tag{7.1}$$

where the survival times have been placed in ascending order so that $t_{(1)} \leq t_{(2)} \leq \cdots \leq t_{(n)}$, for n is the total number of individuals under study and r the runs through the positive integers such that $t_{(r)} \leq t$ and $t_{(r)}$ is uncensored.

A table of the form shown below (Table 7.3) is used in the calculation of the product-limit survival estimate.

TABLE 7.3

General Calculations for Product-Limit Survival Estimate

Ordered Survival Times	Rank	Rank (r) (Uncensored Observations)	Number in Sample (n)	$\dfrac{n-r}{n-r+1}$	$\hat{S}(t)$
$t_{(1)}$	1	1	n		
$t_{(2)}{}^a$	2	/	$n-1$	/	/
$t_{(3)}$	3	3	$n-2$		
.	.	.	.		
$t_{(n)}$	n	n	1		

[a] Censored.

The last column of the table is filled in after calculation of $\frac{n-r}{n-r+1}$. Note that the estimate of the survival function is available only for the noncensored times t. These computations are illustrated using cystic ovary data in Example 7.1 below.

Example 7.1   Cystic Ovary Data

The Kaplan–Meier (product-limit) estimates of the survival function for the cystic ovary data are calculated separately for each treatment group as shown in Table 7.4.

TABLE 7.4

Kaplan–Meier Survival Estimate for Cystic Ovary Data

Treatment	Ordered Survival Times	Rank	Rank (Uncensored Observations)	Number in Sample	$\frac{n-r}{n-r+1}$	$\hat{S}(t)$
1	4	1	1	7	6/7	0.85
	6	2	2	6	5/6	(0.83)(0.85) = 0.71
	8	3	3	5	4/5	(0.80)(0.71) = 0.56
	8	4	4	4	3/4	(0.75)(0.56) = 0.42
	9	5	5	3	2/3	(0.66)(0.42) = 0.28
	10	6	6	2	1/2	(0.50)(0.28) = 0.13
	12	7	7	1	0	0
2	7	1	1	6	5/6	0.83
	12	2	2	5	4/5	(0.80)(0.83) = 0.66
	15	3	3	4	3/4	(0.75)(0.66) = 0.49
	16	4	4	3	2/3	(0.66)(0.49) = 0.33
	18	5	5	2	1/2	(0.50)(0.33) = 0.16
	22[a]	6	/	1	/	/
3	18[a]	1	/	7	/	/
	19	2	2	6	5/6	0.83
	20[a]	3	/	5	/	/
	22[a]	4	/	4	/	/
	24	5	5	3	2/3	(0.66)(0.83) = 0.55
	27[a]	6	/	2	/	/
	30[a]	7	/	1	/	/

[a]Censored.

The following SAS code reads the data and produces the Kaplan–Meier survival estimates. The "censor" variable takes value 1 if failure and 0 if not.

```
data cyst;
input cow treat time censor @@;
datalines;
1 1 4 1 2 1 6 1 3 1 8 1 4 1 8 1
5 1 9 1 6 1 10 1 7 1 12 1 8 2 7 1
9 2 12 1 10 2 15 1 11 2 16 1 12 2 18 1
13 2 22 0 14 3 19 1 15 3 24 1 16 3 18 0
17 3 20 0 18 3 22 0 19 3 27 0 20 3 30 0
;
proc lifetest data=cyst plots=(s) graphics;
time time*censor(0);
strata treat;
symbol1 v=none color=black line=1;
symbol2 v=none color=black line=2;
symbol3 v=none color=black line=3;
run;
```

Selected SAS output:

Stratum 1: treat = 1

Product-Limit Survival Estimates

Time	Survival	Failure	Survival Standard Error	Number Failed	Number Left
0.0000	1.0000	0	0	0	7
4.0000	0.8571	0.1429	0.1323	1	6
6.0000	0.7143	0.2857	0.1707	2	5
8.0000	—	—	—	3	4
8.0000	0.4286	0.5714	0.1870	4	3
9.0000	0.2857	0.7143	0.1707	5	2
10.0000	0.1429	0.8571	0.1323	6	1
12.0000	0	1.0000	0	7	0

Stratum 2: treat = 2

Product-Limit Survival Estimates

Time	Survival	Failure	Survival Standard Error	Number Failed	Number Left
0.0000	1.0000	0	0	0	6
7.0000	0.8333	0.1667	0.1521	1	5
12.0000	0.6667	0.3333	0.1925	2	4
15.0000	0.5000	0.5000	0.2041	3	3
16.0000	0.3333	0.6667	0.1925	4	2
18.0000	0.1667	0.8333	0.1521	5	1
22.0000[a]	—	—	—	5	0

[a] This survival time is censored observation.

Stratum 3: treat = 3

Product-Limit Survival Estimates

Time	Survival	Failure	Survival Standard Error	Number Failed	Number Left
0.0000	1.0000	0	0	0	7
18.0000[a]	—	—	—	0	6
19.0000	0.8333	0.1667	0.1521	1	5
20.0000[a]	—	—	—	1	4
22.0000[a]	—	—	—	1	3
24.0000	0.5556	0.4444	0.2485	2	2
27.0000[a]	—	—	—	2	1
30.0000[a]	—	—	—	2	0

[a] These survival times are censored observations.

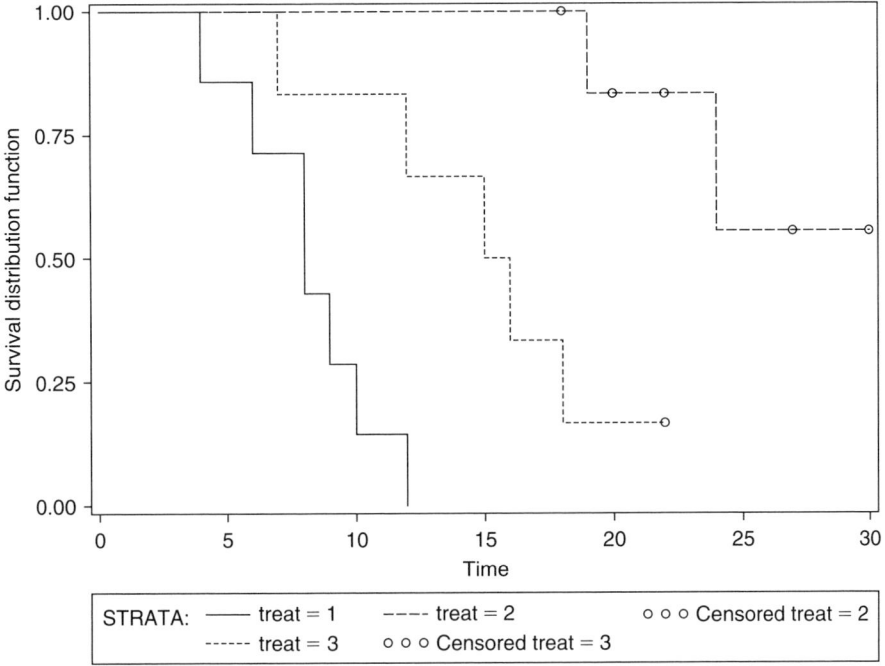

FIGURE 7.1
Survival curves for the treatment groups of the cystic ovary data.

The plots = (s) option in the PROC LIFETEST statement produces survival curves for the three groups overlaid on the same graph as shown in Figure 7.1.

Notes

1. We have included the tables of the estimated survival probabilities. Note that the survival function is only estimated at death times that are not censored. The SAS output also includes the summary statistics concerning sample size and percentage of censored observations, etc. not displayed here.

2. Adding a "strata" statement to the SAS program results in the calculations being performed within each level of the strata variable.

3. The last observation was censored, so the estimate of the mean survival time is biased.

4. The Kaplan–Meier survival curves indicate that, compared to the placebo group, the time of cyst disappearance is shorter with treatment 1 and longer with treatment 2.

The following R code sets up the data and performs the analysis:

```
cow <- c(1:20)
treat <- c(rep(1,7),rep(2,6),rep(3,7))
```

```
time <- c(4,6,8,8,9,10,12,7,12,15,16,18,22,19,24,18,20,22,27,30)
censor <- c(rep(1,12),0,1,1,rep(0,5))
cyst <- data.frame(cow,treat,time,censor)

fit <- survfit(Surv(time, censor) ~ treat, data=cyst)
summary(fit)
plot(fit)
```

To determine whether there is a significant difference between groups in a dataset, a statistical test must be used for comparison of survival curves. Without any prior knowledge of the distribution that may be appropriate for the data, a nonparametric (distribution-free) test is preferable. A test designed for this purpose is the log-rank test by Peto and Peto (1972).

7.3.1.3 *Nonparametric Techniques for Group Comparisons*

7.3.1.3.1 *The Log-Rank Test*

Suppose that we have two treatment groups A and B and it is of interest to compare the survival in these two groups. For a hypothesis test of

H_0: no difference in survival between the two groups

versus

H_A: difference in survival between the two groups

The test statistic is given by

$$\chi^2 = \frac{U_L^2}{V_L} \tag{7.2}$$

where

$$U_L = \sum_{j=1}^{r} (d_{1j} - e_{1j})$$

$$V_L = \sum_{j=1}^{r} \frac{n_{1j} n_{2j} d_j (n_j - d_j)}{n_j^2 (n_j - 1)} = \sum_{j=1}^{r} v_j$$

for $n_{1j}, n_{2j}, d_{1j}, d_{2j}, e_{1j},$ and e_{2j} are defined as follows:

$t_{(j)} = j$th death time (regardless of group)
$n_{1j} = $ number at risk in group A just before time $t_{(j)}$
$n_{2j} = $ number at risk in group B just before time $t_{(j)}$
$d_{1j} = $ number of deaths in group A at time $t_{(j)}$
$d_{2j} = $ number of deaths in group B at time $t_{(j)}$
$e_{1j} = $ expected number of individuals dying in group A at time $t_{(j)}$
$e_{2j} = $ expected number of individuals dying in group B at time $t_{(j)}$

where

$$e_{kj} = \frac{n_{kj}d_j}{n_j}$$

for $k = 1, 2$ so that n_j = total number at risk in both groups just before $t_{(j)}$ and d_j = total number of deaths in both groups at $t_{(j)}$.

The test statistic is calculated by constructing a table of the following nature (Table 7.5):

TABLE 7.5

Calculations for Log-Rank Test Statistic

Death Time	d_{1j}	n_{1j}	d_{2j}	n_{2j}	d_j	n_j	$e_{1j} = n_{1j}d_j/n_j$	$d_{1j} - e_{1j}$ (1)	v_{1j} (2)
$t_{(1)}$									
$t_{(2)}$									
$\vdots$									
$t_{(n)}$									

Under the null hypothesis of no differences between groups A and B, the test statistic is distributed as $\chi^2_{(1)}$.

Example 7.2   The Breast Cancer Data

The following SAS program with strata = pag statement calculates the log-rank test to determine whether differences are present in survival for patients with a high proliferative AgNOR index (pag = 1) and those with a low index (pag = 0).

```
data cancer;
input id censor time pag mag age tsize;
datalines;
1 0 130 0 0 57 0
2 0 136 1 1 67 0
. . . . . . .
73 0 100 1 1 50 1
;

proc lifetest data=cancer plots=(s) graphics;
time time*censor(0);
strata pag;
symbol1 v=none color=black line=1;
symbol2 v=none color=black line=2;
run;
```

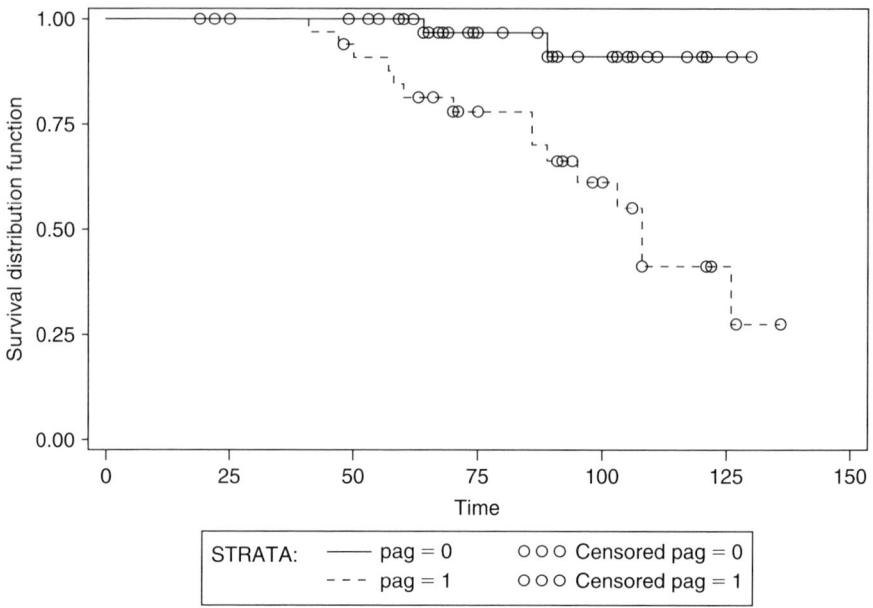

FIGURE 7.2
The Kaplan–Meier curves for the two groups of the breast cancer recurrence data.

The SAS output showing the log-rank and the other tests for the equality of survival functions is displayed below:

Test of Equality over Strata

Test	χ^2	DF	$Pr > \chi^2$
Log-rank	10.3104	1	0.0013
Wilcoxon	8.6344	1	0.0033
-2 Log(LR)	12.7162	1	0.0004

The p-value for the log-rank test ($p = 0.0013$) indicates that there are significant differences in the two groups with respect to survival. This is in agreement with the survival graph shown in Figure 7.2, which implied substantially better survival for the low index group (pag $= 0$).

Note that SAS also provides Wilcoxon and -2 Log(LR) tests of equality over the strata. The Wilcoxon test statistic has a similar form to the log-rank; however, the Wilcoxon test weights each term in the summation over the various death times by the number of individuals alive at that death time, thus giving less weight to terms where few women had not experienced breast cancer recurrence. For general use, the log-rank test is most appropriate when the assumption of proportional hazards between treatment groups holds. The topic of proportional hazards will be discussed subsequently.

The following R code may be used to perform the analysis and compute the log-rank test.

```
cancer <- read.table("x:/xxx/cancer.txt",header=T)
fit <- survfit(Surv(time, censor) ~ pag, data=cancer)
summary(fit)
plot(fit)
survdiff(Surv(time, censor) ~ pag,data=cancer,rho=0)
```

7.3.1.3.2 *✴Log-Rank Test for More than Two Groups*

Often it is desirable to make comparisons of the survival between three or more groups; in this case, an extension of the log-rank test is used. If there are q groups we wish to make comparisons between, then the following are calculated for each group $i = 1, \ldots, q$:

$$U_{Li} = \sum_{j=1}^{r} \left(d_{ij} - \frac{n_{ij}d_j}{n_j} \right)$$

$$U_{Wi} = \sum_{j=1}^{r} n_j \left(d_{ij} - \frac{n_{ij}d_j}{n_j} \right)$$

The vectors

$$U_L = \begin{bmatrix} U_{L1} \\ U_{L2} \\ \vdots \\ U_{Lq} \end{bmatrix}$$

and

$$U_W = \begin{bmatrix} U_{W1} \\ U_{W2} \\ \vdots \\ U_{Wq} \end{bmatrix}$$

are then formed. In addition, the variances and covariances are needed and are given by the formula:

$$V_{Lii'} = \sum_{j=1}^{r} \frac{n_{ij}d_j(n_j - d_j)}{n_j(n_j - 1)} \left(\delta_{ii} - \frac{n_{ij}}{n_j} \right)$$

where $\delta_{ii'}$ is such that

$$\delta_{ii'} = \begin{cases} 1 & \text{if } i = i' \\ 0 & \text{otherwise} \end{cases}$$

The variance–covariance matrix is then given by

$$V = \begin{bmatrix} V_{L11} & V_{L12} & \cdots & V_{L1i} \\ V_{L21} & V_{L22} & \cdots & V_{L2i} \\ \vdots & \vdots & \ddots & \vdots \\ V_{Li1} & V_{Li2} & \cdots & V_{Lii} \end{bmatrix}$$

where $V_{Lij} = \text{Cov}(U_{Li}, U_{Lj})$ and $V_{Lii} = \text{Var}(U_{Li})$.

To test a null hypothesis of

H_0: no difference in survival between all groups

versus

H_A: difference in survival between at least two groups

the test statistic given by

$$\chi^2 = U_L' V_L^{-1} U_L \qquad\qquad (7.3)$$

has a $\chi^2_{(q-1)}$ distribution under the null hypothesis, where q is the number of strata.

For calculation of the stratified log-rank test in SAS, the same strata statement is used as for calculation of the log-rank test between two groups. A stratified test will be performed automatically for variables having more than two levels.

Example 7.1 (Continued)

The following SAS program with the "strata = group" statement calculates the log-rank test to determine whether differences are present in time of cyst disappearance for cows treated with hormone treatment 1, hormone treatment 2, and the control. The relevant portion of the output is as shown:

Test of Equality over Strata

Test	χ^2	DF	Pr > χ^2
Log-rank	21.2401	2	<0.0001
Wilcoxon	17.8661	2	0.0001
−2 Log(LR)	10.6663	2	0.0048

In this case, the p-value for the log-rank test ($p = 0.0001$) indicates that there are significant differences in the three groups with respect to time until cyst disappearance.

The R code to produce log-rank test to compare three groups is displayed below:

```
survdiff(Surv(time, censor) ~ treat,data=cyst,rho=0)
```

7.3.2 Parametric Methods

All parametric methods involve the specification of a distributional form for the probability density function $f(t)$. This in turn specifies the survival function $S(t)$ and the hazard function $h(t)$ using the relationships previously defined. The two parametric models to be discussed are the Exponential and the Weibull. Their survival and hazard functions are given and their properties are reviewed. Much of the work in this section can be found in Lawless (1982).

7.3.2.1 Exponential Model

An Exponential density function is given by

$$f(t) = \lambda \exp(-\lambda t) \qquad t \geq 0, \quad \lambda > 0$$

and zero elsewhere.

Therefore,

$$S(t) = \exp(-\lambda t) \qquad t \geq 0, \quad \lambda > 0 \tag{7.4}$$

and

$$h(t) = \lambda$$

Note that the hazard function is independent of time, implying that the instantaneous conditional failure rate does not change within a lifetime. This is also referred to as the memory-less property of the Exponential distribution, since the age of an individual does not affect their probability of future survival. When $\lambda = 1$, the distribution is referred to as the unit Exponential.

In practice, most failure times do not have a constant hazard of failure, and thus the application of the Exponential model for survival analysis is limited. The Exponential model is in fact a special case of a more general model that is widely applicable: the Weibull model.

7.3.2.2 Weibull Model

A continuously distributed random variable is said to have a Weibull distribution if its probability density function is given by

$$f(t) = \alpha \gamma (\alpha t)^{\gamma - 1} \exp[-(\alpha t)^{\gamma}] \qquad t \geq 0 \quad \text{and} \quad \alpha > 0, \gamma > 0$$

The survival function is given by

$$S(t) = \exp[-(\alpha t)^{\gamma}] \tag{7.5}$$

Moreover, the hazard function is $h(t) = \alpha \gamma (\alpha t)^{\gamma - 1}$ and

$$\ln[-\ln S(t)] = a + bt^* \tag{7.6}$$

The above linear equation has $a = \gamma \ln \alpha$, $b = \gamma$, and $t^* = \ln(t)$.

For the Weibull distribution, α and γ are the scale and shape parameters, respectively. The specific case of $\gamma = 1$ defines the Exponential model with constant hazard previously discussed, $\gamma > 1$ implies a hazard that increases with time and $\gamma < 1$ yields a hazard decreasing with time. It is evident that the Weibull distribution is widely applicable since it allows modeling of populations with various types of failure risk.

Example 7.2 (Continued)

Here we fit the Exponential as well as the Weibull model to the breast cancer data using "proc lifereg" in SAS. The SAS code followed by the selected output is shown below:

(a) Exponential Model

```
* Fitting Exponential regression model;
proc lifereg data=cancer;
model time*censor(0)= pag age tsize/ dist=exponential;
run;
```

Model Information

Dataset	WORK.CANCER
Dependent variable	Log(time)
Censoring variable	censor
Censoring value(s)	0
Number of observations	73
Noncensored values	17
Right censored values	56
Left censored values	0
Interval censored values	0
Name of distribution	Exponential
Log likelihood	−36.73724081

Analysis of Parameter Estimates

Parameter	DF	Estimate	Standard Error	95% Confidence Limits		χ^2	Pr > χ^2
Intercept	1	6.6328	1.3522	3.9825	9.2831	24.06	<0.0001
pag	1	−2.1811	0.7550	−3.6609	−0.7013	8.35	0.0039
age	1	0.0107	0.0204	−0.0293	0.0506	0.28	0.5999
tsize	1	0.3938	0.4945	−0.5754	1.3631	0.63	0.4258
Scale	0	1.0000	0.0000	1.0000	1.0000		
Weibull shape	0	1.0000	0.0000	1.0000	1.0000		

(b) Weibull Model

```
* Fitting Weibull regression model;
proc lifereg data=cancer;
```

model time*censor(0)= pag age tsize/ dist=weibull;
run;

Model Information

Dataset	WORK.CANCER
Dependent variable	Log(time)
Censoring variable	censor
Censoring value(s)	0
Number of observations	73
Noncensored values	17
Right censored values	56
Left censored values	0
Interval censored values	0
Name of distribution	Weibull
Log likelihood	−26.88658984

Analysis of Parameter Estimates

Parameter	DF	Estimate	Standard Error	95% Confidence Limits		χ^2	$Pr > \chi^2$
Intercept	1	5.1084	0.4737	4.1799	6.0369	116.28	<0.0001
pag	1	−0.6610	0.2812	−1.2121	−0.1100	5.53	0.0187
age	1	0.0058	0.0070	−0.0080	0.0196	0.67	0.4125
tsize	1	0.0347	0.1622	−0.2831	0.3525	0.05	0.8305
Scale	1	0.3205	0.0653	0.2150	0.4777		
Weibull shape	1	3.1204	0.6354	2.0935	4.6510		

Note that the model statement specifies the dependent variable as time*censor(0), where time is the variable in the analysis recording the failure or censoring time, censor is an indicator variable denoting whether or not a failure time is censored, and the number in brackets indicates the coded value of the censor variable indicating that an observation was censored.

As was noted using the log-rank test and the survival curves, a significant difference exists in the failure times between those with a high AgNOR proliferative index and those with a low index, both when the failure times are modeled to be Exponential and when they are modeled as Weibull.

This is reflected in the *p*-values of 0.0039 and 0.0187 for the Exponential and Weibull models, respectively. The other variables included in the model, age and tumor size, appear to have little effect on the time of breast cancer recurrence. The log-likelihood values of −36.74 and −26.89 indicate that the Weibull distribution is slightly better at modeling the breast cancer recurrence times. This may be due to the fact that the previously discussed restrictions imposed by an Exponential model (i.e., a constant hazard rate) may not be valid when examining disease recurrence. In such a situation, a distribution with a hazard function that changes over time is preferable.

The R code to fit the Exponential and Weibull models to breast cancer data is

```
# Fitting Exponential regression model
summary(survreg(Surv(time, censor) ~ pag + age + tsize, cancer,
dist='exponential'))
# Fitting Weibull regression model
summary(survreg(Surv(time, censor) ~ pag + age + tsize, cancer, dist=
'weibull'))
```

linear. exponential $<$ $\frac{\log(survival)}{time}$

7.3.2.3 Graphical Assessment of Model Adequacy

weibull $<$ $\frac{\log(survival)}{\log(time)}$

The fit of the Exponential and Weibull models to the breast cancer data may also be assessed graphically. We expect to see a straight line relationship between log(survival) and time if the Exponential model is adequate and log($-$log(survival)) and log(time) if the Weibull model is adequate as shown by Equations 7.4 and 7.6. Recall that the survival functions for the Exponential and Weibull models were given, respectively, by

$$S(t) = \exp(-\lambda t) \quad \text{for Exponential}$$
$$S(t) = \exp[-(\alpha t)^{\gamma}] \quad \text{for Weibull}$$

We rearrange the equations to obtain linear functions of t. Taking the log of each side in the Exponential model gives

$$\log[S(t)] = -\lambda t$$

which is now a linear function of t, so that a graph of the log of the survival estimates versus time should be linear if the Exponential model is adequate. Similarly, rearranging the Weibull survival function gives

$$\log\{-\log[S(t)]\} = a + bt^{*}$$

where $a \equiv \gamma \log \alpha$, $b \equiv \gamma$, and $t^{*} \equiv \log(t)$.

Again, we have a linear function of t, so that a graph of the log of the negative-log (survival) estimates versus log of time should be linear if the Weibull model is adequate.

The following SAS program constructs the desired plots for the breast cancer data.

```
* Graphical assessment of model adequacy;
proc lifetest data=cancer outsurv=a;
time time*censor(0);
run;

data graph; set a;
log_s=log(survival);
log_logS=log(-log(survival));
```

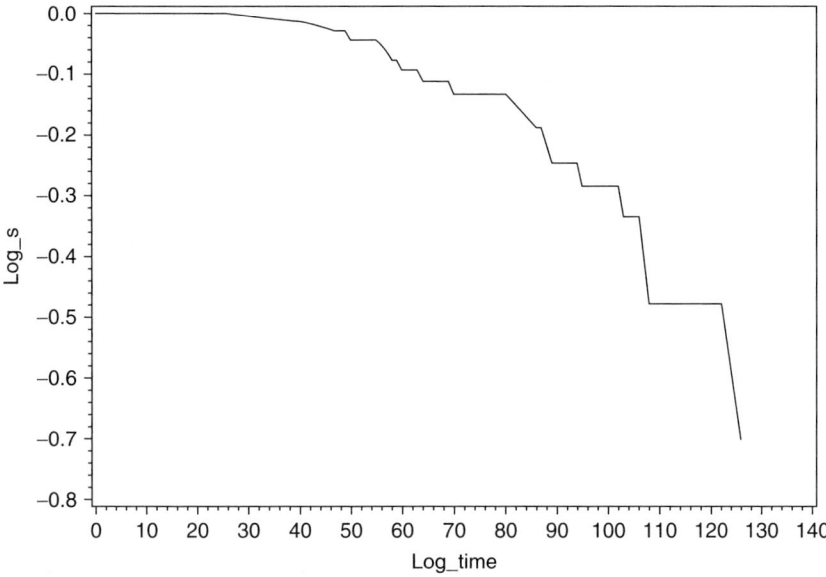

FIGURE 7.3
Log-survival against time to see if Exponential model is adequate.

```
log_time=log(time);
run;

proc gplot data=graph;
symbol value=none i=join;
plot log_s*time log_logs*log_time;
run; quit;
```

The resulting plots of the adequacy of the Exponential and Weibull models for breast cancer data are shown in Figures 7.3 and 7.4, respectively.

A straight line relationship indicates no departures from model adequacy. The two figures indicate that the Weibull model is more suitable than the Exponential model for the breast cancer data, as was also indicated by the log-likelihood value.

The R code to produce Figures 7.3 and 7.4 is

```
fit <- survfit(Surv(time, censor), data=cancer)
plot(fit$time,log(fit$surv),type="l")
plot(log(fit$time),log(-log(fit$surv)),type="l")
```

7.3.3 Semiparametric Models

7.3.3.1 Cox Proportional Hazards Model

One positive feature of the parametric methods previously discussed is that specification of a form for the probability density function allows the

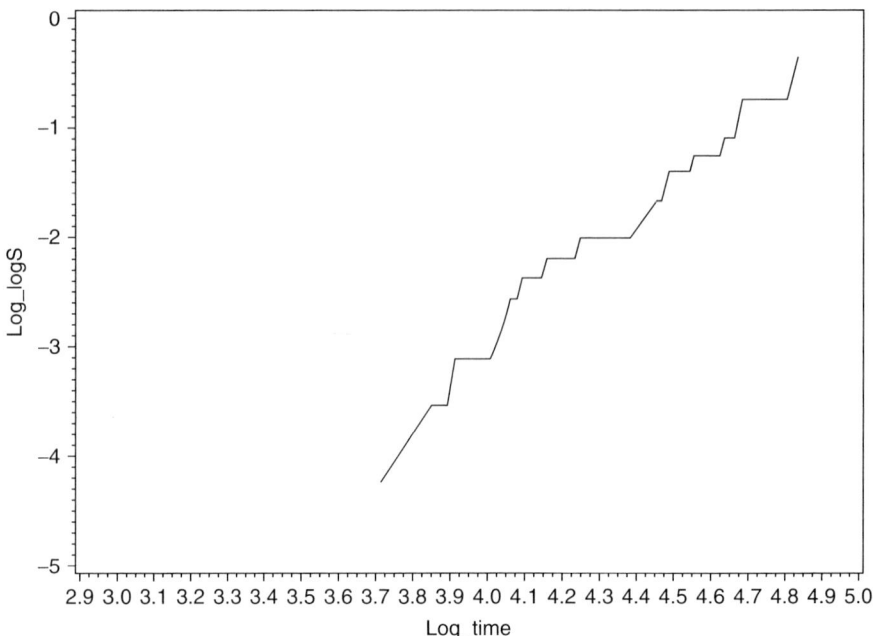

FIGURE 7.4
Plot of log[−log(survival)] versus time showing the adequacy of the Weibull model.

likelihood to be constructed. Maximum likelihood estimates and standard errors may then be obtained for all parameters in the model. However, the drawback in parametric modeling lies in the fact that it may not be desirable to specify a probability distribution function for a particular set of data, making nonparametric calculations more attractive. The ideal situation would involve no distributional restrictions on the density, yet maximum likelihood estimates of regression parameters (and thus treatment effects) would be readily available. An analysis with such properties may be performed using the Cox proportional hazards model (Cox, 1972).

As its name implies, the proportional hazards model is constructed by assuming that the hazard function of the ith individual is the product of a baseline hazard common to all individuals, denoted by $h_0(t)$, and a function of the covariate vector, $x_i = (x_{i1}, x_{i2}, \ldots, x_{ip})$ for that individual, $\varphi(x)$:

$$h_i(t) = h_0(t)\varphi(x_i) \tag{7.7}$$

Since rearrangement yields the hazard ratio or relative hazard to be the nonnegative function

$$\varphi(x_i) = \frac{h_i(t)}{h_0(t)} \tag{7.8}$$

The covariate function is specified to be $\varphi(x_i) = \exp(x_i \beta)$.

Further rearrangement shows that

$$\log\left(\frac{h_i(t)}{h_0(t)}\right) = \beta_1 x_{i1} + \cdots + \beta_p x_{ip}$$

Therefore, the proportional hazards model is a linear model for the log hazard ratio.

7.3.3.2 Estimation of Regression Parameters

Cox (1972) introduced the method of partial likelihood to estimate the regression parameters and avoid the specification of the baseline hazard function $h_0(t)$. The partial likelihood for the proportional hazards model is given by

$$L(\beta) = \prod_{j=1}^{r} \frac{\exp(\beta' x_{(j)})}{\sum_{l \in R(t_i)} \exp(\beta' x_{(l)})}$$

where $R(t_{(j)})$ is the risk set (individuals alive) at the jth ordered death time, $t_{(j)}$. Thus the likelihood takes the product over the jth ordered death times of terms of the form:

$$L(\beta) = \frac{\exp(\beta' x_{(j)})}{\sum_{l \in R(t_i)} \exp(\beta' x_{(l)})}$$

$$= \Pr \begin{pmatrix} \text{failure occurs to observed} \\ \text{individual given the risk set} \\ R(t_i) \text{ and a failure at } t_{(i)} \end{pmatrix} \quad (7.9)$$

As can be seen, $L_i(\beta)$ is the ratio of the hazard for the individual who died at the ith ordered death time divided by the sum of hazards for the individuals who were at risk when the ith ordered death occurred. Note that individuals with censored failure times do not contribute a term to the likelihood; however, they are included in the risk sets. Hence $L(\beta)$ may be expressed as

$$L(\beta) = \prod_{i=1}^{n} \left[\frac{\exp(\beta' x_{(i)})}{\sum_{l \in R(t_{(j)})} \exp(\beta' x_l)} \right]^{\delta_i} \quad (7.10)$$

where

$$\delta_i = \begin{cases} 1 & \text{if the } i\text{th individual fails during the study} \\ 0 & \text{if the failure time of the } i\text{th individual is censored} \end{cases}$$

Taking the product over the j uncensored failure times in Equation 7.9 is equivalent to taking the product over the n censored and uncensored failure times in Equation 7.10 due to the indicator variable δ_i.

Note that the likelihood 7.10 is referred to as a partial likelihood due to the fact that it is based on the product of probabilities of failure rather than official density functions. Maximum likelihood estimation of the regression parameters β occurs by treating the partial likelihood given in Equation 7.10 as a true likelihood, so that differentiation of the log and subsequent maximization is possible. Variance estimates are found using the matrix of partial second derivatives. Newton–Rhapson techniques are required for the maximization.

7.3.3.3 Treatment of Ties in the Proportional Hazards Model

The proportional hazards model implicitly assumes (due to its continuous nature) that the exact time of failure or censoring is known for each individual under study. For this situation, there are no ties in failure times. Such accuracy is not usually encountered in practice, where frequently survival times are only available for the nearest day, week, or month. This may result in tied failure times in the data. Several methods exist for dealing with tied failure times in the Cox proportional hazards model. Two will be discussed here.

Note that in the treatment of ties, it is assumed that

(i)   there are r distinct deaths at $t_{(j)}$, where $j = 1, \ldots, r$;
(ii) there may be d_j deaths at $t_{(j)}$; and
(iii) $s_j = x_1 + x_2 + \cdots + x_{d_j}$, where $j = 1, \ldots, r$ and $x_1, x_2, \ldots, x_{d_j}$ are the covariate vectors of the individuals dying at $t_{(j)}$.

In addition, it is assumed that if an uncensored failure and a censored failure (i.e., a death and a drop-out) occur at the same time, the uncensored failure occurs first, so that the discussion below focuses on ties in uncensored failure times.

Breslow (1972) suggested the following approximation to the partial likelihood function to account for tied failure times in the data:

$$\prod_{j=1}^{r} \frac{\exp(\beta' s_j)}{\left[\sum_{l \in R(t_{(j)})} \exp(\beta' x_l) \right]^{d_j}}$$

where all possible sequences of deaths are summed for the respective component of the likelihood function. Breslow's approximation is simple to compute and has the advantage of being quite accurate when the number of ties at a given death time is small.

Example 7.2 (Continued)

We fit the Cox proportional hazards model to the breast cancer data using SAS.

```
proc phreg data=cancer;
model time*censor(0)= pag age tsize/ ties=efron;
run;
```

The partial output is

Model Fit Statistics

Criterion	Without Covariates	With Covariates
−2 LOG L	120.924	108.462
AIC	120.924	114.462
SBC	120.924	116.961

Analysis of Maximum Likelihood Estimates

Variable	DF	Parameter Estimate	Standard Error	χ^2	Pr > χ^2	Hazard Ratio
pag	1	2.09807	0.75574	7.7071	0.0055	8.150
age	1	−0.01894	0.02163	0.7668	0.3812	0.981
tsize	1	−0.17756	0.50822	0.1221	0.7268	0.837

Once again, the pag variable for proliferate AgNOR index implies there is a significant difference ($p = 0.0055$) between survival for those with high and low scores, and that the variables age and tumor size are not predictive of breast cancer recurrence ($p = 0.3812$ and $p = 0.7268$, respectively). In addition, the positive parameter estimate of pag implies that the hazard of breast cancer recurrence becomes larger as the level of pag increases, meaning a greater hazard for the pag $= 1$ group versus pag $= 0$. The hazard ratio of 8.150 for the pag variable indicates the hazard of breast cancer recurrence is eight times greater in the high AgNOR proliferative index group.

The R code to fit the model is

coxph(Surv(time, censor) ~ pag + age + tsize, cancer)

7.4 Modeling Correlated Survival Data

As with all types of response variables, techniques must be available for analyses performed on correlated time to event data. The complexity of studies involving multiple treatment centers, family members, and measurements repeatedly made on the same individual requires methods to account for correlation in the data. Such is the case for any type of response, be it continuous, binary, or a time to event. Use of the multivariate normal distribution allows correlation to be accounted for in continuous data where techniques are well established. For the situation of binary responses, work over the past few decades has resulted in tests adjusted for correlation in the data. However, for the time to event case, methods of accounting for correlation in the data have only recently been developed. Two methods with existing programs in computer software packages are currently available: the marginal approach and frailty models. They will be discussed subsequently and their properties contrasted. Situations in which each method is desirable are discussed.

7.4.1 Marginal Models (GJE Approach)

The Generalized Jackknife Estimator (GJE) (Therneau, 1993) produces robust parameter estimates and variances. The score residual matrix, denoted by B, and Fisher's information matrix are required to obtain these types of robust variance estimates. The motivation for the GJE approach is now discussed. The partial likelihood function $L(\beta)$ in Equation 7.10 is differentiated with respect to β_r, the rth parameter that yields

$$\frac{\partial \log L(\beta)}{\partial \beta_r} = \sum_{i=1}^{N} \delta_i(x_{ri} - a_{ri})$$

$$= \sum_{i=1}^{N} \delta_i S_{ri} \qquad r = 1, \dots, p$$

where

$$a_{ri} = \frac{\sum_{\ell \in R_i} x_{ri} \exp(x_\ell' \hat{\beta})}{\sum_{\ell \in R_i} \exp(x_\ell' \hat{\beta})}$$

The implication that $\partial \log L(\beta)/\partial \beta_r$ is the difference between the rth covariate x_{ri}, and a weighted average of values of the explanatory variable over individuals at risk at the failure time of the ith individual. The information matrix is obtained through differentiation a second time and is seen to be

$$-\frac{\partial^2 \log L(\beta)}{\partial \beta_r \partial \beta_s} = \sum_{i=1}^{N} \delta_i \left[\frac{\sum_{\ell \in R_i} x_{rt} x_{st} \exp(x_\ell' \hat{\beta})}{\sum_{\ell \in R_i} \exp(x_\ell' \hat{\beta})} - a_{ri} a_{st} \right] \qquad r, s = 1, \dots, p$$

If B is the vector with rth component $B_r = \partial \log L(B)/\partial \beta_r$ and A is the matrix with the entry in the rth row, sth column being $-\partial^2 \log L(\beta)/\partial \beta_r \partial \beta_s$, then the traditional sandwich estimate is given by

$$V(\hat{\beta}) = H'H$$

where

$$H = BA^{-1}$$

For the GJE, the matrix B (containing one row per patient per cluster) is collapsed into $\tilde{B}$ with one row per cluster, where the row for the cluster has been summed over patients in that cluster. The result is then the GJE robust variance estimate is given by

$$\widetilde{V}(\hat{\beta}) = \widetilde{H}'\widetilde{H}$$

where

$$\widetilde{H} = \widetilde{B}A^{-1}$$

Note that $\widetilde{V}$ underestimates V when the number of clusters is small.

7.4.2 Random Effects Models (Frailty Models)

The notion of frailty provides a convenient way to introduce random effects, association, and unobserved heterogeneity into models for survival data. In its simplest form, a frailty is an unobserved random proportionality factor that modifies the hazard function of an individual or of related individuals. In essence, the frailty concept goes back to the work of Greenwood and Yule (1920) on "accident proneness." The term frailty itself was introduced by Vaupel et al. (1979) in univariate survival models, and the model was substantially promoted by its application to multivariate survival data in a seminal article by Clayton (1978) (without using the notion "frailty") on chronic disease incidence in families.

Frailty models are extensions of the proportional hazards model that is best known as the Cox model (Cox, 1972), the most popular model in survival analysis. Normally, in most clinical applications, survival analysis implicitly assumes a homogeneous population to be studied. This means that all individuals sampled in that study are subject, in principle, to the same risk (e.g., risk of death and risk of disease recurrence). In many applications, the study population cannot be assumed to be homogeneous but must be considered as a heterogeneous sample, i.e., a mixture of individuals with different hazards. For example, in many cases it is impossible to measure all relevant covariates related to the disease of interest, sometimes because of economical reasons, sometimes the importance of some covariates is still unknown. The frailty approach is a statistical modeling concept that aims to account for heterogeneity, caused by unmeasured covariates. In statistical terms, a frailty model is a random effects model for time-to-event data, where the random effect (the frailty) has a multiplicative effect on the baseline hazard function. One can distinguish two broad classes of frailty models:

1. Models with a univariate survival time as endpoint
2. Models that describe multivariate survival endpoints (e.g., competing risks, recurrence of events in the same individual, and occurrence of a disease in relatives).

In the first case, a univariate (independent) lifetime is used to describe the influence of unobserved covariates in a proportional hazards model (heterogeneity). The variability of survival data is split into a part that depends on risk factors, and is therefore theoretically predictable, and a part that is initially unpredictable, even when all relevant information is known. A separation of these two sources of variability has the advantage that heterogeneity can explain some unexpected results or give an alternative interpretation of some results, for example, crossing-over effects or convergence of hazard functions of two different treatment arms (see Manton and Stallard, 1981) or leveling-off effects—that means the decline in the increase of mortality rates, which could result in a hazard function at old ages parallel to the x-axis (Aalen and Tretli, 1999). More interesting, however, is the second case when multivariate survival times are considered. There one aims to account for the dependence in clustered event times, for example, in the lifetimes of patients in study centers in a multicenter clinical trial, caused by center-specific conditions (see Andersen et al., 1999). A natural way to model dependence of clustered event times is through the introduction of a cluster-specific random effect—the frailty. This random effect explains the dependence in the sense that had we known the frailty, the events would be independent. In other words, the lifetimes are conditionally independent, given the frailty. This approach can be used for survival times of related individuals like family members or recurrent observations on the same person. The extension of the Cox regression model that incorporates frailty component is

$$h(t|v_i) = v_i h_0(t) \exp(\beta x_{ij}) = h_0(t) \exp(\beta x_{ij} + z_i) \tag{7.11}$$

showing that $v_i = \exp(z_i)$ actually behaves as an unknown covariate for the ith cluster in the model.

Using previous relationships between the survival and hazard function, we have the conditional survival function as

$$S(t|v_i) = \exp[-v_i H_0(t) \exp(\beta x_{ij})]$$

and the conditional likelihood as

$$L(\gamma, \beta|v_i) = \prod_{i=1}^{k} \prod_{j=1}^{n_j} (h(t_{ij}|v_i)^{\delta_{ij}} S(t_{ij}|v_i))$$

Note that for the Weibull failure time distribution with $\alpha = 1$, the cumulative baseline hazard is

$$H_0(t|z) = \exp[\gamma \log(t) + x\beta + z]$$

where there are k clusters, the ith one being of size n_i. Substitution gives

$$L(\gamma, \beta|v_i) = \prod_{i=1}^{k} \prod_{j=1}^{n_j} \{[h_0(t)v_i \exp(\beta X_{ij})]^{\delta_{ij}} \exp[-v_i H_0(t) \exp(\beta X_{ij})]\} \tag{7.12}$$

The marginal (i.e., independent of v_i) likelihood, $L(\gamma, \beta)$, is obtained through integration of the random effect distribution. In the following subsections, we illustrate the methodology when the frailty distributions are conveniently chosen.

7.4.2.1 Weibull Model with Gamma Frailty

A common assumption is for the random effect to follow a gamma distribution with mean 1 and variance τ, i.e.,

$$g(v_i) = \frac{v_i^{1/\tau - 1} \exp(-v_i/\tau)}{\Gamma(1/\tau)\tau^{1/r}}$$

Therefore, $E(v_i) = 1$ and $var(v_i) = \tau$. The failure times are assumed to follow Weibull distribution with baseline hazard function $h_0(t) = f(t)/S(t) = \alpha\gamma(\alpha t)^{\gamma-1}$.

The marginal likelihood is then obtained as

$$L(\gamma, \beta, \tau) = \prod_{i=1}^{k} \prod_{j=1}^{n_j} \int_0^\infty L(\gamma, \beta|v_i)g(v_i)\, dv_i \qquad (7.13)$$

Inference on the regression parameters, baseline hazard parameter, and dispersion parameter is then possible using maximum likelihood procedures. Newton–Rhapson methods are used for the optimization of the likelihood function and obtaining the parameters' estimates.

Example 7.3 Ventilating Tube Data

Because a SAS Macro is not available yet, a FORTRAN program was written to obtain the maximum likelihood estimates shown in the marginal likelihood above (Equation 7.13) for the ventilating tube data. It was desired to examine the significance of treatment in delaying time to tube failure after accounting for correlation within ears. Note that maximum likelihood estimates are obtained for the cluster-level treatment effect β, the Weibull baseline hazard parameter γ, and the dispersion parameter τ, but not for within-cluster covariates due to the fact that each child received the same medicine in each ear. The results are as shown:

Parameters	β	γ	τ
Estimates	−4.19	2.00	2.75

To examine the significance of treatment effect, the estimate of the standard error of β is required and was found to be 0.479, so that $\hat{\beta}/S_{\hat{\beta}} = -8.75$, implying the treatment substantially decreases time to tube failure after adjusting for the correlation between ears ($p = 0.000$).

For the sake of comparison, we fitted the data with the Cox regression model, accounting for the correlation between ears using the "aggregate" option in the model statement. The SAS code for the data step and the PHREG procedure is

```
data ear;
input subject treat ear time censor;
cards;
1001 1 1 3.10 1
1001 1 2 4.80 0
. . .
. . .
2017 2 2 8.70 1
;

proc phreg data=ear covs(aggregate) covm;
model time*censor(0)= treat;
id subject;
run;
```

The partial output is

Testing Global Null Hypothesis: BETA=0

Test	χ^2	DF	$Pr > \chi^2$
Likelihood ratio	4.3407	1	0.0372
Score (model-based)	4.4225	1	0.0355
Score (sandwich)	3.8127	1	0.0509
Wald (model-based)	4.3788	1	0.0364
Wald (sandwich)	3.5996	1	0.0578

Analysis of Maximum Likelihood Estimates with *parameter*
Model-Based Variance Estimate

Variable	DF	Parameter Estimate	Standard Error	χ^2	$Pr > \chi^2$	Hazard Ratio
treat	1	−0.35292	0.16865	4.3788	0.0364 *small*	0.703

Analysis of Maximum Likelihood Estimates with
Sandwich Variance Estimate

Variable	DF	Parameter Estimate	Standard Error	Std Err Ratio	χ^2	$Pr > \chi^2$	Hazard Ratio
treat	1	−0.35292	0.18601	1.103	3.5996	0.0578	0.703

It is well known that parametric survival regression models have more power than semiparametric models such as Cox regression. From the output, we find that both models provide the same interpretation for the treatment effect, which is the reduction of the hazard of failure. The *p*-value provided by the parametric gamma frailty model is much smaller than the one obtained from the Cox regression model after accounting for the possible correlation between ears.

Frailty models have a great deal of potential in accounting for correlation arising in clustered survival data (Hougaard, 1995). Although the gamma frailty distribution has been examined here, other possibilities include the inverse Gaussian and log normal. The inverse Gaussian appears to be particularly well suited to the situation in which survival times are positively skewed as well as correlated. However, these types of models have the drawback of being difficult to fit due to complex distributional structure, and divergence is not uncommon when attempting to maximize the likelihood.

The R code to read the data and fit the gamma frailty model is shown below.

```
ear <- read.table("x:/xxx/ear.txt",header=T)
fit <- coxph(Surv(time, censor)~ treat + frailty(subject, dist='gamma'), ear)

summary(fit)
```

The results of fitting the model are

```
Call:
coxph(formula = Surv(time, censor) ~ treat + frailty(subject,
    dist = "gamma"), data = ear)

  n= 156
            coef se(coef) se2 Chisq DF p
treat -0.506 0.228  0.177  4.93  1.0  0.026
frailty(subject, dist = "  42.24  24.7  0.015

    exp(coef) exp(-coef) lower .95 upper .95
treat  0.603       1.66      0.386      0.943

Iterations: 7 outer, 40 Newton–Raphson
    Variance of random effect= 0.267 I-likelihood = -584.8
Degrees of freedom for terms= 0.6 24.7
Rsquare= 0.348 (max possible= 0.999 )
Likelihood ratio test= 66.7 on 25.3 df, p=1.36e-05
Wald test = 4.93 on 25.3 df, p=1
```

7.4.2.2 Weibull Model with Log-Normal Frailty (Hierarchical Likelihood Approach)

In this case, we assume that conditional on the frailty $v_i = \exp(z_i)$, where the random variable $z_i \sim N(0, \sigma^2)$. This means that v_i has a log-normal distribution with mean $e^{\sigma^2/2}$ and variance $e^{\sigma^2}(e^{\sigma^2} - 1)$. Here the random variables z_i are assumed to be unknown parameters, where $i = 1, 2, \ldots, k$. Therefore, likelihood function is not exact in a statistical sense and is considered as pseudolikelihood, since these variables are not observed.

The regression effect is modeled through $\alpha = e^{-x\beta - z}$. The hierarchical likelihood is thus written as

$$L(\beta, \gamma, z_i, \sigma^2) = \prod_{i=1}^{k} \prod_{j=1}^{n_i} [h(t_{ij}|z_i)]^{\delta_{ij}} S(t_{ij}|z_i) g(z_i) \qquad (7.14)$$

where $g(z) = (2\pi\sigma^2)^{-1/2} \exp(-z^2/\sigma^2)$.

Taking the logarithm of Equation 7.14 and differentiating with respect to $(\beta, \gamma, z_i, \sigma^2)$, we get the likelihood estimates. The estimates of z_i, where $i = 1, 2, \ldots, k$, are called the empirical Bayes' estimates.

We illustrate this approach through the following example.

Example 7.4   Culling Cows Data (Weibull Model with Frailty Component)

```
data herd;
input herdid cowed time censor parity herdsiz milk disease;
cards;
1 1 2.081 1 1.350 -1.082 1.129 0.
1 2 1.766 1 0.386 -1.082 0.629 0.

. . . . . . . .

72 25 1.054 0 -1.060 0.308 2.061 0.
;

* Accounting for clustering using PHREG;
proc phreg data=herd covs(aggregate) covm;
model time*censor(0) = disease parity milk herdsiz;
id herdid;

run;
```

Analysis of Maximum Likelihood Estimates with Model-Based
Variance Estimate

Variable	DF	Parameter Estimate	Standard Error	χ^2	Pr > χ^2	Hazard Ratio
disease	1	0.10554	0.06756	2.4403	0.1183	1.111
parity	1	−1.54452	0.04298	1291.5677	<0.0001	0.213
milk	1	−0.01719	0.02524	0.4642	0.4957	0.983
herdsiz	1	−0.02015	0.02861	0.4961	0.4812	0.980

nonmodel-based. approach

Analysis of Maximum Likelihood Estimates
with Sandwich Variance Estimate

Variable	DF	Parameter Estimate	Standard Error	Std Err Ratio	χ^2	$Pr > \chi^2$	Hazard Ratio
disease	1	0.10554	0.06486	0.960	2.6480	0.1037	1.111
parity	1	-1.54452	0.17335	4.034	79.3871	<0.0001	0.213
milk	1	-0.01719	0.07052	2.794	0.0594	0.8074	0.983
herdsiz	1	-0.02015	0.06151	2.150	0.1073	0.7432	0.980

higher SE

Remarks

Note that the SAS program fits the Cox proportional hazard regression model accounting for clustering using the option "aggregate" in the model statement. The "covm" option produces model-based standard errors. The parameter estimates under both options are the same, but the standard errors are substantially higher with the nonmodel-based approach. However, both techniques indicate that parity is the only factor that correlates significantly with time to death. The negative sign means that increased parity lowers the risk of a cow being culled.

The R code to fit the model is

```
herd <- read.table("x:/xxx/herd.txt",header=T)
summary(coxph(Surv(time, censor) ~
disease+parity+milk+herdsiz+cluster(herdid), herd))
```

We fit Weibull model with frailty components

```
*Weibull model with frailty components;
proc nlmixed data=herd;
bounds gamma > 0;
linp = b0+b1*parity*b2*milk+b3*herdsiz*b3*(disease-2) +z;
alpha = exp(-linp);
G_t = exp(-(alpha*time)**gamma);
g = gamma*alpha*((alpha*time)**(gamma-1))*G_t;
LL = (censor=0)*log(g)+(censor=1)*log(G_t);
model time ~ general(LL);
random z ~ normal(0,exp(2*logsig)) subject=cluster out=EB;
predict 1-G_t out=cdf;
run;
```

The selected SAS output is

Parameter Estimates

Parameter	Estimate	Standard Error	DF	t-Value	Pr > |t|	Alpha	Lower	Upper
gamma	7.1135	0.4138	71	17.19	<0.0001	0.05	6.2883	7.9387
b0	0.8741	0.05817	71	15.03	<0.0001	0.05	0.7581	0.9901
b1	0.2096	0.01637	71	12.80	<0.0001	0.05	0.1770	0.2423
b2	0.0257	0.03022	71	0.85	0.3978	0.05	−0.0345	0.0859
b3	−0.0021	0.01166	71	−0.18	0.8567	0.05	−0.0254	0.0211
log-sig	−10.2387	464.88	71	−0.02	0.9825	0.05	−937.18	916.70

Remarks

From the SAS output, the estimate of the shape parameter is $\hat{\gamma} = 7.1135$, and the estimate of the variance of the frailty component is $\hat{\sigma}^2 = 0.0095$. Similar to the PHREG procedure, the only significant covariate is parity. The sign of the estimated regression coefficient of parity under this model is positive, meaning that increased parity increases the survival time of a randomly selected cow. This interpretation is similar to the interpretation under the above PHREG model.

7.5 Sample Size Requirements for Survival Data

Suppose that all subjects are followed for the same fixed period of time (say 2 years), we would simply compare the proportions of patients with the outcome of interest, and sample size formulas to compare two independent proportions apply (see Chapter 2). The development of this section is based on material presented in Lee and Wang (2003).

Not all studies have equal follow-up times for all subjects, so one should use survival analysis methods.

We have shown that in randomized trials the usual statistic for comparing two survival functions is the nonparametric log-rank test. It does not make any assumptions about the survival distributions in the groups.

Even when the log-rank test is intended for analysis, often assumptions about the survival functions are made when determining the appropriate sample size.

To compute sample size any of the following is needed:

1. The estimated proportions of subjects in each group who are "event-free" at a fixed time

2. The estimated hazard ratio ($h = e^\beta$, where β is the Cox model coefficient corresponding to the treatment effect) and estimated control group probability of survival at a fixed time
3. The estimated median survival times or exponential hazard rates in each group.

7.5.1 Sample Size Based on Log-Rank Test

This calculation assumes that patients are followed for a *fixed length of time* (t), and the hazard ratio (h) is constant over time. Suppose that we have two treatment groups, if p_i denotes the proportion of subjects who are event-free at time t for group i, where $i = 1, 2$, then

$$h = \frac{\ln(p_1)}{\ln(p_2)}$$

and the sample size per group is

$$n = \frac{(z_{\alpha/2} + z_\beta)^2 (h + 1)^2}{(2 - p_1 - p_2)(h - 1)^2}$$

Example 7.5

We need to determine if a new drug for treatment of lung cancer lengthens the survival time. All patients in the trial will be followed for 2 years. Find sample size needed for an $\alpha = 0.05$ level test to have 80% power to detect $h = 2$ if the 2-year survival rate under standard therapy is $p_1 = 0.30$

$$h = 2 = \frac{\ln(0.30)}{\ln(p_2)} \Rightarrow p_2 = 0.55$$

$$n = \frac{(1.96 + 0.84)^2 (2 + 1)^2}{(2 - 0.30 - 0.55)(2 - 1)^2} = 62$$

7.5.2 Exponential Survival and Accrual

This calculation assumes that patients enter the study at a uniform rate until the trial ends in t years, and the survival curves are exponential with parameter λ_i, the hazard for group i, where $i = 1, 2$.
The sample size per group is

$$n = \frac{(z_{\alpha/2} + z_\beta)^2 [\phi(\lambda_1) + \phi(\lambda_2)]}{(\lambda_1 - \lambda_2)^2}$$

where $\phi(\lambda) = \lambda^3 t / (\lambda t + e^{-\lambda t} - 1)$.

If the survival curves are exponential, the hazard for group i can be estimated using

$$\lambda_i = -\frac{1}{t_{50}} \ln(0.5)$$

where t_{50} is the median survival time for group i.

Or, if you have λ for the control group, and h use

$$h = \frac{\lambda_1}{\lambda_2}$$

to determine $\lambda_2 = \lambda_1/h$.

Example 7.6

In the previous example, suppose the trial lasts 2 years and the survival curves are exponential. The median survival with the standard drug is 1 year, corresponding to

$$\lambda_1 = -\ln(0.5) = 0.693$$

$$h = 1.5 = \frac{0.693}{\lambda_2} \Rightarrow \lambda_2 = 0.462$$

$$\phi(\lambda_1) = \frac{(0.693)^3 \times 2}{(0.693)2 + e^{-0.693 \times 2} - 1} = 1.046 \quad \phi(\lambda_2) = 0.615$$

$$n = \frac{(1.96 + 1.28)^2[1.046 + 0.615]}{(0.693 - 0.462)^2} = 324$$

7.5.3   Sample Size Requirements for Clustered Survival

In this section, we present a simple sample size formula for log-rank statistics applied to clustered survival data with variable cluster sizes and arbitrary treatment assignments within clusters. This formula is based on the asymptotic normality of log-rank statistics under certain local alternatives. The derived sample size expression reduces to the formula given in cases of no clustering or within-clustering independence. The results presented here are based on the work by Schoenfeld (1983), and Gangnon and Kosorok (2004).

We assume that

1. We have n clusters and the average cluster size is m.
2. The entire cluster is randomized as a whole (i.e., no within-cluster randomization).
3. The log hazard ratio is denoted by ϑ.

4. $P_1 = n_1/n$ is the proportion of clusters receiving the first treatment, and $P_2 = 1 - P_1$ the proportion of clusters receiving the second treatment.
5. $D \equiv$ probability of observing an event, hence the required number of events $k = mnd$ is estimated as

$$k = \frac{(Z_{\alpha/Z} + Z_\beta)^2}{P_1 P_2 \theta^2}[1 + (m-1)\rho] \quad n = \frac{(Z_{\alpha/Z} + Z_\beta)[1 + (m-1)\rho]}{mDP_1 P_2 \theta^2}$$

here ρ is the intraclass correlation.

Note that in most settings, it is difficult to specify ρ in advance, because ρ depends on the censoring distribution and the dependence between event times within a cluster. The sample size should be based on a conservative choice of ρ, such as the largest ρ-value for clustered data.

Remark

If the cluster size $m = 2$, and one unit receives treatment (1), and the other receives treatment (2), the sample size formula is

$$n = \frac{2(Z_{\alpha/2} + Z_\beta)^2}{D\theta^2}(1 - \rho)$$

In this case, one should choose the smallest possible value for ρ to get a conservative estimate of n (the number of pairs).

Example 7.7

In a cluster randomized trial, we want to determine if a new drug for treating a familial disease lengthens the survival time. The follow-up period is 3 years. We need to estimate the number of clusters for an $\alpha = 0.05$ level test to have 90% power to detect a hazard ratio of 2. Assume an average cluster size $m = 5$, and intracluster correlation $\rho = 0.5$, and equal number of clusters in both arms ($P_1 = P_2 = 1/2$). We may also expect 10% subjects to be censored.

Here, $D = 90\%$, $\vartheta = \ln(2) = 0.69$

$$n = \frac{(1.96 + 1.28)^2[1 + 4(0.5)]}{(5)(0.25)(0.9)(0.69)^2} = 27$$

That is we need 27 clusters to be randomized in each arm.

Exercises

7.1   The data below show survival times (in months) of patients with Hodgkin's disease who were treated with nitrogen mustards. Group A patients received little or no prior therapy, whereas Group B patients received heavy prior therapy. Asterisked observations are censoring times.

Group A   1.20, 1.11, 4.96, 5.25, 5.40, 5.92, 8.89, 10.98, 11.18, 13.11, 14.21,
          16.33, 19.77, 21.08, 21.84*, 22.07, 31.38*, 32.62*, 36.18*, 44.99
Group B   1.01, 2.82, 3.61, 5.20, 5.49, 6.72, 7.31, 8.08, 9.11, 14.49*, 16.85,
          18.92*, 26.59*, 30.26*, 46.74*

   (a) Obtain and compare product-limit estimates for two groups. Does
       there appear to be a difference in the 1-year survival probability for
       the two types of patients?
   (b) Do any parametric models whereby one might compare the two
       distributions suggest themselves?
   (c) Use (hazard) plots of the empirical hazard function $\hat{H}(t)$ to examine
       and compare the two life distributions.

7.2   The following data are remission times, in weeks, for a group of 30
leukemia patients in a certain type of therapy; asterisked observations are
censoring times: 1, 1, 2, 5, 5, 6, 6, 6, 7, 8, 9, 9, 10, 12, 13, 14, 18, 20, 24, 26, 29,
32^*, 42, 45^*, 55^*, 59, 66, 73^*, 86^*, 100.
   (a) Estimate the mean remission time (1) using the nonparametric method,
       and (2) assuming that the underlying distribution of remission times
       is Exponential. Obtain and compare confidence intervals for the mean
       using the two methods.
   (b) Similarly compare estimates of $S(26)$, the probability of a remission
       lasting more than 26 weeks, using the nonparametric product-limit
       estimate and the Exponential model, respectively.

7.3   The data in the following table are from a more comprehensive set given
by Krall et al. (1975). The problem is to relate survival times for multiple
myeloma patients to a number of prognostic variables. The data given here
show survival times, in months, for 65 patients and include measurements
on each patient for the following five independent variables:
   x_1 Logarithm of a blood urea nitrogen measurement at diagnosis
   x_2 Hemoglobin measurement at diagnosis
   x_3 Age at diagnosis
   x_4 Sex: 0, male; 1, female
   x_5 Serum calcium measurement at diagnosis
   Asterisks denote censoring times. The data are given in the table at the end
of this chapter.
   1. Examine the relationship of these variables to survival time by fitting
      and examining Exponential regression model.
   2. Fit Exponential models with $\theta_x = x\beta$. Does this yield any different con-
      clusions other than those obtained in part (1)? Compare the fit of this
      model with that of part (1).
   3. Analyze the data using Weibull model. Does this provide any evidence
      against the Exponential model of part (1)?

7.4   Fit the EARS DATA using the log-normal frailty in SAS. The code is given by

```
proc nlmixed data=ear;
bounds gamma > 0;
linp = b0+b1*(treat-2) +z;
alpha = exp(-linp);
G_t = exp(-(alpha*time)**gamma);
g = gamma*alpha*((alpha*time)**(gamma-1))*G_t;
LL = (censor=0)*log(g)+(censor=1)*log(G_t);
model time ~ general(LL);
random z ~ normal(1,exp(2*logsig)) subject=subject out=EB;
predict 1-G_t out=cdf;
run;
proc print data=eb;
run;
```

Interpret the results obtained from this model to the results obtained from the other fitting procedures.

7.5   For the example on sample size for clustered survival data, what is the required number of events needed to achieve the study objectives?

Data for Exercise 7.3

t	x_1	x_2	x_3	x_4	x_5	t	x_1	x_2	x_3	x_4	x_5
1	2.218	9.4	67	0	10	26	1.230	11.2	49	1	11
1	1.940	12.0	38	0	18	32	1.322	10.6	46	0	9
2	1.519	9.8	81	0	15	35	1.114	7.0	48	0	10
2	1.748	11.3	75	0	12	37	1.602	11.0	63	0	9
2	1.301	5.1	57	0	9	41	1.000	10.2	69	0	10
3	1.544	6.7	46	1	10	42	1.146	5.0	70	1	9
5	2.236	10.1	50	1	9	51	1.568	7.7	74	0	13
5	1.681	6.5	74	0	9	52	1.000	10.1	60	1	10
6	1.362	9.0	77	0	8	54	1.255	9.0	49	0	10
6	2.114	10.2	70	1	8	58	1.204	12.1	42	1	10
6	1.114	9.7	60	0	10	66	1.447	6.6	59	0	9
6	1.415	10.4	67	1	8	67	1.322	12.8	52	0	10
7	1.978	9.5	48	0	10	88	1.176	10.6	47	1	9
7	1.041	5.1	61	1	10	89	1.322	14.0	63	0	9
7	1.176	11.4	53	1	13	92	1.431	11.0	58	1	11
9	1.724	8.2	55	0	12	4*	1.945	10.2	59	0	10
11	1.114	14.0	61	0	10	4*	1.924	10.0	49	1	13
11	1.230	12.0	43	0	9	7*	1.114	12.4	48	1	10
11	1.301	13.2	65	0	10	7*	1.532	10.2	81	0	11
11	1.508	7.5	70	0	12	8*	1.079	9.9	57	1	8
11	1.079	9.6	51	1	9	12*	1.146	11.6	46	1	7

(Continued)

(*Continued*)

t	x_1	x_2	x_3	x_4	x_5	t	x_1	x_2	x_3	x_4	x_5
13	0.778	5.5	60	1	10	11*	1.613	14.0	60	0	9
14	1.398	14.6	66	0	10	12*	1.398	8.8	66	1	9
15	1.602	10.6	70	0	11	13*	1.663	4.9	71	1	9
16	1.342	9.0	48	0	10	16*	1.146	13.0	55	0	9
16	1.322	8.8	62	1	10	19*	1.322	13.0	59	1	10
17	1.230	10.0	53	0	9	19*	1.322	10.8	69	1	10
17	1.591	11.2	68	0	10	28*	1.230	7.3	82	1	9
18	1.447	7.5	65	1	8	41*	1.756	12.8	72	0	9
19	1.079	14.4	51	0	15	53*	1.114	12.0	66	0	11
19	1.255	7.5	60	1	9	57*	1.255	12.5	66	0	11
24	1.301	14.6	56	1	9	77*	1.079	14.0	60	0	12
25	1.000	12.4	67	0	10						

References

Aalen, O.O. and Tretli, S. (1999). Analyzing incidence of testis cancer by means of a frailty model. *Cancer Causes and Control*, 10, 285–292.

Abraham, B. and Ledolter, J. (1983). *Statistical Methods for Forecasting*, Wiley, New York.

Agresti, A. (1990). *Categorical Data Analysis*, Wiley, New York.

Ahn, C. and Odom-Maryon, T. (1995). Estimation of a common odds ratio under binary cluster sampling. *Statistics in Medicine*, 14, 1567–1577.

Akaike, H. (1973). Information theory and extension of the maximum likelihood principle, in *Second International Symposium on Information Theory*, Petrov, B.N. and Csaki, F., Eds., *Budapest, Akademiai Kaido*, pp. 267–281.

Andersen, P.K., Klein, J.P., and Zhang, M.-J. (1999). Testing for centre effects in multi-centre survival studies: A Monte Carlo comparison of fixed and random effects tests. *Statistics in Medicine*, 18, 1489–1500.

Anderson, T.W. (1971). *The Statistical Analysis of Time Series*. Wiley, New York.

Andrews, D. and Herzberg, A. (1985). *Data: A Collection of Problems from Many Fields for the Students and Research Workers*, Springer-Verlag, New York.

Bartlett, M. (1946). On the theoretical justification of sampling properties of an autocorrelated time series. *Journal of Royal Statistical Society, B*, 8, 27–41.

Bishop, Y.M., Fienberg, S.E., and Holland, P.W. (1975). *Discrete Multivariate Analysis*. MIT Press, Cambridge, MA.

Bloomfield, P. (1976). *Fourier Analysis of Time Series: An Introduction*, Wiley InterScience, New York.

Box, G.E.P. and Jenkins, G.M. (1970). *Time Series Analysis, Forecasting, and Control*, Holden Day, San Francisco.

Box, G.E.P. and Pierce, D.A. (1970). Distribution of residual autocorrelations in autoregressive-integrated moving average time series models. *Journal of the American Association*, 70, 1509–1526.

Breslow, N. (1972). Contribution to the discussion of a paper by D.R. Cox. *Journal of the Royal Statistical Society, B*, 34, 216–217.

Breslow, N., Day, N., Halvorsen, K., Prentice, R., and Sabai, C. (1978). Estimation of multiple relative risk functions in matched case–control studies. *American Journal of Epidemiology*, 108, 299–307.

Bryk, A.S. and Raudenbush, S.W. (1992). *Hierarchical Linear Models: Applications and Data Analysis Methods*, Sage, Newbury Park, CA.

Cameron, A.C. and Trivedi, P.K. (1998). *Regression Analysis of Count Data*, Cambridge University Press, UK.

Clayton, D.G. (1978). A model for association in bivariate life tables and its application in epidemiological studies of familial tendency in chronic disease incidence. *Biometrika*, 65, 141–151.

Cochran, W.G. (1937). Problems arising in the analysis of a series of similar experiments. *Journal of the Royal Statistical Society*, 4(1), 102–118.

Cochran, W.G. (1977). *Sampling Techniques*, 3rd edition. Wiley, New York.

Collett, D. (2003). *Modeling Binary Data*, 2nd edition, Chapman & Hall/CRC Press, London.

Collings, B.J. (1981). The negative binomial distribution: An alternative to the Poison. Unpublished Ph.D. thesis. University of North Carolina at Chapel Hill.

Collings, B.J. and Margolin, B.H. (1985). Testing goodness of fit for the Poisson assumption when observations are not identically distributed. *Journal of American Statistical Association*, 74, 411–418.

Connor, R.J. (1987). Ample size for testing differences in proportions for the paired sample design. *Biometrics*, 43(1), 207–211.

Consul, P.C. and Jain, G.C. (1973). A generalization of the Poisson distribution. *Technometrics*, 15, 791–799.

Cornfield, J. (1978). Randomization by group: A formal analysis. *American Journal of Epidemiology*, 108, 100–102.

Cox, D.R. (1970). *Analysis of Binary Data*, Chapman & Hall, London.

Cox, D.R. (1972). Regression models and life-tables (with discussion). *Journal of the Royal Statistical Society*, B, 34, 187–220.

Cox, D.R. and Snell, E. (1989). *Analysis of Binary Data*, 2nd edition, Chapman & Hall, London.

Crowder, M. and Hand, D. (1990). *Analysis of Repeated Measures*, Chapman & Hall, London.

Cryer, J. (1986). *Time Series Analysis*, Duxbury Press, Boston.

Dean, C., Lawless J.F., and Wilmot, G.E. (1989). A mixed Poisson-inverse Gaussian regression model. *Canadian Journal of Statistics*, 17, 171–182.

DeCosse, J.J., Miller, H.H., and Lesser, M.L. (1989). Effect of wheat fiber and vitamins C and E on rectal polyps in patients with familial adenomatous polyposis. *Journal of the National Cancer Institute*, 81, 1290–1297.

Diggle, P. (1988). An approach to the analysis of repeated measures. *Biometrics*, 44, 959–971.

Diggle, P. (1989). Testing for random dropouts in repeated measurement data. *Biometrics*, 45, 1255–1258.

Diggle, P. (1990). *Time Series: A Biostatistical Introduction*, Oxford Science Publication, Oxford.

Diggle, P., Liang, K.-Y., and Zeger, S. (1994). *The Analysis of Longitudinal Data*, Oxford Science Publications, Oxford.

Donald, A. and Donner, A. (1987). Adjustments to the Mantel–Haenszel chi-squared statistic and odds ratio estimator when the data are clustered. *Statistics in Medicine*, 6, 491–499.

Donner, A. (1982). An empirical study of cluster randomization. *International Journal of Epidemiology*, 11, 283–286.

Donner, A. (1989). Statistical methods in ophthalmology: An adjusted chi-squared approach. *Biometrics*, 45, 605–611.

Donner, A., Eliasziw, M., and Klar, N. (1994). A comparison of methods for testing homogeneity of proportions in teratologic studies. *Statistics in Medicine*, 13, 1253–1264.

Donner, A., Birkett, N., and Buck, C. (1981). Randomization by cluster-sample size requirements and analysis. *American Journal of Epidemiology*, 144, 905–914.

Draper, N. and Smith, H. (1981). *Applied Regression Analysis*, 2nd edition, Wiley, New York.

Duffy, S.W., Tabar, L., Vitak, B., Yen, M.F., Warwick, J., Smith R.A., and Chen, H.H. (2003). The Swedish Two-County Trial of mammographic screening: Cluster randomization and end point evaluation. *Annals of Oncology*, 14, 1196–1198.

Durbin, J. and Watson, G. (1951). Testing for serial correlation in least squares regression II. *Biometrika*, 38, 159–178.

Elston, R.C. (1977). Response to query: Estimating "heritability" of a dichotomous trait. *Biometrics*, 33, 232–233.

Emslie, C., Gremshaw, J., and Templeton, A. (1993). Do clinical guidelines improve general-practice management and referral of infertile couples? *British Medical Journal*, 306, 1728–1731.

Firth, D. (1991). Generalized linear models, in *Statistical Theory and Modeling*, Hinkley, D., Reid, N., and Snell, E.J. Eds., Chapman & Hall, London.

Fisher, R. (1932). *Statistical Methods for Research Workers*, 4th edition, Oliver and Boyd, Edinburgh.

Fitzmaurice, G.M. (1995). A caveat concerning independence estimating equations with multivariate binary data. *Biometrics*, 51, 309–317.

Fleiss, J. (1979). Confidence intervals for the odds ratio in case-control studies: The state of the art. *Journal of Chronic Diseases*, 32, 69–77.

Fleiss, J. (1981). *Statistical Methods for Rates and Proportions*, Wiley, New York.

Frison, I. and Pocock, S.J. (1992). Repeated measures in clinical trials: Analysis using mean summary statistics and its implications for design. *Statistics in Medicine*, 11, 1685–1704.

Gangnon, R.E. and Kosorok, M.R. (2004). Sample size formula for clustered survival data using weighted log-rank statistics. *Biometrics*, 91(2), 263–275.

Gail, M. (1973). The determination of sample sizes for trials involving several independent 2×2 tables. *Journal of Chronic Diseases*, 26, 669–673.

Gart, J.J. and Thomas, D. (1982). The performance of three approximate confidence limit methods for the odds ratio. *American Journal of Epidemiology*, 115, 453–470.

Geisser, S. (1963). Multivariate analysis of variance of a special covariance case. *Journal of the American Statistical Association*, 58, 660–669.

Greenwood, M. and Yule, G.U. (1920). An inquiry into the nature of frequency distributions representative of multiple happenings with particular reference to he occurrence of multiple attacks of disease or repeated accidents. *Journal of the Royal Statistical Society*, 83, 255–279.

Haldane, J. (1956). The estimation and significance of the logarithm of a ratio of frequencies. *Annals of Human Genetics*, 20, 309–311.

Hauck, W. (1979). The large sample variance of the Mantel–Haenszel estimator of a common odds ratio. *Biometrics*, 35, 817–819.

Hayes, R.J. and Bennett, S. (1999). Simple sample size calculation for cluster randomized trials. *International Journal of Epidemiology*, 28, 319–326.

Hosmer, D. and Lemeshow, S. (1989). *Applied Logistic Regression*, Wiley, New York.

Hougaard, P. (1995). Frailty models for survival data. *Lifetime Data Analysis*, 1, 255–273.

Huber, P.J. (1967). The behavior of maximum likelihood estimators under nonstandard conditions, *Proceedings of the Fifth Berkeley Symposium on Mathematical Statistics and Probability*, Vol. A, University of California Press, Berkeley, pp. 221–233.

Janardan, K.G., Kerster, H.W., and Schaeffer, D.J. (1979). Biological applications of the Lagrangian Poisson distribution. *BioScience* 29(10), 599–602.

Jewell, N. (1984). Small-sample bias of point estimators of the odds ratio from matched sets. *Biometrics*, 40, 421–435.

Jewell, N. (1986). On the bias of commonly used measures of association for 2×2 tables. *Biometrics*, 42, 351–358.

Jones, R.H. (1993). *Longitudinal Data with Serial Correlation: A State-Space Approach*, Chapman & Hall, London.

Kalman, R. (1960). A new approach to linear filtering and prediction problems. *Transactions of ASME Journal of Basic Engineering*, 82, 35–45.

Kaplan, E.L. and Meier, P. (1958). Nonparametric estimation from incomplete observations. *Journal of the American Statistical Association*, 53, 457–481.

Katz, J., Carey, V., Zeger, S., and Sommer, L. (1993). Estimation of design effects and diarrhea clustering within household and villages. *American Journal of Epidemiology*, 138(11), 994–1006.

Kendall, M. and Ord, K. (1990). *Time Series*, 3rd edition, Edward Arnold, London.

Kempthorne, O. and Tandon, O.B. (1953). The estimation of heritability by regression offspring on parent. *Biometrics*, 9, 90–100.

Kerry, S.M. and Bland, J.M. (1998). The intracluster correlation coefficient in cluster randomization. *British Medical Journal*, 316, 1455.

Kleinbaum, D., Kapper, L., and Muller, K. (1988). *Applied Regression Analysis and Other Multivariable Methods*, PWS-Kent, Boston.

Kolmogorov, A. (1939). Sur L'interpolation et L'extrapolation des suites stationnaires. *C.R. Academy of Sciences*, Paris, 208, 2043–2045.

Kolmogorov, A. (1941). Interpolation and extrapolation von stationären Zufälligen Folgen. *Bulletin of the Academy Sciences (Nauk), USSR, Ser. Math.*, 5, 3–14.

Korn, E.L. and Whittemore, A.S. (1979). Methods for analyzing panel studies of acute health effects of air pollution. *Biometrics*, 35, 795–802.

Krall, J.M., Uthoff, V.A., and Harley, J.B. (1975). A step-up procedure for selecting variables associated with survival. *Biometrics*, 31, 49–57.

Laird, N. (1988). Missing data in longitudinal studies. *Statistics in Medicine*, 7, 305–315.

Laird, N.M. and Ware, J.H. (1982). Random effects models for longitudinal data. *Biometrics*, 38, 963–974.

Lambert, D. (1992). Zero-inflated Poisson regression with an application to defects in manufacturing. *Technometrics*, 34, 1–14.

Lawless, J.F. (1982). *Statistical Models and Methods for Lifetime Data*, Wiley, New York.

Le, C.T. and Lindgren, B.R. (1996). Duration of ventilating tubes: A test for comparing two clustered samples of censored data. *Biometrics*, 52, 328–334.

Lee, E. and Wang, J.W. (2003). *Statistical Methods for Survival Data*, 3rd edition, Wiley, New York.

Liang, K.Y. and Zeger, S.L. (1986). Longitudinal data analysis using generalized linear models. *Biometrika*, 73, 13–122.

Liang, K.Y. and Zeger, S.L. (1993). Regression analysis for correlated data. *Annual Review of Public Health*, 14, 43–68.

Lindsay, J. (1993). *Models for Repeated Measurements*, Oxford Science Publications, Oxford.

Littell, R.C., Milliken, G.A., Stroup, W.W., and Wolfinger, R.D. (1996). *SAS System for Mixed Models*. SAS Institute, Cary, NC.

Little, R. and Rubin, D. (1987). *Statistical Analysis with Missing Data*. Wiley, New York.

Ljung, G.M. and Box, G.E.P. (1978). On the measure of lack of fit in time series models. *Biometrika*, 65, 297–304.

MacDonald, B. (1993). Estimating logistic regression parameters for bivariate binary data. *Journal of the Statistical Society, B*, 55(2), 391–397.

Mantel, N. (1973). Synthetic retrospective studies and related topics. *Biometrics*, 29, 479–486.

Mantel, N. and Haenszel, W. (1959). Statistical aspects of the analysis of data from retrospective studies of disease. *Journal of the National Cancer Institute*, 22, 719–748.

Manton, K.G. and Stallard, E. (1981). Methods for evaluating the heterogeneity of aging processes in human populations using vital statistics data: Explaining the black/white mortality crossover by a model of mortality selection. *Human Biology*, 53, 47–67.

McCullagh, P. and Nelder, J. (1989). *Generalized Linear Models*, 2nd edition, Chapman & Hall, London.

Miall, W.E. and Oldham, P.D. (1955). A study of arterial blood pressure and its inheritance in a sample of the general population. *Clinical Science*, 14(3), 459–488.

Miettenen, O.S. (1968). The matched pairs design in the case of all-or-none responses. *Biometrics*, 24, 339–352.

Mosteller, F. and Tukey, J. (1977). *Data Analysis and Regression: A Second Course in Statistics*, Addison-Wesley, Reading, MA.

Murray, D.M., Perry, C.L., and Griffin, G. (1992). Results from a statewide approach to adolescent tobacco use prevention. *Preventive Medicine*, 21, 449–472.

Neuhaus, J.M., Kalbfleisch, J.D., and Hauck, W.W. (1991). A comparison of cluster-specific and population-averaged approaches for analyzing correlated binary data. *International Statistical Review*, 59, 25–35.

Oakes, M. (1986). *Statistical Inference*, Epidemiology Resources Inc., Chestnut Hills, MD.

Paul, S.R. (1982). Analysis of proportions of affected fetuses in teratological experiments. *Biometrics*, 38, 361–370.

Peto, R. and Peto, J. (1972). Asymptotically efficient rank invariant procedures. *Journal of the Royal Statistical Society, A*, 135, 185–207.

Pinheiro, J.C. and Bates, D.M. (2000). *Mixed Effects Models in S and S-Plus*, Springer, New York.

Potthoff, R.F. and Roy, S.N. (1964). A generalized multivariate analysis of variance model useful especially for growth curve problems. *Biometrika*, 51, 313–326.

Prentice, R. (1976). Use of the logistic model in retrospective studies. *Biometrics*, 32, 599–606.

Prentice, R. (1988). Correlated binary regression with covariates specific to each binary observation. *Biometrics*, 44, 1033–1048.

R 2.3.1 (2006). *A Language and Environment*, R Development Core Team, Stanford University, California.

Rao, J.N.K. and Scott, A.J. (1992). A simple method for the analysis of clustered binary data. *Biometrics*, 48, 577–585.

Robins, J., Breslow, N., and Greenland, S. (1986). Estimators of the Mantel–Haenszel variance consistent in both sparse data and large-strata limiting models. *Biometrics*, 42, 311–323.

Roizman, B., Hoggan, D., and Cornfield, J. (1960). Linear and parabolic estimates of the titers of Herpes Simplex from pock counts on the chorioallantoic membrane of embryonated eggs. *Virology*, 11, 572–589.

Rubin, D. (1976). Inference and missing data. *Biometrika*, 63, 581–592.

Rubin, D. (1994). Modeling the drop-out mechanism in repeated measures studies. *9th International Workshop on Statistical Modeling*, Exeter, UK.

Russell, M.A.H., Merriman, R., Stapleton, J., and Taylor, W. (1983). Effect of nicotine chewing gum as an adjunct to general practitioners advice against smoking. *British Medical Journal*, 286, 1782–1785.

SAS Institute (1995). *PROC GENMOD*. SAS Institute, Cary, NC. Available in release 6.12 of SAS/STAT.

SAS Institute (1996). *GLMMIX*. SAS Institute, Cary, NC. SAS Macro for version 6.08 or later obtainable from SAS Institute Technical Support.

Schall, R. (1991). Estimation in generalized linear models with random effects, *Biometrika*, 78, 719–727.

Schlesselman, J. (1982). *Case-Control Studies Design, Conduct, Analysis*, Oxford University Press, Oxford.

Schwarz, G. (1978). Estimating the dimension of a model. *Annals of Statistics*, 6, 461–464.

Schoenfeld, D.A. (1983). Sample size formula for the proportional hazards regression model. *Biometrics*, 38, 499–503.

Shoukri, M.M., Asyali, M.H., Van Dorp, R., and Kelton, D. (2004). The Poisson Inverse Gaussian distribution regression model in the analysis of clustered counts data. *Journal of Data Science*, 2, 17–32.

Shumway, R. (1982). Discriminant analysis for time series, in *Handbook of Statistics*, Vol. II, Classification, Pattern Recognition and Reduction of Dimensionality, Kirshnaiah, P.R., Ed., North Holland, Amsterdam, pp. 1–43.

Singer, J.D. (1998). Using SAS PROC MIXED to fit multilevel models, hierarchical models, and individual growth models. *Journal of Educational and Behavioral Statistics*, 23, 323–355.

Snedecor, G. and Cochran, W.G. (1981). *Statistical Methods*, 8th edition, Iowa State University Press, Ames, Iowa.

Stukel, T.A. (1993). Comparison of methods for the analysis of longitudinal data. *Statistics in Medicine*, 12, 1339–1351.

Tabar, L., Fagerberg, C.J., Gad, A., Baldetorp, L., Holmberg, L.H., Grontoft, O., Ljungquist, U., Lundstrom, B., Manson, J.C., and Eklund, G. (1985). Reduction in mortality from breast cancer after mass screening with mammography. *Lancet*, 1(8433), 829–832.

Tarone, R. (1979). Testing the goodness of fit of the binomial distribution. *Biometrika*, 66(3), 585–590.

Thall, P.F. and Vail, S.C. (1990). Some covariance models for longitudinal count data with over-dispersion. *Biometrics*, 46, 657–671.

Therneau, T. (1993). Using a multiple-events Cox model. *Proceedings from the Biometrics Section of the American Statistical Association*, pp. 1–14.

Thomas, D. and Gart, J.J. (1977). A table of exact confidence limits for differences and ratios of two proportions and their odds ratios. *Journal of the American Statistical Association*, 72, 386–394.

Vaupel, J.W., Manton, K.G., and Stallard, E. (1979). The impact of heterogeneity in individual frailty on the dynamics of mortality. *Demography*, 16, 439–454.

Walter, S. (1985). Small-sample estimation of log odds ratios from logistic regression and fourfold tables. *Statistics in Medicine*, 4, 437–444.

Walter, S. and Cook, R. (1991). A comparison of several point estimators of the odds ratio in a single 2×2 contingency table. *Biometrics*, 47, 795–811.

Ware, J.H., Lipsitz, S., and Speizer, F.E. (1988). Issues in the analysis of repeated categorical outcomes. *Statistics in Medicine*, 7, 95–107.

Wedderburn, R. (1974). Quasi-likelihood functions, generalized linear models and the Gauss-Newton method. *Biometrika*, 61, 439–447.

Weil, C.S. (1970). Selection of the valid number of sampling units and a consideration of their combination in toxicological studies involving reproduction, teratogenesis or carcinogenesis. *Food and Cosmetics Toxicology*, 8, 177–182.

Williams, D.A. (1975). The analyses of binary responses from toxicological experiments involving reproduction and teratogenicity. *Biometrics*, 31, 949–952.

Whittemore, A.S. (1981). Sample size for logistic regression with small response probability. *Journal of American Statistical Association*, 76, 27–32.

Whittle, P. (1983). *Prediction and Regulations*, 2nd edition, University of Minnesota Press, Minneapolis.

Willeberg, P. (1980). The analysis and interpretation of epidemiological data. *Veterinary Epidemiology and Economics, Proceedings of the 2nd International Symposium*, Geering, W.A. and Chapman, L.A., Eds., Canberra, Australia.

Wilmot, G.E. (1987). The Poisson-Inverse Gaussian distribution as an alternative to the negative binomial. *Scandinavian Journal of Statistics*, 14(1), 113–127.

Wilson, S.R. and Gordon, I. (1986). Calculating sample sizes in the presence of confounding variables. *Applied statistics*, 35(2), 207–213.

Wolfinger, R. and O'Connell, M. (1993). Generalized linear mixed models: A pseudo-likelihood approach. *Journal of Statistical Computation and Simulation*, 48, 233–243.

Woolf, B. (1955). On estimating the relationship between blood group and disease. *Annals of Human Genetics*, 19, 251–253.

World Health Organization (2000). *Acluster 2.1: Design and Analysis of Cluster of Cluster Randomization Trial*, Geneva, Switzerland.

Yule, G. (1927). On a method of investigating periodicities in disturbed series, with special reference to Wolfer's sunspot numbers. *Philosophical Translations*, A226, 267–298.

Zeger, S. and Liang, K.Y. (1986). Longitudinal data analysis for discrete and continuous outcomes. *Biometrics*, 42, 121–130.

Zeger, S. and Karim, M.R. (1991). Generalized linear models with random effects: A Gibbs sampling approach. *Journal of the American Statistical Association*, 86, 79–86.

Zeger, S.L., Liang, K.Y., and Albert, P.A. (1988). Models for longitudinal data: A generalized estimating equation approach. *Biometrics*, 44, 1049–1060.

Index

A

Additive seasonal variation model (ASVM), 163, 169–172

Akaike's information criterion (AIC), 215

Analysis, cluster, *see under* Cluster data

Autocorrelation functions (ACF), 182

Autocovariance and autocorrelation functions, 181–183

Autoregressive integrated moving average (ARIMA) models, 160, 191

modeling seasonality with, 199–203

Autoregressive processes, 184–187

AR(1) model, 184–185

AR(2) model (Yule's process), 185–187

B

Binary outcome data, modeling, 83–131

correlated binary outcome data, modeling, 103–119, *see also under* Correlated binary outcome data

logistic regression model, 86–103, 119–128, *see also under* Logistic regression

Box–Pierce–Ljung (BPL) statistics, 203

Breslow–Day test, 49

C

Categorical explanatory variables, coding and coefficients, interpretation, 88–90

Censoring, 244

types, 244

random censoring, 244–245

Type 1 censoring, 244

Type 2 censoring, 244

Cluster data, analyzing, 1–28

alternative models, fitting, 19–28

ANOVA table, 5

basic features, 2–7

conventional methods, 6

data layout, 3

failures in, 3

generalized linear models, 15–19, *see also separate entry*

PROC MIXED for, 21–28

regression analysis for, 11–15, *see also under* Regression analysis

sample and design issues, 7–11

smokeless tobacco use among schoolchildren, 2

Clustered binary data

Pearson's χ^2, approaches to adjust, 57–67, *see also separate entry*

sample size requirements for, 75–77

cluster sizes greater than or equal to 2, comparative studies for, 76

paired sample design, 75–76

statistical analysis of, 56–75

Clustered count data, analysis, 133–157

count data random effects models, 140–149

count data, overdispersion in, 139–140

model inference and goodness of fit, 138–139

Poisson regression, 134–138

Clustering, *see also individual entries*

cluster-specific logistic regression models, 104, 106–108

definition and basics, 1

multiple levels of, 115–119

Cochran and Orcutt procedure, 177

Cohort vs case–control models, 38, 119–121

Common odds ratio

confidence interval on the, 50–51

inference on, 67–75

significance test of, 47–50

uncorrected chi-squared test of, 72

Confidence interval construction, 59

Correlated binary outcome data, modeling, 103–119

clustering, multiple levels of, 115–119